Thymus Involvement In Immunity And Disease

Papers by
W. D. Biggar, T. Mandel, Mary A. Ritter, Osias Stutman, J. Kruger, Olli Ruuskanen, David L. Rosenstreich, Y. Takada, M. C. Raff, Ulf Ernstrom, Arthur Bankhurst, H. F. Jeejeebhoy, Michael L. Howe, B. P. MacLaurin, L. Stavy, Hermann Wagner, J. F. A. P. Miller, I. Gery, Stella C. Knight, Jennifer Aird, Linda Poole Merke, Stanley Burrows, William E. DeMuth, Jr., David Osoba, E. J. Yunis et al.

MSS Information Corporation
655 Madison Avenue, New York, N.Y. 10021

Library of Congress Cataloging in Publication Data
Main entry under title:

Thymus involvement in immunity and disease.

   1. Thymus gland--Addresses, essays, lectures.
2. Immunity--Addresses, essays, lectures. 3. Thymus gland--Diseases--Addresses, essays, lectures.
I. Biggar, W. D. [DNLM: 1. Thymus gland--Immunology --Collected works. WK 400 T549 1973]
RC663.T49   1973   612'.43'08   72-13558
ISBN 0-8422-7068-X

Copyright © 1973
by MSS Information Corporation
All Rights Reserved

TABLE OF CONTENTS

Cell Types and Their Differentiation in the Thymus Gland. 9

Morphological and Functional Studies of Fetal Thymus Transplants in Mice .... Biggar, Stutman and Good   10

Differentiation of Foetal Mouse Thymus: Ultrastructure of Organ Cultures and of Subcapsular Grafts .... Mandel and Russell   25

Functional Maturation of Lymphocytes within Embryonic Mouse Thymus .... Ritter   41

Immunocompetence of Embryonic Hemopoietic Cells after Traffic to Thymus. .... .Stutman and Good·   45

Immunologic and Anatomic Consequences of Calf Thymosin Injection in Rats   Krüger, Goldstein and Waksman   48

Immunological Studies of the Thymus Gland 59

The Fate of Thymocytes: A Study of Kinetics of Thymocytes Using High Alkaline Phosphatase Activity as an Endogenous Label ... Ruuskanen and Kouvalainen   60

The Uropod-Bearing Lymphocyte of the Guinea Pig: Evidence for Thymic Origin ...... Rosenstreich, Shevach, Green and Rosenthal   72

Role of the Thymus in the Recovery of Hemolytic Plaque Formation after X-Irradiation ...... Takada Takada and Ambrus   84

Thymus-Derived Lymphocytes: Their Distribution and Role in the Development of Peripheral Lymphoid Tissues of the Mouse .... Raff and Owen   89

Thymus-Derived Lymphocytes in Blood, Lymph and Lymphoid Organs after Intrathymic Labelling with ^{3}H-Thymidine. .... Ernström, Larsson and Linna   99

Surface Immunoglobulins on Thymus and Thymus-Derived Lymphoid Cells .... Bankhurst, Warner and Sprent   109

Decreased Longevity of Mice Following Thymectomy
  in Adult Life .... Jeejeebhoy   120
Isogeneic Lymphocyte Interaction: Recognition of
  Self Antigens by Cells of the Neonatal
    Thymus .... Howe, Goldstein and Battisto   122

**Thymus-Derived Lymphocytes and Their Function
  in Immunity**   129

Thymus Origin of Lymphocytes Reacting and
  Stimulating Reaction in Mixed Lymphocyte
    Cultures: Studies in the Rat ...... MacLaurin   131
Capacity of Thymic Cells to Effect Target Cell
  Lysis Following Treatment with
    Concanavalin A .... Stavy, Treves
                                   and Feldman   142
Cell-Mediated Immune Response *in Vitro*: II. The
  Role of Thymus and Thymus-Derived
    Lymphocytes ..... Wagner, Harris and Feldmann   148
Thymus-Derived Cells as Killer Cells in Cell-Mediated
  Immunity .... Miller, Brunner, Sprent, Russell
                                     and Mitchell   160
Potentiation of Cultured Mouse Thymocyte Responses
  by Factors Released by Peripheral Leucocytes.. Gery
                               Gershon and Waksman   163
Ontogeny of Cellular Immunity: Development in
  Rat Thymocytes of Mixed Lymphocyte Reactivity
    to Allogeneic and Xenogeneic Cells .... Knight
                                    and Thorbecke   166
Thymus Dependence of the Immune Response:
  Response to the Haptenic Determinant NIP in
    Mice .... Aird   176

The Thymus and Pathogenic States   185

Effects of Infant Thymectomy and Antilymphocyte
  Serum on Xenotransplantation of a Human
    Leukemia in the Hamster .... Merk and Adams   186
Thymoma Associated with
    Pancytopenia .... Burrows and Carroll   196
Malignant Thymoma in a Child..... DeMuth and Smith   200
Thymic Function, Immunologic
    Deficiency, and Autoimmunity .... Osoba   204
Thymus, Immunity and Autoimmunity ..... Yunis
                              Stutman and Good   221

CREDITS AND ACKNOWLEDGEMENTS

Aird, Jennifer, "Thymus Dependence of the Immune Response: Response to the Haptenic Determinant NIP in Mice," *Immunology*, 1971, 20:617-624.

Bankhurst, Arthur D.; Noel L. Warner; and John Sprent, "Surface Immunoglobulins on Thymus and Thymus-Derived Lymphoid Cells," *The Journal of Experimental Medicine*, 1971, 134:1005-1015.

Biggar, W.D.; Osias Stutman; and Robert A. Good, "Morphological and Functional Studies of Fetal Thymus Transplants in Mice," *The Journal of Experimental Medicine*, 1972, 135:793-807.

Burrows, Stanley; and Robert Carroll, "Thymoma Associated with Pancytopenia," *Archives of Pathology*, 1971, 92:465-468.

DeMuth, Jr., William E.; and James Smith, "Malignant Thymoma in a Child," *The American Surgeon*, 1971, 37:742-745.

Ernström, Ulf; Bengt Larsson; and Juhani Linna, "Thymus-Derived Lymphocytes in Blood, Lymph and Lymphoid Organs after Intrathymic Labelling with ^{3}H-Thymidine," *Scandinavian Journal of Haematology*, 1971, 8:141-150.

Gery, I.; R.K. Gershon; and B.H. Waksman, "Potentiation of Cultured Mouse Thymocyte Responses by Factors Released by Peripheral Leucocytes," *The Journal of Immunology*, 1971, 107:1778-1780.

Howe, Michael L.; Allan L. Goldstein; and Jack R. Battisto, "Isogeneic Lymphocyte Interaction: Recognition of Self Antigens by Cells of the Neonatal Thymus," *Proceedings of the National Academy of Sciences*, 1970, 67:613-619.

Jeejeebhoy, H.F., "Decreased Longevity of Mice Following Thymectomy in Adult Life," *Transplantation*, 1971, 12:525-526.

Knight, Stella C.; and G. Jeanette Thorbecke, "Ontogeny of Cellular Immunology: Development in Rat Thymocytes of Mixed Lymphocyte Reactivity to Allogeneic and Xenogeneic Cells," *Cellular Immunology*, 1971, 2:91-100.

Krüger, J.; A.L. Goldstein; and B.H. Waksman, "Immunologic and Anatomic Consequences of Calf Thymosin Injection in Rats," *Cellular Immunology*, 1970, 1:51-61.

MacLaurin, B.P., "Thymus Origin of Lymphocytes Reacting and Stimulating Reaction in Mixed Lymphocyte Cultures: Studies in the Rat," *Clinical and Experimental Immunology*, 1971, 10:649-659.

Mandel, T.; and Pamela J. Russell, "Differentiation of Foetal Mouse Thymus: Ultrastructure of Organ Cultures and of Subcapsular Grafts," *Immunology*, 1971, 21:659-674.

Merk, Linda Poole; and Richard A. Adams, "Effects of Infant Thymectomy and Antilymphocyte Serum on Xenotransplantation of a Human Leukemia in the Hamster," *Cancer Research*, 1972, 32:1580-1583.

Miller, J.F.A.P.; K.T. Brunner; J. Sprent; P.J. Russell; and G.F. Mitchell, "Thymus-Derived Cells as Killer Cells in Cell-Mediated Immunity," *Transplantation Proceedings*, 1971, 3:915-917.

Osoba, David, "Thymic Function, Immunologic Deficiency, and Autoimmunity," *The Medical Clinics of America*, 1972, 56:319-335.

Raff, M.C.; and J.J.T. Owen, "Thymus-Derived Lymphocytes: Their Distribution and Role in the Development of Peripheral Lymphoid Tissues of the Mouse," *European Journal of Immunology*, 1971, 1:27-30.

Ritter, Mary A., "Functional Maturation of Lymphocytes within Embryonic Mouse Thymus," *Transplantation*, 1971, 12:279-282.

Rosenstreich, David L.; Ethan Shevach; Ira Green; and Alan S. Rosenthal, "The Uropod-Bearing Lymphocyte of the Guinea Pig: Evidence for Thymic Origin," *The Journal of Experimental Medicine*, 1972, 135:1037-1048.

Ruuskanen, Olli; and Kauko Kouvalainen, "The Fate of Thymocytes: A Study of Kinetics of Thymocytes Using High Alkaline Phosphatase Activity as an Endogenous Label, *Scandinavian Journal of Haematology*, 1972, 9:174-185.

Stavy, L.; A.J. Treves; and M. Feldman, "Capacity of Thymic Cells to Effect Target Cell Lysis Following Treatment with Concanavalin A," *Cellular Immunology*, 1972, 3:623-628.

Stutman, Osias; and Robert A. Good, "Immunocompetence of Embryonic Hemopoietic Cells after Traffic to Thymus," *Transplantation Proceedings*, 1971, 3:923-925.

Takada, Yumiko; Akikazu Takada; and Julian L. Ambrus, "Role of the Thymus in the Recovery of Hemolytic Plaque Formation after X-Irradiation," *Proceedings of the Society for Experimental Biology and Medicine*, 1971, 138:216-220.

Wagner, Hermann; Alan W. Harris; and Marc Feldmann, "Cell-Mediated Immune Response *in Vitro*. II. The Role of Thymus and Thymus-Derived Lymphocytes," *Cellular Immunology*, 1972, 4:39-50.

Yunis, E.J.; O. Stutman; and R.A. Good, "Thymus, Immunity and Autoimmunity," *Annals of the New York Academy of Sciences*, 1971, 183:205-220.

PREFACE

In recent years it has been shown that the thymus plays an active role in the ontogenetic development of cellular immunity. The precursor cells are influenced by the thymus microenvironment, either directly or by hormonal substance secreted by this gland. They then differentiate into lymphoid cells which have the ability to reject foreign and malignant cells, defend against microbial invasion, and collaborate with other types of lymphocytes. In fact, individuals born without a functioning thymus usually die within a few months. This observation has also been confirmed in experimental animals where it was learned that thymectomy leads to a "runting" or wasting disease, resulting in the death of the animal. Death is due to various infections and malignancies which arise in these thymectomized animals.

It has also become clear that the thymus is often the focal point of many disease states. Not only do malignancies often arise within cells of the thymus, but other abnormalities of this gland appear to predispose an individual to a particular disease. These findings have provided useful clues for the clinician in the management and treatment of patients suffering from thymus associated disease states. It is anticipated that future experimental studies will continue to provide new concepts to aid the clinician in an understanding of many related thymus disease processes. Ultimately, these studies should provide the expertise needed to alter and direct thymus-dependent lymphocytes.

This volume reviews recent literature on the thymus and its role in immunity. The topics have been selected to provide a clear and concise picture of the diffuse information now available. As editor, I have tried to present the data dealing with the thymus as the gland which directs the differentiation of precursor bone marrow cells into mature lymphocytes. A section is also included which explores the thymus' role in the immune response in terms of these differentiated cells. Furthermore, the volume considers those pathogenic states in which thymus involvement is suspected. It is presented with the hope that it may clarify the present state of knowledge in this area and give direction to future studies.

Ronald Acton, Ph.D.
December, 1972

Cell Types and Their Differentiation

MORPHOLOGICAL AND FUNCTIONAL STUDIES OF FETAL THYMUS TRANSPLANTS IN MICE*

By W. D. BIGGAR, OSIAS STUTMAN, AND ROBERT A. GOOD

The thymus gland develops as an epithelial anlage of the third and fourth pharyngeal pouches (1). Detailed ontogenic studies of the developing thymus have been important, not only for understanding its role in the biology of the host's bodily defenses, but also in the immunological analysis of congenital thymic abnormalities and immunodeficiency diseases of man.

The behavior of a thymus graft after transplantation into a secondary host has received much attention (2–11). When a neonatal thymus is transplanted under the renal capsule of a syngenic host rapid and severe necrosis results (7). After this, lymphoid proliferation occurs and restoration of a normal thymus architecture is seen 7–8 days after transplantation (3, 4). The initial regenerative phase is accomplished by donor cells, but by 3 wk after transplantation the graft is repopulated by host cells (8–11). In contrast, lymphoid proliferation and differentiation does not occur in allogenic thymus grafts after the early transplant period of necrosis and rejection is usually complete by 12–14 days (6).

The grafting of thymus tissue under the renal capsule has the distinct advantage of allowing a detailed morphological analysis of both the graft and the host response. Successful immunological reconstitution of neonatally thymectomized mice can be achieved in a high proportion of mice grafted with syngenic thymic tissue (3, 12). Similarly, thymus grafts with minor, non–$H-2$ histocompatibility differences are usually successful in reconstituting a significant percentage of neonatally thymectomized mice and the success of such grafting varies with the strains of mice used (12). In contrast, allogenic thymus grafts across major $H-2$ histocompatibility barriers often fail to achieve immunological reconstitution and frequently induce a severe and fatal graft-vs.-host disease (GVH)[1] (12). The capacity of thymus grafts to induce GVH was further defined by producing GVH with the implantation of parental thymus grafts into neonatally thymectomized F_1 hybrid mice (13).

---

* Aided by grants from The National Foundation–March of Dimes, US Public Health Service (AI-08677 and AI-00798).

[1] *Abbreviations used in this paper*: GVH, graft-vs.-host disease; SRBC, sheep erythrocytes; UMC, University of Minnesota colony sublines.

Children with a congenital absence of the thymus have an immunological deficiency similar to that produced by neonatal thymectomy in mice (14, 15). Thymus transplants, taken from fetuses early in gestation, have given apparent successful reconstitution of cell-mediated immunity in two of these patients (16, 17). Concern has been raised as to the capacity of a primitive "wet membrane" of fetal thymic tissue to have any influence in the immunological reconstitution of these patients (18, 19). The following experiments were undertaken to examine the capacity of the murine fetal thymus, taken early in gestation, to withstand transplantation and develop normally under the renal capsule of a syngenic host. Furthermore, the capacity of embryonic thymus grafts with minor and major histocompatibility differences to develop and restore immunologically, neonatally thymectomized mice was studied.

Materials and Methods

Mice.—Inbred mice of the A/Jax, C3H, C57BL/1, DBA/2, CBA/H, and (C3H × A)F_1 strains were used. The inbred strains of mice originated from the colonies of the late Doctors J. J. Bittner and C. Martinez. A detailed description of the strains has been reported (20); they are designated as the University of Minnesota colony sublines (UMC).

Thymus Grafting.—Donor thymuses were removed aseptically from 13-day-old fetuses and transferred to cold normal saline. For the morphological studies of thymus transplantation the left kidney of the recipient mouse was exposed through a flank incision under Nembutal anesthesia. A single lobe of thymus was introduced under the renal capsule by means of fine forceps. The skin was closed with wound clips. For the restoration experiments, two to five thymus grafts were injected intraperitoneally into 6-day-old neonatally thymectomized mice. Fetal thymuses were obtained from 14–18-day-old embryos. Adult thymuses were obtained from three 15–30-day-old mice.

Neonatal thymectomy was performed using a standard technique for our laboratory (21). Skin grafting from DBA/2 donors was performed between 75 and 100 days of age using a technique previously described (22). Skin graft rejection in less than 15 days was considered normal. Approximately 30 days after skin grafting the mice were given 0.2 ml of a 20% suspension of sheep erythrocytes (SRBC) intraperitoneally. Sera were titrated for anti-SRBC hemagglutinins in saline 9 days after challenge. These were expressed as the logarithim to the base 2 of the reciprocal of the final dilution showing macroscopically visible agglutination. Titers greater than 7 were considered significant. At 250 days the mice were sacrificed and examined under the dissecting microscope for thymic remnants in the neck. Mice with thymic remnants were excluded.

Histology.—The recipient mice were sacrificed at various time intervals after thymus transplantation and the kidneys removed. The tissues were fixed in Formalin and 5-μ sections were cut and stained with hematoxylin and eosin. Serial sections were prepared on each thymus graft.

RESULTS

Development of Syngenic Fetal Thymus Grafts.—The growth and development of the fetal thymus grafted into a normal syngenic host had several characteristic stages (Figs. 1–8).

At 13 days' gestation the mouse thymus is virtually devoid of lymphocytes (23). 24 hr after grafting a 13-day-old fetal thymus under the renal capsule, a healthy-appearing graft was observed. No evidence of the necrosis and hemorrhage described for newborn or young adult grafts (7) was encountered. The primary cell at this stage is the stromal reticular-epithelial cell. Occasional lymphocytes and mitotic figures were seen throughout the graft. These probably represent the very early stages of lymphoid stem cell division and differentiation which lead to the development of a normal-appearing thymus.

48 hr after grafting the thymus had increased considerably in size. Microscopic examination showed many more lymphocytes (Fig. 4). These were actively proliferating cells as evidenced by the many mitotic figures seen in the section. Clear evidence of a vascularization was seen in that area of the grafted thymus next to the kidney parenchyma (Fig. 4). In contrast, the area adjacent to the renal capsule did not appear to be vascularized.

7 days after grafting, the fetal thymus contained densely packed lymphocytes and had the characteristic appearance of thymus cortex. Early evidence of lobulation was seen. A peripheral thin layer of large pale-appearing cells was seen adjacent to the kidney parenchyma (Fig. 5).

The thymus graft continued to grow rapidly. 12 days after grafting a well-differentiated cortex and medulla were seen (Fig. 7). Normal-appearing Hassall's corpuscles were present in the medulla (Fig. 8). Mitotic activity remained high. A clear line of demarcation existed between the thymus and kidney. No apparent cellular infiltration was seen in the renal cortex as compared with the normal kidney.

Thymus Development across Non–H-2 Histocompatibility Barriers.—Thymuses from fetal (13–15 days) CBA/H mice were grafted into normal 30-day-old C3H mice. These thymus grafts underwent a normal stage of early proliferation and differentiation. No necrosis was seen after transplantation. The lymphoid proliferation continued with differentiation into a normal medulla and cortex, Hassall's corpuscles, lobulation, and normal cellular morphology. No differences between the development of these grafts compared with syngenic grafts were observed until 20–25 days.

In some animals evidence of rejection appeared as early as 25 days posttransplantation (Fig. 9). These signs of rejection first appeared in the periphery of the graft. A round cell infiltrate was present in the area between the thymus and kidney. In addition the renal cortex appeared to contain an increased number of lymphoid cells; however, in some mice evidence of rejection of such thymus transplants did not appear until 50–60 days.

Thymus Development across H-2 Histocompatibility Barriers.—When 13-day-old fetal A thymuses were transplanted into normal C3H and C57BL/1 mice, early acute rejection was not seen. During the 1st wk after transplantation the graft underwent early growth and intense lymphoid proliferation. By 8–10 days after grafting growth and development ceased and rejection of the graft began. By 12–14 days graft rejection was extensive and usually complete by 15–20 days. Cell destruction was widespread, and polymorphonuclear leukocytes, cellular debris, fragmented and pycnotic nuclei were seen (Fig. 11).

In contrast to the fetal thymus graft, neonatal A strain thymus grafts trans-

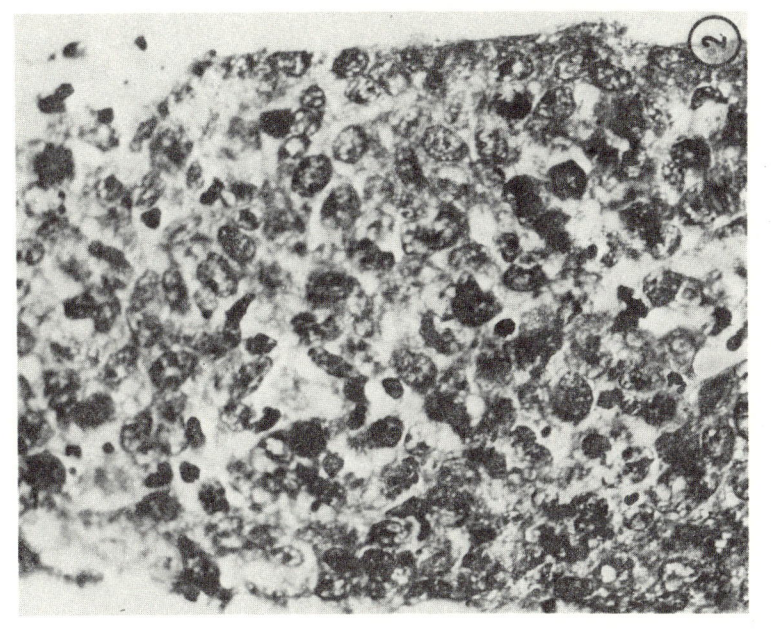

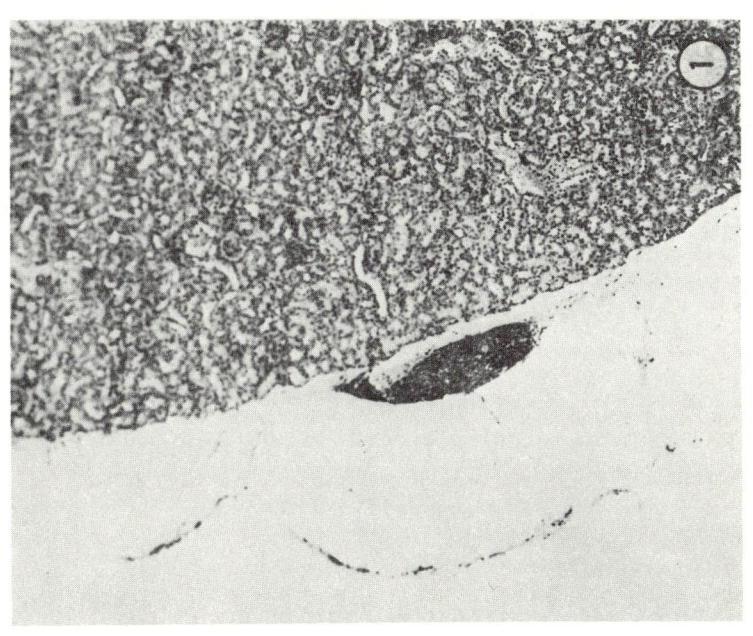

FIG. 1. Subcapsular thymus graft from a 13-day-old A fetal donor 24 hr after grafting into a normal 30-day-old syngenic host. No necrosis is seen. × 50.
FIG. 2. Higher magnification of Fig. 1. The cellular architecture is intact. Large reticular-epithelial cells predominate and occasional mitotic figures are present. × 600.

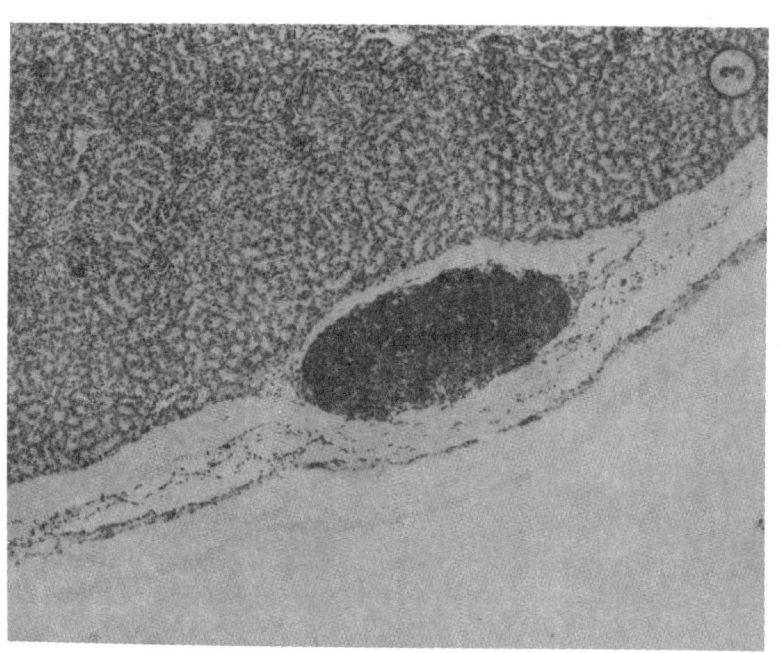

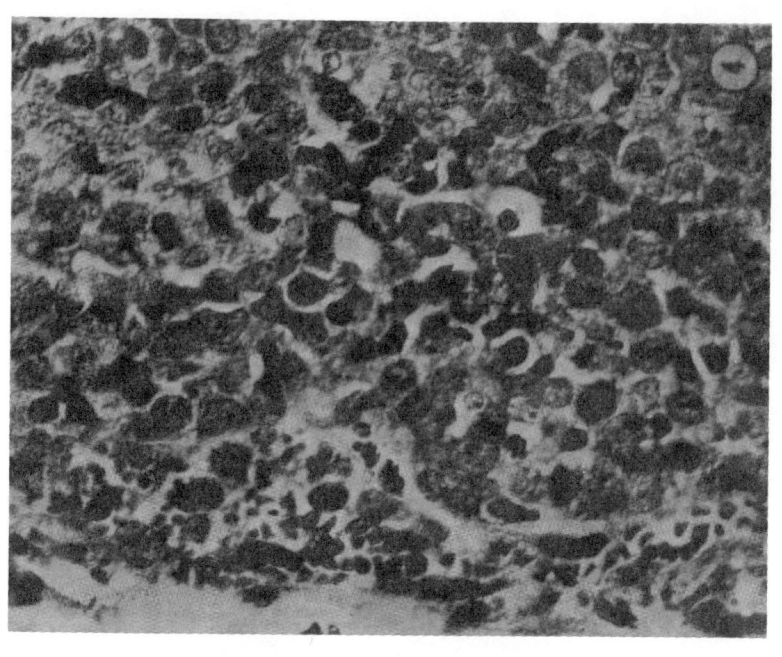

FIG. 3. Subcapsular thymus graft from a 13-day-old A fetal donor 48 hr after grafting into a normal 30-day-old syngenic host. Considerable growth of the thymus has occurred. No necrosis is evident. × 50.

FIG. 4. Higher magnification of Fig. 3. The predominant cell is the large reticular-epithelial cell. Thymocytes have appeared. Vessels are seen containing red blood cells. × 600.

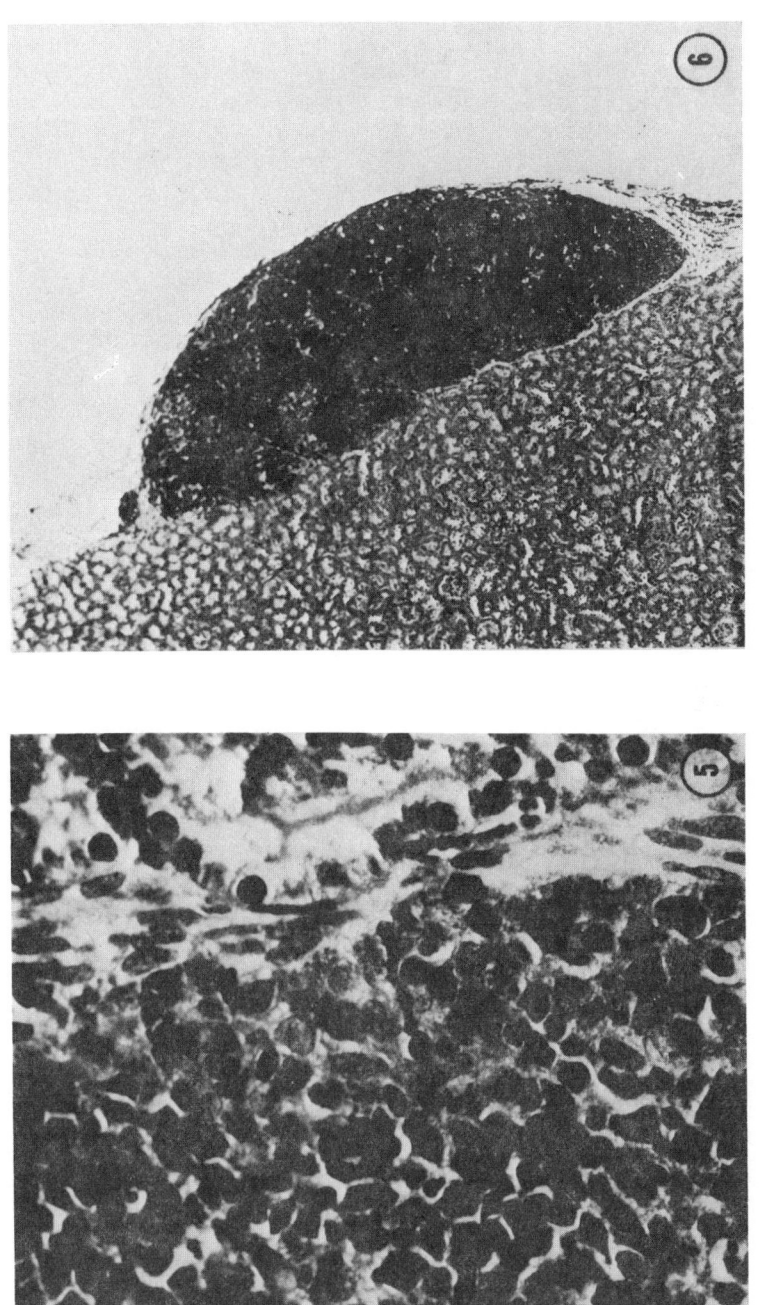

FIG. 5. Subcapsular thymus graft from a 13-day-old A fetal donor 72 hr after grafting into a normal 30-day-old syngenic host at the junction of thymus graft and kidney cortex. Many large, medium, and small thymocytes are packed within the reticular-epithelial framework (large clear nuclei). × 600.

FIG. 6. Subcapsular thymus graft from a 13-day-old A fetal donor 7 days after grafting into a normal 30-day-old syngenic host. The thymus, primarily cortex, shows early differentiation into a medullary zone. × 50.

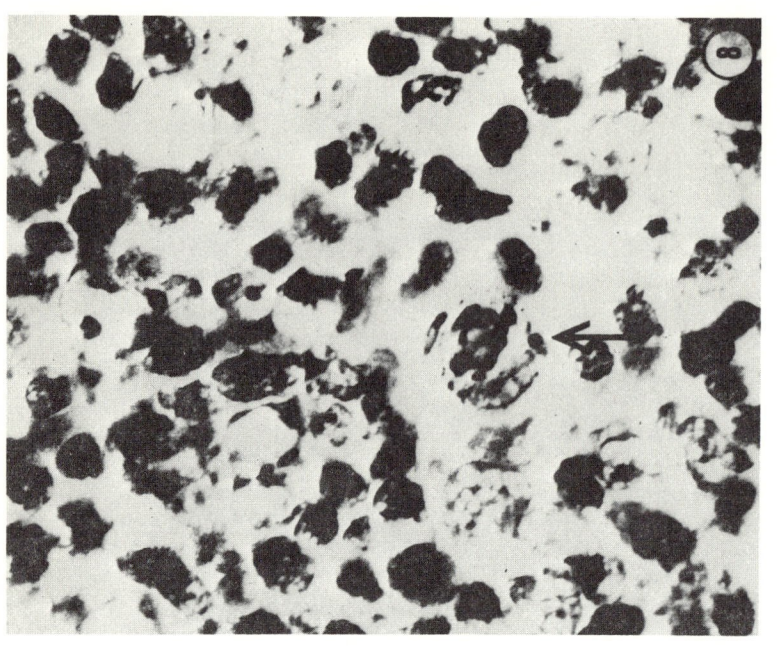

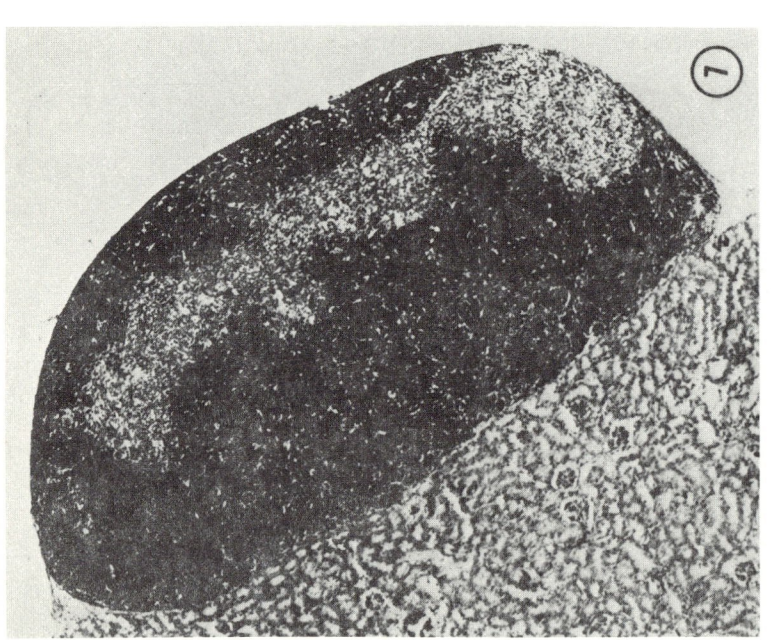

FIG. 7. Subcapsular thymus graft from a 13 day old A fetal donor 12 days after grafting into a normal 30-day-old syngenic host. A well differentiated cortex and medulla are present. × 50.

FIG. 8. Subcapsular thymus graft from a 13 day old A fetal donor 12 days after grafting to a normal 30-day-old syngenic host. A normal Hassall's corpuscle is seen surrounded by epithelial reticular cells and thymocytes. × 100 oil.

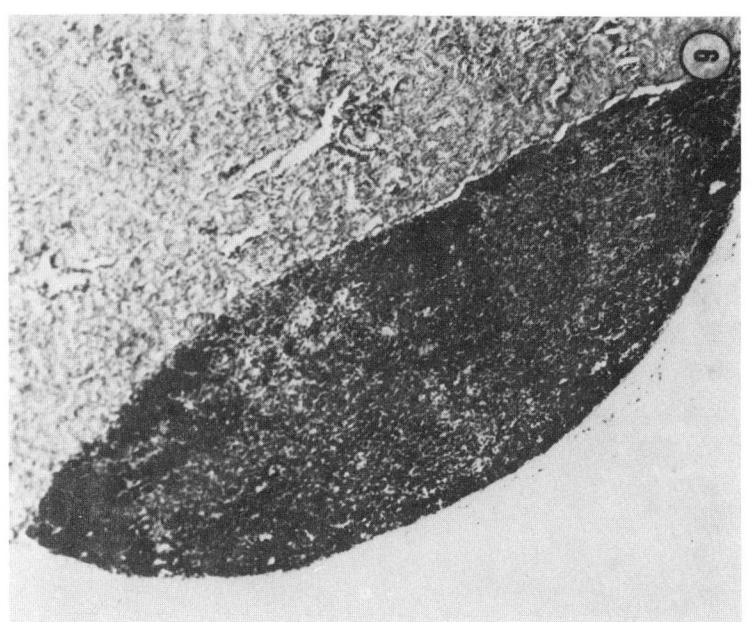

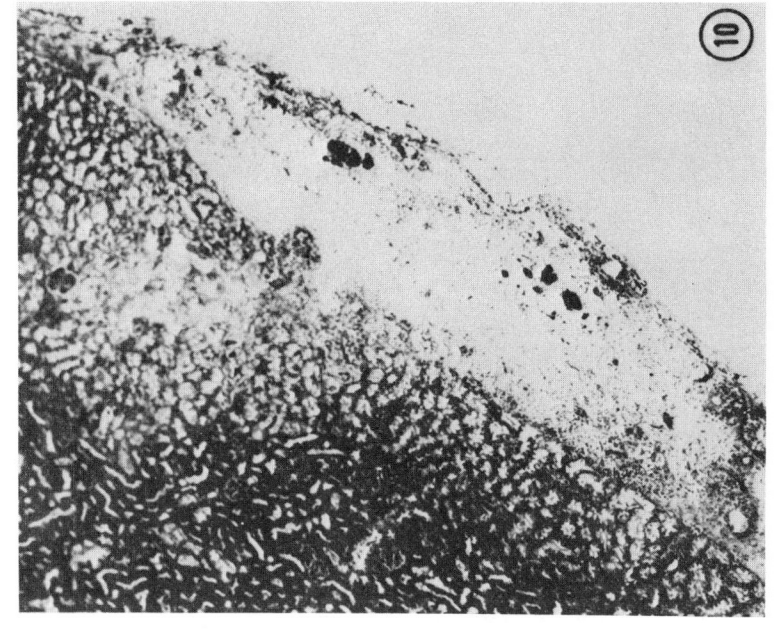

FIG. 9. Subcapsular thymus graft from a 13-day-old CBA/H fetal donor 180 days after grafting into a normal 30-day-old C3H host. The thymus shows evidence of rejection with preservation of thymic architecture. × 50.

FIG. 10. Subcapsular thymus graft from a neonatal A donor 48 hr after grafting into a normal 30-day-old C57BL/1 host. Extensive necrosis and loss of thymic architecture is evident. × 50.

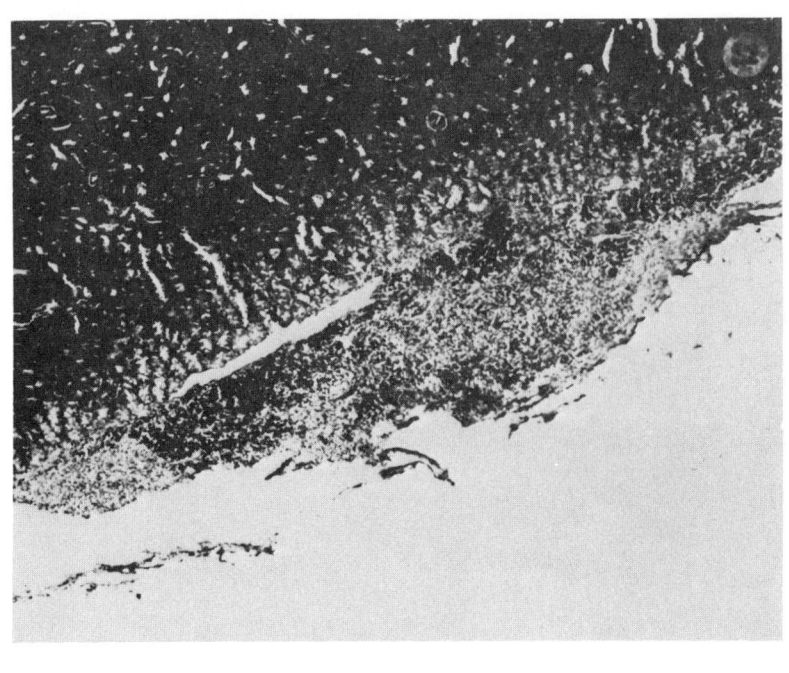

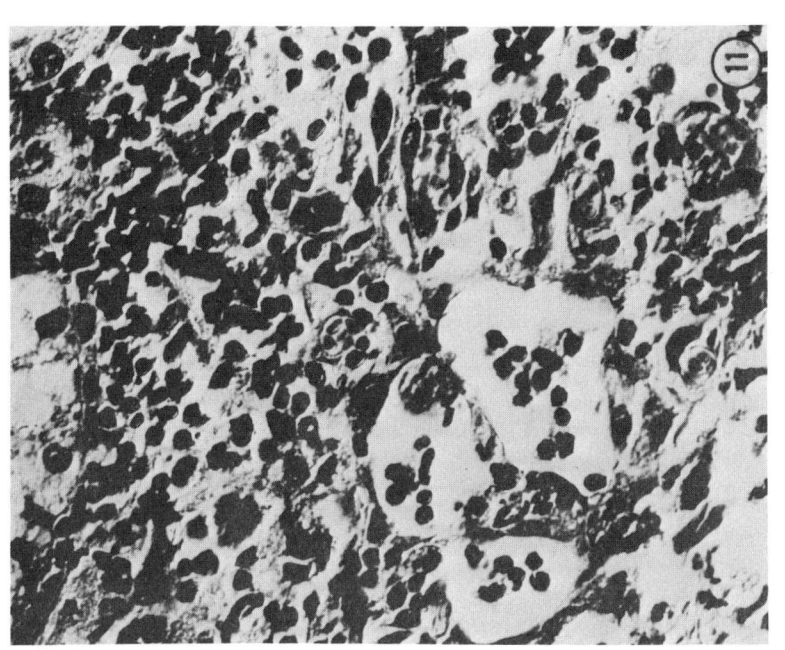

Fig. 11. Subcapsular thymus graft from a 13-day-old A fetal donor 15 days after grafting into a normal 30-day-old syngenic host. Cell destruction is extensive. Pycnotic lymphocytes, polymorphonuclear leukocytes, fragmented nuclei, cellular debris, and hemorrhage are present. × 600.

Fig. 12. Subcapsular thymus graft from a neonatal A donor 12 days after grafting into a normal 30-day-old C57BL/1 host. No repopulation of the graft is evident and rejection is almost complete. × 50.

planted into normal 30-day-old C3H or C57BL/1 hosts underwent rapid and acute necrosis (Fig. 10). 24–48 hr after grafting intense hemorrhagic necrosis was seen. Pycnotic lymphocytes, polymorphonuclear leukocytes, fragmented nuclei, cellular debris, and hemorrhages were present. An intense round cell infiltrate of small lymphocytes and histiocytes was seen in the renal cortex and at the junction of the thymus graft and kidney cortex. Progressive fibrosis and scarring ensued. Rejection was complete by 8–12 days (Fig. 12). Morphological analysis of thymus grafts under the renal capsule is summarized in Table I.

Immune Restoration of Thymectomized Mice using Different Thymus Grafts.— Table II shows the capacity of the various thymus grafts to restore neonatally

TABLE I
Morphologic Analysis of Renal Subcapsular Fetal and Adult Thymus Grafts*

	Syngenic		Allogenic non-H-2 different		Allogenic H-2 different	
	Fetal	Adult	Fetal	Adult	Fetal	Adult
Early necrosis	0/7	5/5	0/5	5/5	0/5	5/5
Acceptance graft‡	9/11	9/10	9/10	10/10	0/10	0/10
Normal rejection§	0/10	0/10	0/10	0/8	5/9	10/10
Late rejection‖	0/5	0/5	5/5	5/5	0/8	0/5

* Morphological studies were done on renal subcapsular thymus grafts examined at various time intervals. Recipients were normal C3H and C57BL/1 mice who were transplanted with syngenic, allogenic non–H-2 different (CBA/H into C3H), and allogenic H-2 different (A into C57BL/1) thymus grafts.
‡ Normal-appearing thymus 60 days after transplantation.
§ Rejection of thymus graft in less than 15 days.
‖ Rejection of thymus graft in greater than 30 days.

thymectomized mice. The parameters of restoration studied were the capacity to form antibodies in response to an antigenic challenge with SRBC, the capacity to reject a third-party skin graft, and to survive 250 days. The 250-day survival of mice grafted with syngenic fetal thymuses was almost equal to that of mice grafted with adult thymuses (75 vs. 85%, respectively). A high percentage of mice given fetal grafts had a good SRBC response (80%) and normal skin graft rejection (100%). When parental strain thymus grafts were given, the fetal thymus proved to be far superior in immunologic reconstitution than were grafts of adult thymuses. 72% of the mice grafted with parental fetal thymuses survived 250 days whereas only 33% of the mice grafted with parental adult thymuses survived that long. Furthermore, the results of syngenic fetal and parental fetal grafts were similar.

When thymus grafting was across a major H-2 histocompatibility barrier (A to C3H) the fetal thymus again was more effective than the adult thymus. 43% of the mice given fetal grafts survived 250 days. All these mice had normal skin graft rejection and 47% had a good antibody response to SRBC. These results stand in marked contrast to those of mice given adult allogenic thymus where only 5% survived 250 days.

DISCUSSION

The observations presented here clearly demonstrate that a fetal thymus transplanted under the renal capsule of a syngenic host develops into a morpho-

TABLE II

Restoration of 6-Day-Old Neonatally Thymectomized Mice Grafted with Fetal or Adult Thymus*

Thymus donor	Recipient	No. surviving 250 days	No. with normal SRBC response‡	No. with normal skin graft rejection§
(C3H × A)F$_1$ adult	(C3H × A)F$_1$	12/14 (85%)	10/12 (84%)	12/12 (100%)
(C3H × A)F$_1$ fetal	(C2H × A)F$_1$	44/59 (75%)	12/15 (80%)	12/12 (100%)
A adult	(C3H × A)F$_1$	5/13 (33%)	Not done	4/5 (80%)
A fetal	(C3H × A)F$_1$	31/43 (72%)	11/15 (74%)	12/12 (100%)
A adult	C3H	1/20 (5%)	Not done	0/1 (0%)
A fetal	C3H	19/44 (43%)	9/19 (47%)	10/10 (100%)
None	(C3H × A)F$_1$	0/20 (0%)	3/20 (15%)	1/18 (5.5%)

* Neonatally thymectomized (C3H × A)F$_1$ and C3H mice grafted intraperitoneally at 6 days of age. Fetal thymus was obtained from 15–18-day-old embryos. Adult thymus was obtained from 30–40-day-old mice. Recipients were given two to five thymuses.

‡ SRBC agglutination titer (log$_2$) greater than 7 was considered normal.

§ Rejection of DBA/2 skin grafts in less than 15 days was considered normal.

logically normal thymus. At 13 days of gestation, the thymus is comprised primarily of reticular-epithelial stromal cells derived from the third and fourth pharyngeal pouches (1, 23). These stromal cells have a round or oval irregular nucleus and a spherical nucleolus. The nucleus is surrounded by abundant cytoplasm which contains small vacuoles (24). When a neonatal or adult thymus is grafted under the renal capsule of a syngenic host, rapid and massive necrosis occurs throughout the graft during the first 24–48 hr. Only a small number of epithelial and lymphoid cells remain in the periphery (3, 7–11). After phagocytosis of nuclear debris, intense mitotic activity is apparent and normal thymic architecture is restored by 7–8 days (3, 4). The fetal thymus graft on the other hand, appears healthy, contains viable cells, and is free of overt necrosis in the early posttransplant period. The absence of necrosis may be related to the graft size (25), the absence of rapidly dividing thymic lymphocytes, qualitative and/or quantitative differences in cell surface antigens, or to the relative avascularity of the 13-day-old embryonic thymus. 48 hr after transplantation, considerable growth and evidence of vascularization had occurred. The vessels first appeared in the area next to the kidney parenchyma. Active cell proliferation was seen. The lymphoid cells proliferating at this time are probably progeny of stem cells present in the graft at the time of transplantation (25).

The graft continued to grow and to be populated with densely packed lymphocytes. These varied in size and had a deeply stained nucleus surrounded by a small rim of cytoplasm. By 7 days, islands of reticular-epithelial cells were distinguishable as medullas. Contained in these medullary islands were larger lymphocytes with deeply staining nuclei, containing central nucleoli and large clumps of chromatin attached to the dense nuclear membrane. The nucleus was enclosed by a rim of cytoplasm. 12 days after grafting the medullary region appeared to be fully developed and to contain Hassall's corpuscles.

These observations indicate that the primitive fetal thymic anlage, at a stage when reticular-epithelial stromal cells predominate, can withstand the trauma of transplantation. Furthermore, these studies clearly demonstrate that fetal thymus is capable of restoring neonatally thymectomized mice as well as the adult thymus and is superior to the adult thymus when allogenic grafting is done (Table II). The relevance of these data to the treatment of thymic deficiency syndromes in man (16, 17) is obvious. If the thymus graft had been significantly traumatized by the surgical manipulation, delay in its growth and development in the transplanted host would have occurred. The thymus tissue transplanted in these experiments appeared to develop and mature at a rate very similar to that of a normal fetal thymus.

When allogenic thymus was grafted into mice with non–H-2 histocompatibility differences (CBA/H into C3H), a similar early period of rapid growth and development was observed. These grafts appeared to be healthy mature thymuses until approximately 20–25 days after transplantation. At this time, progressive lymphocyte infiltration appeared at the periphery of the graft. The central portion of the grafted thymus remained intact. Progressive cellular infiltration and cellular destruction ensued. By 60–80 days, only a small island of normal-appearing thymus remained. Complete rejection and fibrosis followed; however, in some mice, complete rejection was as late as 180–200 days.

Allogenic fetal thymuses grafted across a major histocompatibility barrier (A into C3H) were rejected a little more slowly than were thymus grafts taken from neontal donors. The thymus grafts from allogenic neonatal donors failed to develop after the early period of necrosis (3, 6, 12). The degree of lymphoid proliferation and graft repopulation related to the immunological capacity of the host. Neonatally thymectomized mice apparently accepted these allogenic non–H-2 identical grafts at the times studied. That nonimmune factors might also influence the capacity of lymphoid cells to proliferate in the adult thymus after transplantation was suggested by the occurrence of acute and severe rejection phenomenon with virtually no latent period (3, 7).

Fetal allogenic thymus grafts were not rejected as rapidly as were the neonatal grafts. These grafts clearly underwent lymphoid proliferation in the early stages after transplantation. By 8–10 days, an intense cellular infiltrate appeared in the renal cortex and the process of rejection followed. The early lymphoid development within the allogenic fetal thymus graft, as compared with the neonatal thymus graft, may be related to quantitative and/or qualitative differences in the tissue-specific surface antigens of fetal cells. Fetal cells are known to contain less H-2 specificity than do similar cells from newborn mice (26). Similarly, surface isoantigens, for example TL, are expressed on thymus cells towards the latter part of gestation (25). Fetal tissues early in gestation might then be expected to reflect the weak antigenic stimulus to the immunocompetent host and a delay of the rejection phenomenon.

These studies have shown that the fetal thymus, obtained early in gestation when it is primarily a reticular-epithelial structure, can withstand the surgical manipulation of transplantation and undergo apparently normal differentiation and maturation under the renal capsule of a secondary syngenic host. It seems possible therefore that a similar process of development and restoration could occur in the patients with a congenital absence of the thymus who are transplanted with fetal thymic tissue (14, 15). Hematopoietic pluripotential prethymic stem cells would migrate to the thymus graft and, under its influence, thymus cell maturation processes and immunocompetence would be achieved (27). These immunologically competent lymphocytes could then traffic from the thymus and restore the peripheral lymphoid tissues. When major histocompatibility differences exist between the donor thymus and host, these developing immunocompetent, thymus-derived lymphocytes could conceivably recognize the grafted thymus as being foreign and thus reject it. Evidence of such a phenomenon has been observed in mice (12, 28). If a similar process applies to man, a patient restored with an HL-A–incompatible thymus graft might be expected to reject that same thymus which restored his cell-mediated immune deficiency. Such a patient might then slowly develop deficiencies of cell-mediated immunity similar to those present before transplantation and thus require retransplantation.

SUMMARY

The fetal thymus at 13 days of gestation withstands transplantation and develops normally under the renal capsule of a syngenic host. Distinct differences were observed between the fetal thymus grafts and grafts from neonatal or adult thymus donors. The fetal thymus graft did not undergo the rapid and severe necrosis observed when adult thymus was grafted. Furthermore, when thymuses were transplanted into allogenic recipients, rejection was delayed.

The fetal thymus was as effective as the adult thymus in restoring syngenic neonatally thymectomized mice and far superior to adult thymus when grafted into allogenic recipients. These observations seem relevant to clinical efforts to restore immunocompetence in patients with congenital absence of the thymus.

We thank Jim Wicks for his excellent technical assistance.

REFERENCES

1. Rugh, R. 1968. The Mouse, Its Reproduction and Development. Burgess Publishing Company, Minneapolis, Minn.
2. Jaffe, H. L. 1926. Autoplastic thymus transplants. *J. Exp. Med.* **44**:523.
3. Dukor, P., J. F. A. P. Miller, W. House, and V. Allman. 1965. Regeneration of thymus grafts. I. Histological and cytological aspects. *Transplantation.* **3**:639.
4. Blackburn, W. R., and J. F. A. P. Miller. 1967. Electron microscopic studies of thymus graft regeneration and rejection. I. Syngeneic grafts. *Lab. Invest.* **16**:66.
5. Blackburn, W. R., and J. F. A. P. Miller. 1967. Electron microscopic studies of thymus graft regeneration and rejection. II. Syngeneic-irradiated grafts. *Lab. Invest.* **16**:833.
6. Blackburn, W. R., and J. F. A. P. Miller. 1968. Electron microscopic studies of thymus graft regeneration and rejection. III. Allogeneic grafts. *Lab. Invest.* **18**:771.
7. Law, L. W., and J. H. Miller, 1950. The influence of thymectomy on the incidence of carcinogen induced leukemia in strain DBA mice. *J. Nat. Cancer Inst.* **2**:425.
8. Metcalf, D., and R. Wakonig-Vaartaja. 1964. Stem cell replacement in normal thymus grafts. *Proc. Soc. Exp. Biol. Med.* **115**:731.
9. Metcalf, D., R. Wakonig-Vaartaja, and T. R. Bradley. 1965. The growth and repopulation of thymus grafts placed under the kidney capsule. *Aust. J. Exp. Biol. Med. Sci.* **43**:17.
10. Schlesinger, M., and D. Hurvitz. 1968. Serological analysis of thymus and spleen grafts. *J. Exp. Med.* **127**:1127.
11. Green, I. 1964. The regeneration of F_1 host cell spleen and thymus at ectopic sites in F_1 animals induced by implantation of parental spleen and thymus. *J. Exp. Med.* **119**:581.
12. Stutman, O., E. J. Yunis, and R. A. Good. 1969. Tolerance induction with thymus grafts in neonatally thymectomized mice. *J. Immunol.* **103**:92.
13. Stutman, O., E. J. Yunis, P. O. Teague, and R. A. Good. 1968. Graft-*versus*-host reactions induced by transplantation of parental strain thymus in neonatally thymectomized F_1 hybrid mice. *Transplantation.* **6**:514.
14. DiGeorge, A. M. 1965. A new concept of the cellular basis of immunity *J. Pediat.* **67**:907. (Abstr.)
15. DiGeorge, A. M. 1968. *In* Immunologic Deficiency Diseases of Man. R. A. Good and D. Bergsma, editors. National Foundation March of Dimes Publisher, New York. 116.
16. Cleveland, W. W., B. J. Fogel, W. T. Brown, and H. E. M. Kay. 1968. Foetal thymic transplant in a case of DiGeorge's syndrome. *Lancet.* **2**:1211.
17. August, C. S., F. S. Rosen, R. M. Filler, C. A. Janeway, B. Markowski, and H. E. M. Kay. 1968. Implantation of a foetal thymus, restoring immunological

competence in a patient with thymic aplasia (DiGeorge's syndrome). *Lancet.* **2**:1210.
18. Dempster, W. J. 1969. Transplanting the thymus. Letter to the Editor. *Lancet.* **1**:468.
19. Dempster, W. J. 1970. Treatment of congenital thymic aplasia by graft of fetal thymus. *Lancet.* **1**:1294.
20. Staats, J., editor. 1969. *In* Inbred Strains of Mice. Jackson Laboratories, Bar Harbor, Maine. 60.
21. Sjodin, K., A. P. Dalmasso, J. M. Smith, and C. Martinez. 1963. Thymectomy in newborn and adult mice. *Transplantation.* **1**:521.
22. Martinez, C., J. M. Smith, J. B. Aust, and R. A. Good. 1958. Acquired tolerance to skin homografts in mice of different strains. *Proc. Soc. Exp. Biol. Med.* **97**:736.
23. Auerbach, R. 1964. *In* The Thymus in Immunobiology. R. A. Good and A. E. Gabrielsen, editors. Hoeber Medical Division. Harper and Row, Publishers, New York. 95.
24. Smith, C. 1964. *In* The Thymus in Immunobiology. R. A. Good and A. E. Gabrielsen, editors. Hoeber Medical Division. Harper and Row, Publishers, New York. 71.
25. Owen, J. J. T., and M. C. Raff. 1970. Studies on the differentiation of thymus-derived lymphocytes. *J. Exp. Med.* **132**:1216.
26. Schlessinger, M. 1964. Serologic studies of embryonic and trophoblastic tissues of the mouse. *J. Immunol.* **93**:255.
27. Stutman, O., and R. A. Good. 1971. Immunocompetence of embryonic hematopoietic cells after traffic to thymus. *Transplant. Proc.* **3**:923.
28. Stutman, O., E. J. Yunis, and R. A. Good. 1969. Reversal of post-thymectomy wasting in mice with immunocompetent cells: Influence of histocompatibility differences. *J. Immunol.* **102**:87.

Differentation of Foetal Mouse Thymus. Ultrastructure of Organ Cultures and of Subcapsular Grafts†

T. Mandel and Pamela J. Russell

INTRODUCTION

Over the past decade the role of the thymus in the development of immune competence has been widely investigated. Although it is clear that thymic lymphocytes are important in both cellular and humoral immunity, very little is known of the events which occur within the thymus and which result in the production of immunologically mature lymphocytes from stem cells. Moore and Owen (1967) showed that stem cells entered the early foetal epithelial thymus from the blood stream and their experiments dispelled the idea that lymphoid cells developed by differentiation from the thymic epithelium (Auerbach, 1960, 1961, 1963; Ball and Auerbach, 1960; Weakley, Patt and Shepro, 1964; Izard, 1966; Sanel, 1967).

Lymphoid stem cells can be identified in the early foetal mouse thymus with the light microscope (Moore and Owen, 1967) and also with the electron microscope (Hoshino, Takeda, Abe and Ito, 1969; Mandel, 1970). *In vivo*, a constant influx of stem cells enters

† This is Publication No. 1478 from the Walter and Eliza Hall Institute.

the thymus throughout life as has been shown by studies of parabiosed mice (Harris, Ford, Barnes and Evans, 1964; Ford, 1966), by the repopulation of thymus grafts (Metcalf and Wakonig-Vaartaja, 1964), and of the thymus in irradiated recipients (Ford and Micklem, 1963). Within the thymic micro-environment the lymphoid stem cells proliferate and differentiate and their progeny leave the thymus (Weissman, 1967) to colonize the thymus-dependent areas of the secondary lymphoid tissue (Parrott, de Sousa and East, 1966) and form part of the recirculating lymphocyte pool (Miller, Mitchell and Weiss, 1967).

The mechanisms which control the intrathymic development of lymphoid stem cells are not understood but it seems likely that epithelial cells play a dominant role. Metcalf (1956) suggested that a lymphopoietic humoral factor was produced by the thymic epithelial cells, and in the guinea-pig thymic cortex mitotic figures of lymphocytes were commonly adjacent to epithelial cells (Mandel, 1969). Others have suggested that the proliferative and competence-inducing functions of the thymus may be under the control of separate factors (Osoba and Miller, 1964). Recently functional thymic epithelial tumours have been produced which have the capacity to restore immunological competence in neonatally thymectomized mice (Stutman, Yunis and Good, 1968; 1969a,b). The thymic epithelial cells thus appear to be closely implicated in the development of immunologically competent cells and their further study is clearly warranted.

In this study we have investigated the development of the early foetal mouse thymus in organ culture under conditions in which the number of stem cells is restricted to those already present in the explanted tissue. The ability of such cultured tissue to reform a thymus *in vivo* was also investigated in syngeneic neonatally thymectomized and sham thymectomized animals. The functional capacity of the cultured organs will be reported separately.

MATERIALS AND METHODS

Thymuses were obtained from 12–13-day-old foetal (C57Bl × CBA)F_1 mice, the gestation stage being determined by noting the appearance of vaginal plugs (Auerbach, 1960). The thymuses were isolated in 50 per cent horse serum in phosphate buffered saline and placed on to a millipore filter well assembly for culture (Auerbach, 1960). The culture medium consisted of Eagles Basal Medium (Commonwealth Serum Laboratories, Melbourne), 10 per cent horse serum (CSL) and 5 per cent chick embryo extract (9 day) to which were added 7 ml of sodium bicarbonate solution (2·8 per cent w/v CSL) per 100 ml and penicillin (50 μg/ml), streptomycin (50 μg/ml), erythromycin (30 μg/ml) and mycostatin (50 μg/ml). The organs were grown in a humidified incubator at 37° in an atmosphere of 5 per cent CO_2 in air with media changes every 3 days.

For electron microscopy, cultures were fixed at daily intervals in ice cold 2½ per cent glutaraldehyde buffered with 0·1 M cacodylate by immersing the culture on the millipore disc into a large excess of fixative. Cultures were sampled at daily intervals for the first 4 days, then less frequently until the 25th day of culture. At least two cultures were examined at each time point.

To study the capacity of the cultures to reform a thymus *in vivo*, single lobes of cultured thymus, maintained *in vitro* for between 14–25 days, were grafted either subcutaneously or beneath the kidney capsule in neonatally thymectomized or sham thymectomized syngeneic mice aged 13–14 days. The grafted thymuses were fixed for light or electron microscopy at daily intervals for the first 4 days, at 1 week and after 6–10 weeks of growth. Subcapsular grafts were separated carefully from the underlying kidney following partial fixation. They were weighed and for ultrastructural study were further diced into pieces less than 1 mm^3 and fully fixed. These tissues were further processed as described previously (Mandel, 1970). For light microscopy the tissues were fixed in 10 per cent formalin and 5 μ paraffin-embedded sections were stained with haematoxylin and eosin. In order to assess the proliferation of the cultured cells counts were made of mitotic figures in 1 μ sections cut from Araldite embedded blocks, stained with toluidine blue and examined with the light microscope. Some cultures were given a 3-hour pulse of tritiated thymidine (1 μCi/culture) before fixation in glutaraldehyde and embedding in Araldite. Thick (1 μ) sections cut from these blocks were dipped in Kodak NTB2 emulsion and exposed for autoradiography. Classification of mitotic figures and labelled cells as either epithelial or lymphocyte was attempted but many cells could not be positively identified with the limited resolution of the light microscope.

RESULTS

Macroscopic appearance of the cultures

Initially the explanted thymuses were ovoid measuring about 0·2–0·3 mm in diameter. They flattened on to the millipore filter and increased markedly in area reaching a maximum size of about 0·5 mm diameter at about the end of the first week. The surface of the cultures initially appeared granular but after a few days they became smooth and shiny. The organs remained intact and very little cellular outgrowth occurred.

Histological appearance of the cultures

The fine structure of the foetal thymuses has been described previously (Mandel, 1970) and served as a basis for comparison with the *in vitro* studies. The 12–13 day thymuses were avascular and were surrounded by loose connective tissue. They were composed of two major cell types; large undifferentiated epithelial cells interspersed with lymphoblasts which could be readily identified ultrastructurally.

During the first 24 hours *in vitro* the tissue showed little obvious change. With the electron microscope epithelial cells and lymphoblasts could again be distinguished largely on the basis of cytoplasmic electron density, the lymphoid cells having a much denser cytoplasm. The nuclei of both cell types were similar in size and shape. Mitotic figures were common and in the majority of cases they were large and open in appearance and were identified as being epithelial (Fig. 1). Mitotic figures of lymphoid cells were rarely identified. A close examination of the epithelial cells showed that they were starting to develop membrane-bounded cytoplasmic bodies (Fig. 2) similar to those described in differentiating cortical epithelial cells *in vivo* in the mouse (Mandel, 1970) and in the guinea-pig (Mandel, 1968a). Desmosomes were again a prominent feature of the epithelial cells and provided a reliable cytological marker for their identification (Fig. 2).

During the first week the principal changes in the thymus were a proliferation and differentiation of the lymphocytes which became the most common cells by the end of the first week (Fig. 3). The majority were typical small to medium lymphocytes identical with those seen in the normal post natal thymus. Mitotic figures were common and most could be identified ultrastructurally as lymphocytic by their small size, dense appearance and absence of desmosomes (Fig. 4). The distinction between dividing lymphocytes and epithelial cells was frequently difficult with the limited resolution of the light microscope.

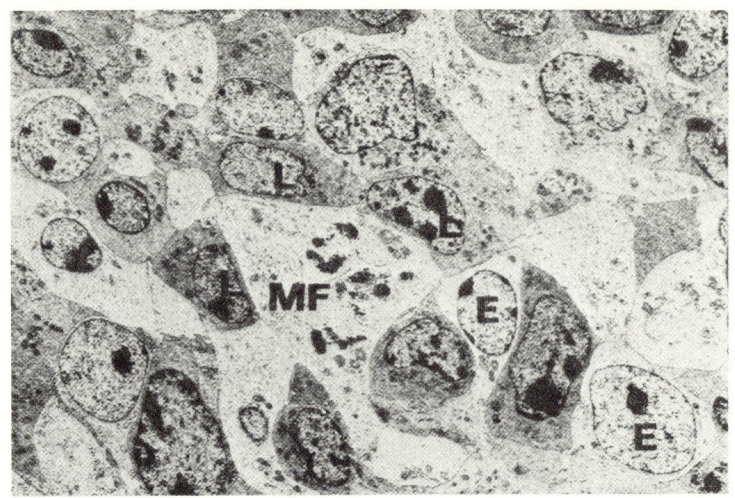

Fig. 1. Electron micrograph of a portion of a 24-hour culture of foetal mouse thymus. The figure shows a mixture of lymphoid cells (L) which are generally large and blast like and have large nuclei with prominent nucleoli and relatively electron dense cytoplasm. The pale cells are epithelial cells (E) and one is seen in division (MF). The epithelial cells and lymphoid cells are of similar overall size. This and all succeeding electron micrographs are of tissue fixed in glutaraldehyde, post-fixed in osmium and stained with uranyl acetate followed by lead citrate. (× 2650.)

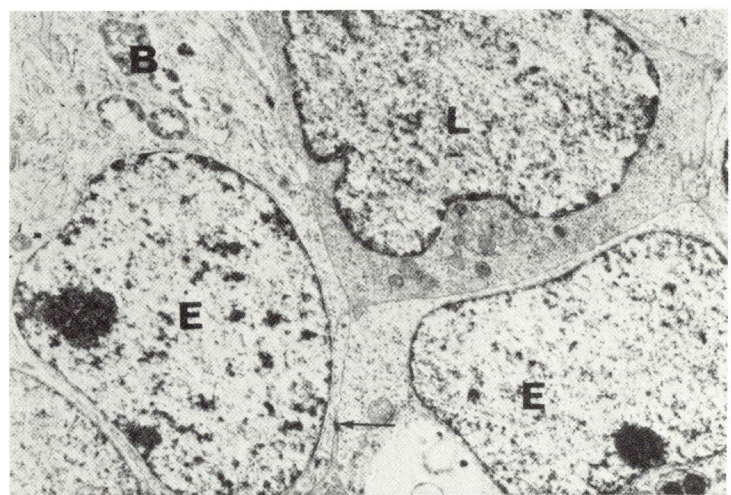

Fig. 2. A higher magnification of a 24-hour culture showing a lymphoblast (L) and portions of epithelial cells (E). Note the denser appearance of the lymphoblast due in part to an accumulation of polyribosomes. One epithelial cell contains some cytoplasmic membrane-bounded bodies (B) which are a characteristic feature of 'cortical' thymic epithelial cells. A small desmosome (arrow) joins two epithelial cells. (× 7850.)

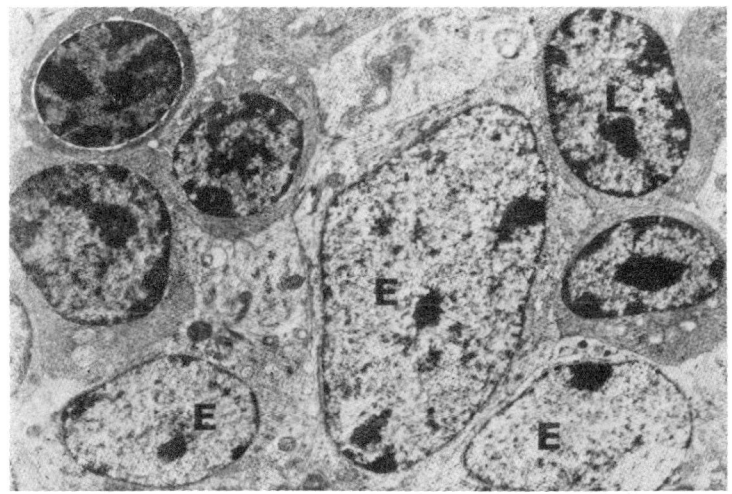

Fig. 3. A portion of a 7-day culture. In contrast with the 24-hour culture and the starting material, there is now a very clear difference in size and appearance between the typical small lymphocytes (L) and the much larger epithelial cells (E). The nuclei of the lymphocytes are rounded and contain condensed and marginated chromatin in contrast to the very large and open epithelial cell nuclei. (× 5560.)

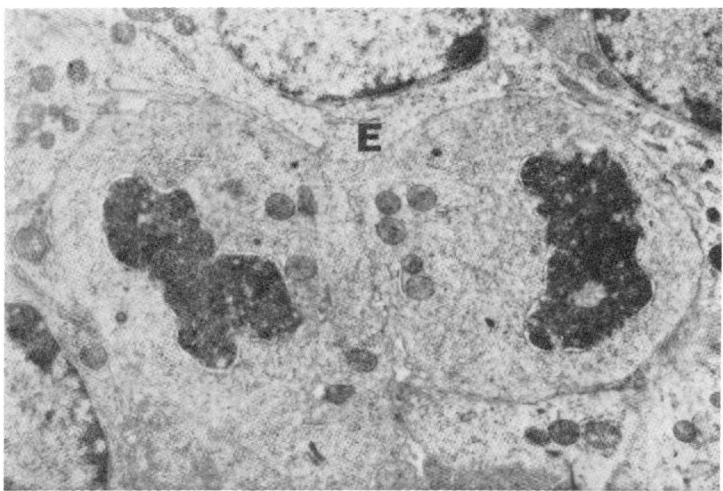

Fig. 4. A dividing lymphocyte from a 96-hour culture. The cell is relatively small and dense with closely aggregated chromosomes. Such mitotic figures formed the majority of those seen during the first 10 days of culture and they could usually be readily distinguished from dividing epithelial cells (compare Fig. 5). The mitotic figure is adjacent to and partially surrounded by an epithelial cell (E). (× 11350.)

Epithelial cells were now larger than the lymphocytes and contained numerous cytoplasmic membrane bounded bodies (Fig. 3). Dividing epithelial cells were also seen and could be positively identified by the presence of desmosomes (Fig. 5). The majority of the cells were intact and appeared to be viable but a few pyknotic epithelial cells and lymphocytes were present.

During the second week the thymuses showed little change in appearance but the numbers of lymphocytes varied widely both from one specimen to another and also within different areas of the same specimen. Most lymphocytes were, however, typically small and medium in size and blasts were rare (Fig. 6). During the third week *in vitro* the proportion of lymphocytes decreased and few lymphoid mitoses were seen. The proportion of dividing

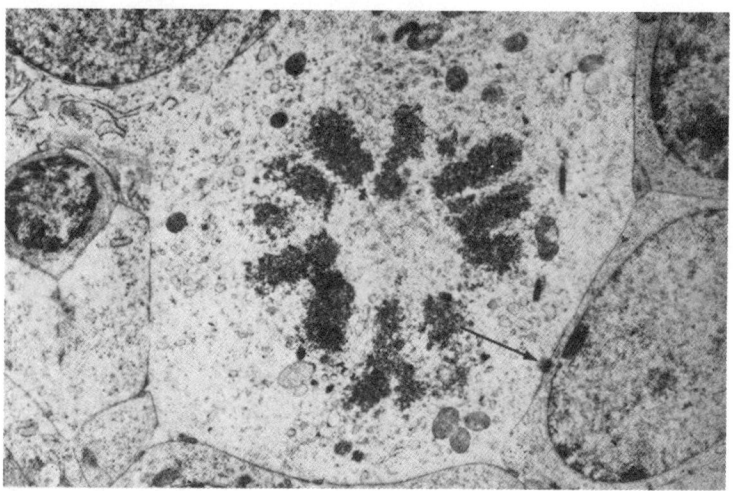

FIG. 5. A dividing epithelial cell from a 72-hour culture. This mitotic figure is large and its chromosomes are widespread. A well-developed desmosome (arrow) links this cell with an adjoining epithelial cell. (× 7800).

cells was smaller than in previous specimens (Table 1) and mitotic figures could usually be identified as being epithelial with the electron microscope. It is important to note, however, that even at this stage numerous apparently viable lymphoid cells were still present (Fig. 7).

Autoradiography and mitotic counts

Since the electron microscope is a poor instrument for screening large volumes of tissue, light microscopy was used to assess the proliferative capacity of the cultured tissue by counts of mitotic figures and tritiated-thymidine labelled cells in 1 μ thick sections. The results of these counts are shown in Table 1. Total rates of cell division could be estimated accurately but the classification of the mitotic figures and labelled cells with the light microscope was frequently difficult. However when the results of the light microscopy

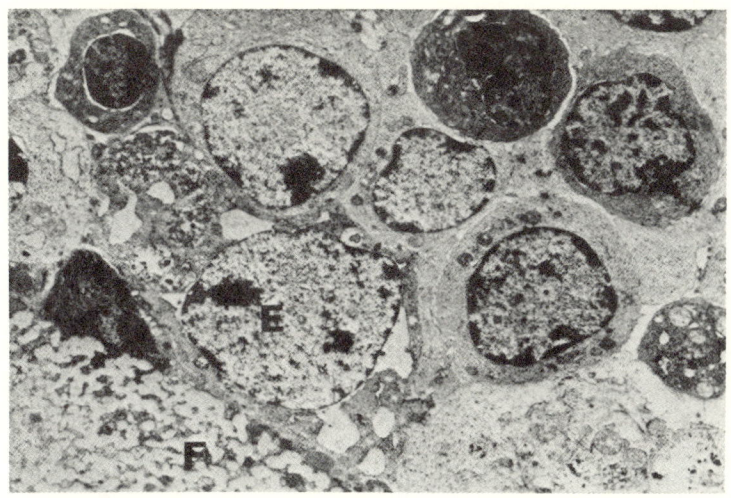

Fig. 6. This portion of a 14-day culture shows large epithelial cells (E) and some smaller dense lymphoid cells (F). A portion of the millipore filter on to which the culture is attached is also visible (F). Cultures at this stage of development were grafted into syngeneic animals. (× 4665.)

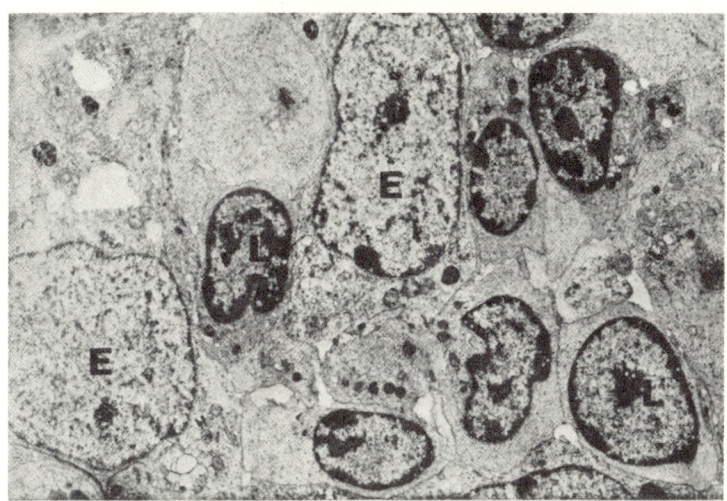

Fig. 7. An 18-day culture showing typical lymphocytes (L) and large epithelial cells (E). This figure represents a lymphoid area of a culture. Other areas of such cultures contained fewer lymphocytes. (× 5100.)

were correlated with the ultrastructural characteristics of mitotic figures, it was apparent that the epithelial cells proliferated throughout the whole period of culture whereas the lymphocytes showed a restricted period of proliferation lasting from the 2nd to about the 10th day.

Macroscopic appearance of grafted cultures

Foetal thymuses cultured for 14 days were grafted into sham thymectomized or neonatally thymectomized syngeneic mice. Subcutaneous cultures, placed in the left flank, and excised about 6 weeks after grafting, resembled lymph nodes in size and appearance but could be identified macroscopically by the presence of the attached piece of millipore filter.

TABLE 1
COUNTS OF LABELLED CELLS AND MITOTIC FIGURES IN THYMUS CULTURES

Time of culture days	Total cells*	Per cent mitotic figures	Total cells†	Per cent labelled
1	2460	1·6	625	31·8
2	6350	0·2	706	40·2
3	7600	0·5	460	26·1
4	8030	1·3	—	—
5	1000	1·5	500	20·8
7	8750	1·2	—	—
10	—	—	600	23·7
12	1496	1·2	670	16·1
14	10,450	0·3	600	16·5
16	1000	0·1	—	—
18	10,000	0·02	—	—

The table shows the percentage of labelled cells and mitotic figures in specimens after various periods of culture. These figures were obtained from counts with the light microscope on 1 μ thick Araldite embedded sections stained with toluidine blue.

* All mitotic figures in at least twenty fields were counted with an oil immersion objective. These were converted to a percentage of the total cells in the same number of fields, this total being calculated from the average cell content of three fields.

† In each case the total cells and labelled cells were counted on the same specimen after a 3-hour pulse of tritiated thymidine.

Subcapsular grafts were readily identified as small pale nodules after 24 hours *in vivo* but they became less apparent during the next 2 days. They started to grow by 4 days and at the end of 1 week were seen as small pale nodules about 1 mm in diameter. When the recipient mice were killed after 6–10 weeks, subcapsular thymuses were usually prominent and weighed from 10 mg to 50 mg. Thus each cultured graft could give rise to an organ which, on occasions, approached in size the thymus of age and sex matched sham thymectomized mice. Since there appeared to be no difference in the structure or growth characteristics of grafts in thymectomized or sham thymectomized mice, the morphology of the grafts in both groups will be described together.

Ultrastructure of grafted cultured thymuses

After 14 days growth *in vitro*, the thymuses consisted mainly of epithelial cells and variable numbers of small lymphocytes. After 24 hours *in vivo*, epithelial cells were the major cell type present and lymphocytes were scarce. There was little evidence of cell damage or death (Fig. 8). The tissue surrounding the grafts was oedematous and consisted of loose connective tissue elements and a granulocytic infiltrate (Fig. 9). However even

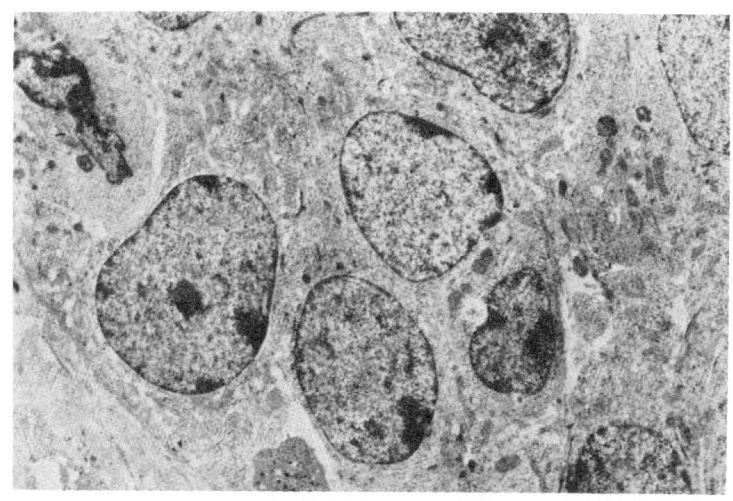

Fig. 8. A portion of a subcapsular graft taken 24 hours after implantation of a 14-day culture. The graft consists of large epithelial cells and appears to be oedematous. (× 4665.)

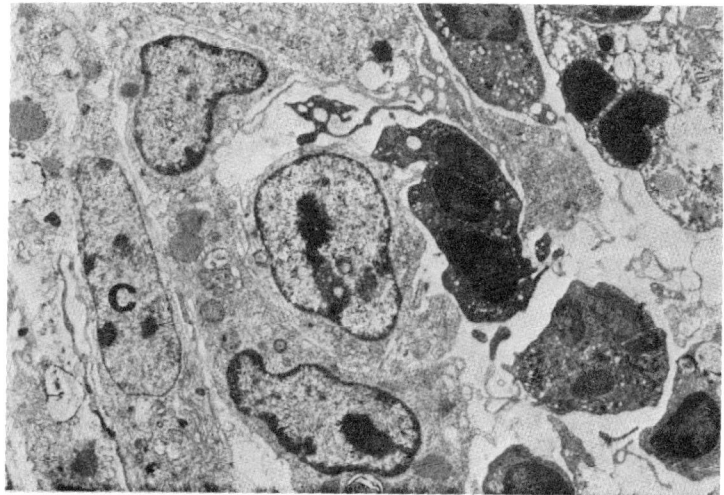

Fig. 9. The edge of a 48-hour graft. Numerous granulocytes are present and the tissue still appears oedematous with wide cell separation. Some connective tissue elements are also present (C). (× 4665.)

during this early period the graft contained mitotic figures (Fig. 10), which were identified as epithelial by the presence of desmosomes. Blood vessels were not present within the grafts at this stage.

During the third day lymphoid cells entered the grafts and were seen interspersed between the epithelial cells. The majority of the lymphoid cells were typical blasts with large nuclei, prominent nucleoli and copious cytoplasm filled with polyribosomes (Fig. 11). Epithelial cells were frequently undifferentiated and again mitotic figures were common. By the fourth day lymphoid cells had started to divide and become more numerous and blood vessels were present in the grafts.

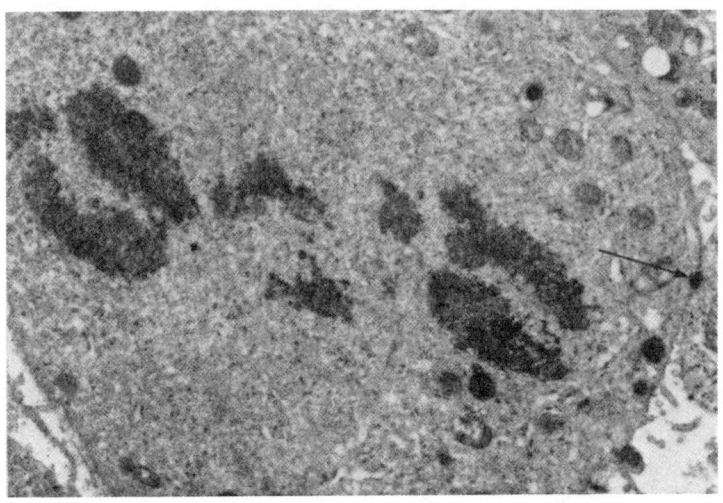

FIG. 10. A mitotic figure of an epithelial cell identified as such by the presence of a desmosome (arrow) in a 48-hour graft. The tissue is still oedematous. (× 11600.)

After 1 week, a typical albeit small thymus was present, and consisted predominantly of a cortex which contained numerous lymphocytes of all sizes (Fig. 12), many of which were in division (Fig. 13). The cortical epithelial cells were identical with those described in the late foetal and post-natal thymic cortex in a previous study (Mandel, 1970). Thus they had large pale nuclei, prominent nucleoli and abundant cytoplasm which extended away from the cell body in long processes (Fig. 13) and contained numerous membrane-bounded bodies. The medullary regions of the grafts could also be identified but occupied only a small proportion of the tissue. The medulla contained less well differentiated epithelial cells but 'cystic' epithelial cells (Mandel, 1970), were usually uncommon and poorly developed (Fig. 14).

Long term (6–10 week) grafts had the morphology of normal post natal mouse thymus. The cortex consisted mainly of small lymphocytes, many of which were in mitosis, and epithelial cells similar to those seen in 1-week grafts and identical to those described in the

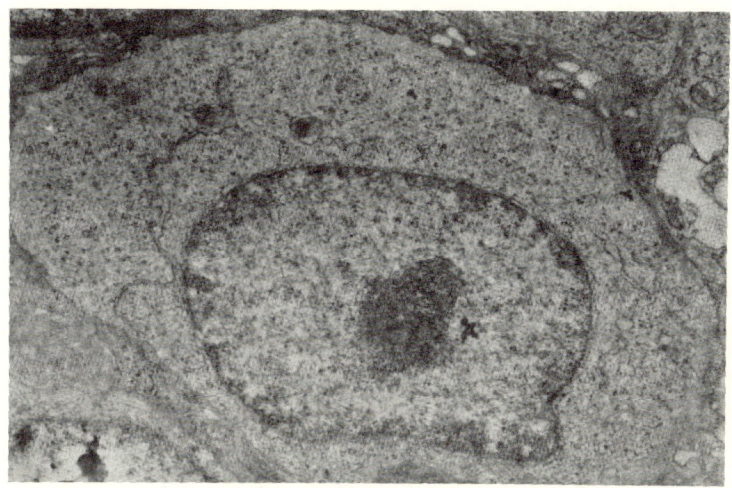

Fig. 11. A large lymphoblast in a 72-hour graft. The cell contains numerous well-developed polyribosomes and a large amount of cytoplasm. Its nucleus is vesicular and contains a prominent nucleolus. (× 9600.)

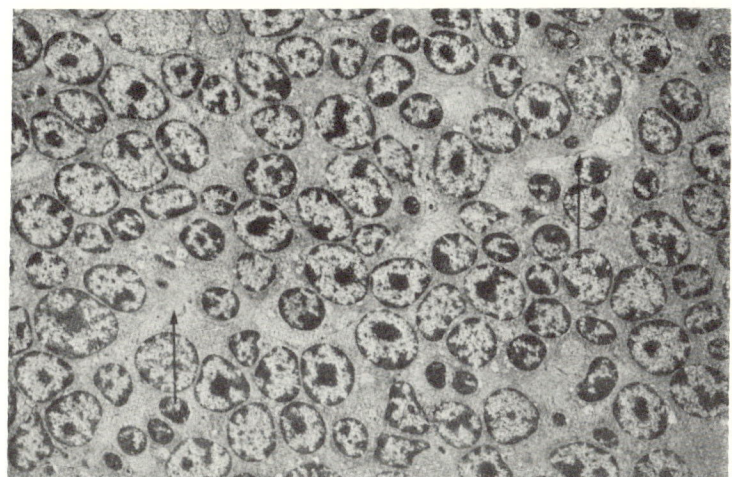

Fig. 12. A low power electron micrograph of the cortex of a 1-week subcapsular graft. The tissue is composed predominantly of closely packed typical small and medium lymphocytes interspersed with epithelial cell processes (arrows). (× 2165.)

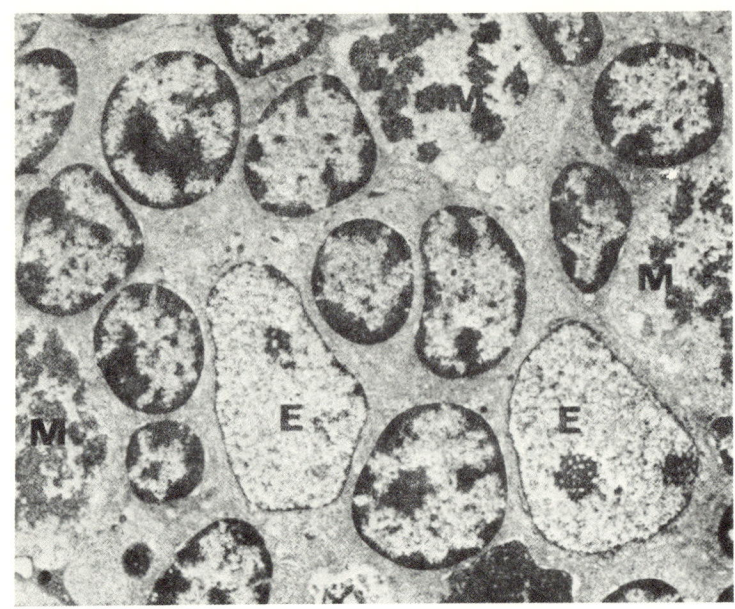

FIG. 13. A detail of the cortex of a 1-week subcapsular graft showing two epithelial cells (E) and numerous typical small lymphocytes. Three mitotic figures (M) of lymphocytes are also seen and two of these are adjacent to epithelial cell cytoplasm. (× 5130.)

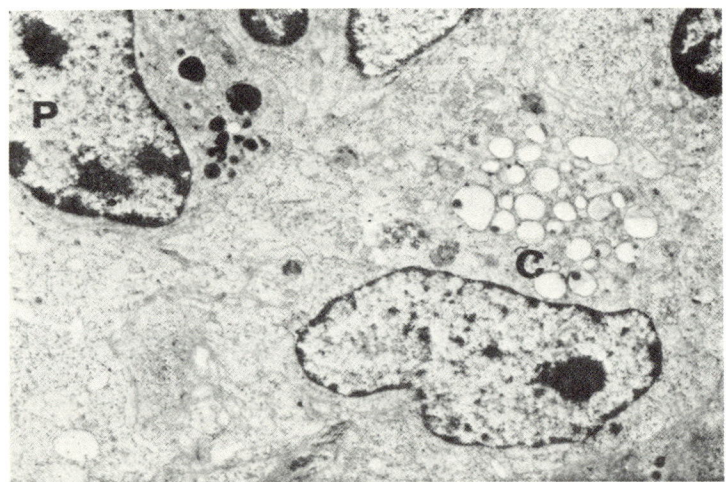

FIG. 14. A portion of the medulla of a 1-week subcapsular graft. A poorly developed 'cystic' epithelial cell (C) is present and shows a collection of small cytoplasmic cystic spaces. A macrophage (P) is also visible and this cell contains numerous phagolysosomes. (× 5565.)

normal post natal thymus. In general there was relatively little medulla when the grafts were compared to normal thymuses from mice of the same age. Ultra-structurally the cells in the medulla were predominantly undifferentiated or poorly differentiated epithelial cells; some rudimentary Hassall's corpuscles were present and possibly the only difference between the medulla of the grafts and the medulla of normal thymuses was a paucity and poor development of the cystic cells

DISCUSSION

The results of this study show that it is possible to maintain foetal mouse thymus in organ culture for extended periods of time. The *in vitro* development of these organs parallels their development *in vivo* (Mandel, 1970), the major difference being in the supply of lymphoid stem cells. In the organ cultures those stem cells initially present underwent proliferation and differentiation but were not supplemented by new stem cells. Similar results have been reported by Owen and Ritter (1969) who showed that the degree of lymphatic development of foetal mouse thymus or embryonic chick thymus cultured in cell tight diffusion chambers on the chorioallantoic membrane was dependent on the number of stem cells initially present. In the present study it was also shown that the cultured thymuses retained their ability to produce a typical lymphoid thymus when grafted into syngeneic recipients. Thus the capacity of the epithelial thymic micro environment to support lymphopoiesis was retained undisturbed even after 25 days *in vitro*. These results differ from those of Reese and Israel (1969) who could not grow neonatal mouse thymus *in vitro* for more than 9 days and still obtain viable thymic tissue following regrafting into syngeneic hosts. Our use of foetal tissue and a different culture system may be responsible for this difference.

The two major cell types present in the explanted foetal thymus showed markedly different growth behaviour *in vitro*. The epithelial cells underwent rapid differentiation and many resembled the 'cortical epithelial cells' of normal mouse thymus (Mandel, 1970). The epithelial cells also proliferated throughout the entire period of culture and their mitotic figures could be identified ultrastructurally. However, the identification both of epithelial mitoses and of [^{3}H]thymidine epithelial cells was frequently difficult with the light microscope though mitoses were seen which resembled those described in the rat thymus and identified as being those of epithelial cells by Sainte-Marie and Leblond (1964).

The mitotic activity of the lymphocytes was in sharp contrast to the epithelial cells. Lymphoid cell proliferation did not occur initially, corresponding to the delay in lymphopoiesis seen *in vivo* (Mandel, 1970). However, between the 2nd and about the 10th days of culture lymphocytes proliferated rapidly and the relatively few lymphoblasts present initially differentiated into numerous typical small lymphocytes. During the latter part of the 2nd week, however, lymphopoiesis decreased sharply. Owen and Ritter (1969) described a similar restricted period of lymphopoiesis and suggested that the stem cells had a limited proliferative capacity. Since the precise identification both of mitotic figures and of labelled cells is frequently difficult with the light microscope an ultrastructural autoradiographic study may be useful for the accurate quantitation of the relative rates of proliferation of the epithelial cells and lymphocytes.

An interesting feature of the development of lymphocytes was the long persistence of these cells *in vitro*. Thus, although most small lymphocytes did indeed die, many were still present even after 3 weeks of culture. It is likely that such cells represent 'thymus derived long lived lymphocytes' which *in vivo* would have migrated out of the thymus and colonized the secondary lymphoid tissues. The functional capacity of these cells is currently being studied. Some support for the maturity of these lymphocytes comes from the study of the grafted tissues. Thus after 24 hours beneath the kidney capsule, there were few lymphocytes left in the grafts and since there was no evidence of their local destruction it is possible that they had migrated from the graft. The use of either chromosome markers or of isotope labelled cells will be required to prove this point.

The subcapsular grafts recapitulated the development of the foetal thymus and showed repopulation characteristics similar to those described by other workers for normal thymus grafts (Miller, 1962; Metcalf and Wakonig-Vaartaja, 1964; Dukor, Miller, House and Allman 1965). In contrast to the ultrastructural studies of Blackburn and Miller (1967), there was no evidence of massive cell death in the cultured grafts. Presumably this difference was due to the very much smaller pieces of tissue used in this study in comparison with the whole neonatal thymuses used by Blackburn and Miller. In the present study it was also possible to identify epithelial cells in mitosis possibly due to the greater concentration of epithelial cells in the cultured thymic tissue. There was also a short delay in appearance of new lymphocytic cells and initially these were blast-like. The rapid development and growth of the graft was striking since within one week of grafting a miniature thymus was already present. The subsequent growth of the grafts indicates that their complement of epithelial cells must have undergone a good deal of proliferation and indeed mitotic figures of these cells were frequently identified particularly during the first week. In this study the lymphocytes in the graft were not formally shown to be of host origin but there is no reason to suspect that this was not the case. As in previous studies (Hoshino *et al.*, 1969; Mandel, 1970) no suggestion of epithelial cell transformation into lymphocytes was seen.

There was no apparent difference in the ultrastructural morphology of the cortex of the grafts when they were compared with normal thymuses. However in the medulla some differences were seen. In particular the 'cystic' epithelial cells which form a major component of normal thymus medulla of a variety of species (Clark, 1963, 1966, 1968; Hoshino, 1963; Ito and Hoshino, 1966; Klug, 1967; Raviola and Raviola, 1967; Gad and Clark, 1968; Mandel, 1968b) were poorly developed and infrequently seen in the grafted tissue. The significance of this observation remains to be evaluated. There was no apparent difference either in the rate of growth or the morphology of the grafts in either thymectomized or sham thymectomized animals, lending further support to the suggestion of Metcalf (1963) that thymic development is autonomous. Studies are in progress in this laboratory aimed at assessing the functional capacity of the grafts and in testing the supernatant fluid from the cultures for evidence of humoral activity. The results of these studies will be reported separately.

ACKNOWLEDGMENTS

The authors are indebted to Professor G. J. V. Nossal and Dr J. F. A. P. Miller for their assistance and support. This investigation was supported by grants from the Jane Coffin Childs Memorial Fund for Medical Research and from the Australian National Health and Medical Research Council. Equipment was supplied by grants from the Australian Research Grant Committee, J. B. Were & Sons and the Potter Foundation. The skilled technical assistance of Miss Leonie Garside and Miss Marie Robinson is gratefully acknowledged.

REFERENCES

AUERBACH, R. (1960). 'Morphogenetic interactions in the development of the mouse thymus gland'. *Develop. Biol.*, **2**, 271.

AUERBACH, R. (1961) 'Experimental analysis of the origin of cell types in the development of the mouse thymus'. *Develop. Biol.*, **3**, 336.

AUERBACH, R. (1963). 'Developmental studies of mouse thymus and spleen.' *Nat. Cancer Inst. Monogr.*, **11**, 23.

BALL, W. D. and AUERBACH, R. (1960). '*In vitro* formation of lymphocytes from embryonic thymus. *Exp. Cell Res.*, **20**, 245.

BLACKBURN, W. R. and MILLER, J. F. A. P. (1967). 'Electron microscopic studies of thymus graft regeneration and rejection. I. Syngeneic grafts.' *Lab. Invest.*, **16**, 66.

CLARK, S. L., JR, (1963). 'The thymus in mice of strain 129/J studies with the electron microscope'. *Amer. J. Anat.*, **112**, 1.

CLARK, S. L., JR (1966). 'Cytological evidences of secretion in the thymus.' *The Thymus*: *Experimental and Clinical Studies*, Ciba Foundation Symposium. pp. 3–30. (Ed. by G. E. W. Wolstenholme and R. Porter), Churchill, London.

CLARK, S. L., JR (1968). 'Incorporation of sulfate by the mouse thymus: its relation to secretion by medullary epithelial cells and to thymic lymphopoiesis.' *J. exp. Med.*, **128**, 957.

DUKOR, P., MILLER, J. F. A. P., HOUSE, W. and ALLMAN, V. (1965). 'Regeneration of thymus grafts. I. Histological and cytological aspects.' *Transplantation*, **3**, 639.

FORD, C. E. (1966). 'Traffic of lymphoid cells in the body.' *The Thymus: Experimental and Clinical Studies*. Ciba Foundation Symposium. (Ed. by G. E. W. Wolstenholme and R. Porter), p. 131–152. Churchill, London.

FORD, C. E. and MICKLEM, H. S. (1963). 'The thymus and lymph-nodes in radiation chimaeras.' *Lancet*, **i**, 359.

GAD, P. and CLARK, S. L., JR (1968). 'Involution and regeneration of the thymus in mice, induced by bacterial endotoxin and studied by quantitative histology and electron miscroscopy.' *Amer. J. Anat.*, **122**, 573.

HARRIS, J. E., FORD, C. E., BARNES, D. W. H. and EVANS, E. P. (1964). 'Cellular traffic of the thymus: experiments with chromosome markers. Evidence from parabiosis for an afferent stream of cells'. *Nature (Lond.)*, **201**, 886.

HOSHINO, T. (1963). Electron microscopic studies of the epithelial reticular cells of the mouse thymus'. *Z. Zellforsch.*, **59**, 513.

HOSHINO, T., TAKEDA, M., ABE, K. and ITO, T. (1969). 'Early development of thymic lymphocytes in mice, studied by light and electron microscopy'. *Anat. Rec.*, **164**, 47.

ITO, T. and HOSHINO, T. (1966). 'Fine structure of the epithelial reticular cells of the medulla of the thymus in the golden hamster.' *Z. Zellforsch.*, **69**, 311.

IZARD, J. (1966). 'Présence de desmosomes entre des cellules épithéliales et des cellules lymphocytaires dans le thymus de cobaye'. *J. Microscopie*, **5**, 361.

KLUG, H. (1967). 'Submikroskopische Zytologie des Thymus von Ambystoma mexicanum.' *Z. Zellforsch.*, **78**, 388.

MANDEL, T. (1968a). 'Ultrastructure of epithelial cells in the cortex of guinea pig thymus.' *Z. Zellforsch.*, **92**, 159.

MANDEL, T. (1968b). 'Ultrastructure of epithelial cells in the medulla of the guinea pig thymus'. *Aust. J. exp. Biol. med. Sci.*, **46**, 755.

MANDEL, T. (1969). 'Epithelial cells and lymphopoiesis in the cortex of guinea pig thymus.' *Aust. J. exp. Biol. med. Sci.*, **47**, 155.

MANDEL, T. (1970). 'Differentiation of epithelial cells in the mouse thymus.' *Z. Zellforsch.*, **106**, 408.

METCALF, D. (1956). 'The thymic origin of the plasma lymphocytosis stimulating factor.' *Brit. J. Cancer*, **10**, 442.

METCALF, D. (1963). 'The autonomous behaviour of normal thymus grafts.' *Aust. J. exp. Biol. med. Sci.*, **41**, 437.

METCALF, D. and WAKONIG-VAARTAJA, R. (1964). 'Stem cell replacement in normal thymus grafts.' *Proc. Soc. exp. Biol. Med.*, **115**, 731.

MILLER, J. F. A. P. (1962). 'Role of the thymus in virus-induced leukaemia.' *Tumour Viruses of Murine Origin*. Ciba Foundation Symposium. (Ed. by G. E. W. Wolstenholme and M. O'Connor). p. 262. Churchill, London.

MILLER, J. F. A. P., MITCHELL, G. F. and WEISS, N. S. (1967). 'Cellular basis of the immunological defect in thymectomized mice.' *Nature (Lond.)*, **214**, 992.

MOORE, M. A. S. and OWEN, J. J. T., (1967). 'Experimental studies on the development of the thymus'. *J. exp. Med.*, **126**, 715.

OSOBA, D. and MILLER, J. F. A. P. (1964). 'The lymphoid tissues and immune responses of neonatally thymectomized mice bearing thymus tissue in millipore diffusion chambers.' *J. exp. Med.*, **119**, 177.

OWEN, J. J. T. and RITTER, M. A. (1969). 'Tissue interaction in the development of thymus lymphocytes.' *J. exp. Med.*, **129**, 431.

PARROTT, D. M. V., DE SOUSA, M. A. B. and EAST, J. (1966). 'Thymus-dependent areas in the lymphoid organs of neonatally thymectomized mice.' *J. exp. Med.*, **123**, 191.

RAVIOLA, E. and RAVIOLA, G. (1967). 'Striated muscle cells in the thymus of reptiles and birds: an electron microscopic study.' *Amer. J. Anat.*, **121**, 623.

REESE, A. J. M. and ISRAEL, M. S. (1969). 'An investigation of a possible humoral factor produced by the thymus in terms of its effect on immunological competence.' *Brit. J. exp. Path.*, **50**, 461.

SAINTE-MARIE, G. and LEBLOND, C. P. (1964). 'Cytologic features and cellular migration in the cortex and medulla of thymus in the young adult rat.' *Blood*, **23**, 275.

SANEL, F. T. (1967). 'Ultrastructure of differentiating cells during thymus histogenesis: a light and electron microscopic study of epithelial and lymphoid cell differentiation during thymus histogenesis in C57 black mice.' *Z. Zellforsch.*, **83**, 8.

STUTMAN, O., YUNIS, E. J. and GOOD, R. A. (1968). 'Carcinogen-induced tumors of the thymus. I.

Restoration of neonatally thymectomized mice with a functional thymoma.' *J. nat. Cancer Inst.*, **41**, 1431.

STUTMAN, O., YUNIS, E. J. and GOOD, R. A. (1969a). 'Carcinogen-induced tumors of the thymus. III. Restoration of neonatally thymectomized mice with thymomas in cell-impermeable chambers.' *J. nat. Cancer Inst.*, **43**, 499.

STUTMAN, O., YUNIS, E. J. and GOOD, R. A. (1969b). 'Carcinogen-induced tumors of the thymus. IV. Humoral influences of normal thymus and functional thymomas and influence of post thymectomy period on restoration.' *J. exp. Med.*, **130**, 809.

WEAKLEY, B. S., PATT, D. I. and SHEPRO, D. (1964). 'Ultrastructure of fetal thymus in the golden hamster.' *J. Morph.*, **115**, 319.

WEISSMAN, I. (1967). 'Thymus cell migration.' *J. exp. Med.*, **126**, 291.

FUNCTIONAL MATURATION OF LYMPHOCYTES WITHIN EMBRYONIC MOUSE THYMUS

Mary A. Ritter

It is now established that the developing embryonic mouse thymus is seeded by blood-borne stem cells derived initially from yolk sac (7–9). These cells then mature structurally within the organ rudiment, developing the morphological appearance of small lymphocytes (9), and later some migrate to the periphery, where they are known to be mediators of cellular immunity (6, 10).

However, it is not known whether this immunocompetence is acquired only after the lymphocytes have reached the periphery, or whether functional maturity develops within the thymus itself. The work described here is a study of the situation in the embryo aimed at elucidating this question.

Using the graft-versus-host response to the injection of parental lymphoid cells into F_1 recipients as an immunologically specific assay system (11), the functional development of prelymphoid (14-day) and early lymphoid (15-day) thymic rudiments was assessed after culture in diffusion chambers (preventing cell inflow and outflow) until temporally equivalent to newborn thymus (5–7 days of culture). The effectiveness of the cultured cells was then compared with that of uncultured 14- and 15-day embryonic thymus cells.

Donor tissue was obtained from CBA/H-T6T6 and CBA/H mice. Diffusion chambers were placed either on the chick chorioallantoic membrane (CAM) (9) or i.p. (3) in male syngeneic mice. The cell suspensions used were: (1) 3×10^6 cultured thymus cells; (2) 3×10^6 noncultured 14- and 15-day embryonic thymus cells; and (3) 3, 10, 20, and 30×10^6 noncultured newborn thymus cells. All cells were injected i.p. in 0.05 ml of medium 199 (tracking under the skin to prevent leakage (1)) into newborn F_1 (CBA/H-T6T6 $\times$ C57BL) recipients. A control series of mice was given medium 199 alone. In each litter, between one and four mice were injected, the uninjected littermates acting as controls. After 8 days, all mice (injected and noninjected) were killed, body and spleen weights recorded, and splenic indices (SIs) calculated for the injected mice based on the method of Simonsen (11):

$$SI = \frac{\text{mean experimental relative spleen weight}}{\text{mean control relative spleen weight}}$$

where relative spleen weight = spleen weight/body weight.

Owing to the limited number of cultured cells available for injection, only small SIs could be obtained, compared with the value of 1.3 and similar figures which have been used in other studies (5, 11). However, the indices obtained were very consistent, giving significance at the 0.1% level and enabling statistically valid conclusions to be drawn from the data.

To avoid nonnormality encountered with ratios, statistical analysis was performed on log-transformed data, giving a normal distribution for $\log_e$ of the SI of 136 control animals. An estimate of the variance was obtained from these data. A weighted analysis was used to control variations in the number of experimental and control mice in each litter. The effects of differ-

TABLE 1. The splenic index observed after injecting various doses of different cell types into newborn F_1 mice

Cell types and dose ($\times 10^6$)	SI[a]	N_1	N_2	Weighted mean[b]	$\log_e$ weighted mean $\pm$ SE[c]	t	P
199							
0	0.99	3	3	1.02	0.0192 ± 0.0126	1.53	$<0.2 > 0.1$
	1.02	2	3				
	0.90	1	1				
	0.98	3	3				
	1.06	2	3				
	1.18	1	3				
	0.91	3	4				
	1.17	2	3				
Normal newborn							
3	0.89	2	2	0.96	-0.0382 ± 0.0202	1.89	$<0.1 > 0.05$
	1.07	2	3				
	0.93	2	3				
10	1.21	2	1	1.32	0.2738 ± 0.0147	18.66	<0.001
	1.14	1	3				
	1.37	3	5				
	1.62	1	4				
	1.11	1	1				
	1.43	1	2				
20	1.14	3	3	1.36	0.3055 ± 0.0158	19.34	<0.001
	1.02	2	2				
	1.57	2	3				
	1.56	2	4				
	1.69	1	2				
30	1.53	4	3	1.43	0.3550 ± 0.0205	17.30	<0.001
	1.29	2	2				
	1.44	1	3				
Embryonic							
3	0.99	1	4	1.05	0.0511 ± 0.0112	4.57	<0.001
	1.01	2	4				
	1.10	2	6				
	1.12	1	5				
	1.02	2	6				
	1.04	2	6				
	1.14	3	5				
	0.99	1	3				
	1.10	2	3				
	1.00	2	5				
CAM-cultured							
3	1.29	2	4	1.22	0.2015 ± 0.0176	11.45	<0.001
	1.14	1	4				
	1.26	1	6				
	1.19	1	7				
I.p. cultured							
3	1.09	1	2	1.15	0.1382 ± 0.0157	8.82	<0.001
	1.19	1	3				
	1.17	1	4				
	1.27	1	5				
	1.03	1	4				

[a] Each value of the splenic index tabulated was determined from a single litter, of which the number N_1 received the cells, while the remaining littermates, N_2, acted as untreated controls.

[b] The weighted mean is the antilog of the computed value $\log_e$ weighted mean.

[c] $\log_e$ weighted mean $= \dfrac{\sum W_j \log_e SI_j}{\sum W_j}$

Variance $= \dfrac{\sigma^2 \sum W_j^2}{(\sum W_j)^2}$

Where $\sigma = 0.035$, from histogram of control $\log_e$ SI distribution,

$W_j = \sqrt{\dfrac{N_1 N_2}{N_1 + N_2}}$

ent experimental treatments were studied by Student's t test. P values were calculated on 120 degrees of freedom, the nearest quoted value to 135 (variance based on 136 control observations). The results, presented in Tables 1 and 2, can be summarized as follows.

1. The SI of mice injected with 199 showed no significant difference from 1. Thus, the operative procedure alone did not cause detectable splenic enlargement.

2. The response to 3×10^6 normal newborn cells does not differ significantly from 1, but 10, 20, and 30×10^6 cells gave increasingly high graft-versus-host responses, all showing a significant difference from 1. Figure 1 gives the dose response curve.

3. Both CAM-cultured and i.p. cultured cells gave a consistent splenomegaly that was significantly greater than 1. The effect was also significantly greater than that produced by the same number of uncultured embryonic cells, by 3×10^6 normal newborn cells, or by medium 199 alone.

The finding that cultured cells produce a greater splenomegaly than do normal embryonic ones demonstrates the acquisition of a significant degree of immunological competence during the culture period. Thus, stem cells can, *solely within the thymic environment*, undergo both structural and functional maturation.

Figure 1 shows a 2-3-fold increase in the effectiveness of cultured cells as compared with normal newborn cells. This may reflect a buildup of immunocompetent cells within the cultured thymus, resulting from barriers to inflow of precursor cells and outflow of competent cells imposed by the diffusion chamber situation.

These results suggest that the immunocompetent cells that have been demonstrated within the adult thymus (*2*, *4*) are cells that have developed functional maturity within the thymic environment prior to migration, rather than lymphocytes initially derived from the thymus that have subsequently acquired immunocompetence in the periphery and have then returned to the thymus.

In conclusion, this evidence indicates an important role for the embryonic thymus in providing a suitable environment for the development of functional immunological maturity. Some lymphocytes leaving the thymus for the first time are therefore already equipped to participate in peripheral immune reactions.

Acknowledgments. I thank Dr. R. W. Hiorns and Miss J. M. Brennan of the Department of Biomathematics, Oxford, for their help with the statistical analysis, and Dr. J. J. T. Owen for many useful discussions.

TABLE 2. The relative effectiveness of different cell inocula in causing splenomegaly[a]

Comparison No.	Group 1	Group 2	t	P
1	CAM-cultured	Embryonic	7.21	<0.001
2	I.p. cultured	Embryonic	4.53	<0.001
3	CAM-cultured	199	8.43	<0.001
4	I.p. cultured	199	5.93	<0.001
5	CAM-cultured	Normal newborn	8.94	<0.001
6	I.p. cultured	Normal newborn	6.90	<0.001
7	CAM-cultured	I.p. cultured	2.68	<0.01

[a] Cells, in doses of 3×10^6, were injected in each case. In all comparisons, significant differences between the two groups were observed, the cell type that produced the greater effect being that tabulated in group 1.

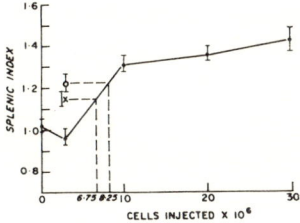

FIGURE 1. The dose response curve for normal newborn thymocytes (●——●). Also shown are the SIs produced by 3×10^6 CAM-cultured (○) and 3×10^6 i.p. cultured cells (×). The values plotted are antilog$_e$ (weighted log$_e$ mean SI ± 95% confidence limits).

REFERENCES

1. Billingham, R. E.; Silvers, W. K. (eds.). 1961. *Transplantation of tissues and cells*. Wistar Institute Press, Philadelphia.
2. Blomgren, H.; Andersson, B. 1969. Exp. Cell Res. *57*: 185.
3. Harrison, G. A.; Owen, J. J. T.; Ritter, M. A. 1968. Nature *219*: 302.
4. Leckband, E. 1970. Fed. Proc. *29*: 621.
5. Michie, D.; Woodruff, M. F. A.; Zeiss, I. M. 1961. Immunology *4*: 413.
6. Miller, J. F. A. P. 1969. p. 4. *In* E. E. Bittar

and N. Bittar (eds.). *The biological basis of medicine*. Academic Press, New York.
7. Moore, M. A. S.; Metcalf, D. 1970. Brit. J. Haematol. *18:* 279.
8. Moore, M. A. S.; Owen, J. J. T. 1967. J. Exp. Med. *126:* 715.
9. Owen, J. J. T.; Ritter, M. A. 1969. J. Exp. Med. *129:* 431.
10. Roitt, I. M.; Greaves, M. F.; Torrigiani, G.; Brostoff, J.; Playfair, J. H. I. 1969. Lancet *1:* 367.
11. Simonsen, M. 1962. Progr. Allergy *6:* 349.

Received 4 March 1971.
Accepted 7 May 1971.

Immunocompetence of Embryonic Hemopoietic Cells After Traffic to Thymus

By OSIAS STUTMAN AND ROBERT A. GOOD

THE TRAFFIC OF CELLS from the bone marrow via the thymus to lymph nodes has been demonstrated, and there is suggestion that during this journey the proliferating cells undergo a process of maturation.[1] Since embryonic hemopoietic liver has traffic patterns similar to those of adult bone marrow (traffic to thymus and from there to lymph nodes)[2] it was of interest to study the traffic patterns of embryonic hemopoietic tissues (yolk sac, blood and liver) and determine if a true maturation process could be implicated.

In all these experiments cell populations with distinct chromosome markers were used. The mice used were CBA, CBA/T6T6 and the CBA/T6 obtained by crossing both sublines. These mice were originally derived from the Harwell (H) sublines and are inbred and syngeneic. CBA/T6T6 have a pair of very small chromosomes,[1] so that dividing cells of any of the three origins can be recognized.

1. Embryonic hemopoietic liver, yolk sac or blood cells migrate to thymus and bone marrow. Hosts were 45-day-old neonatally thymectomized CBA/H grafted subcutaneously (s.c.) or intraperitoneally (i.p.) with a CBA/HT6 from newborn donors and injected i.p. with 5×10^7 hemopoietic liver cells from CBA/HT6T6 embryos (16 to 19 days old). Fifteen to 20 days after treatment, 10-25 per cent liver-type metaphases were

---

Supported by USPHS Grants CA-10445, AI.00798 and AI.08677 and by the National Foundation, March of Dimes.

found in chromosome preparations of the thymus grafts. Liver-type metaphases were also found in bone marrow (3-6%) but were absent from lymph nodes (pooled mesenteric, axilary, cervical and inguinal). When lymph nodes were studied 30-90 days after treatment, liver-type metaphases were now found (5-14%). When 5×10^5 yolk sac cells (from 10- to 12-day embryos) were used, the percentage of yolk sac type metaphases in thymus grafts was two to ten, and in bone marrow 3-8 per cent, 15-20 days after treatment. Yolk sac type metaphases were found in lymph nodes only when studied 30-90 days after treatment and represented 4-15 per cent of the total metaphases scored in the nodes. Comparable results were obtained with embryonic blood cells (15-19 days old.) Table 1 shows the migration of embryonic hemopoietic tissues (including blood) and adult bone marrow cells to thymus grafts. The percentage of dividing cells of the hemopoietic types in the thymus grafts ranged from 10-13 per cent, 20 days after treatment.

2. Requirement of thymus stroma for capacity of embryonic hemopoietic cells to migrate to lymph nodes. This ability of the embryonic cells to migrate to lymph nodes, 30-90 days after administration, was not observed when the thymectomized animals received only liver or yolk sac cells, and it was not dependent on cell dosages, since the traffic pattern was not modified even if 5×10^8 embryonic liver cells or 5×10^6 yolk sac cells were used. Embryonic cells did migrate to bone marrow under these conditions (3-5%). When these bone marrows containing embryonic cells were retransplanted to secondary thymectomized

Table 1.—Chromosome Analysis of IP CBA/HT6 Thymus Grafts in 45-day-old Neonatally Thymectomized CBA/H Mice Injected IP With CBA/HT6T6 Hemopoietic Cells

Cell Type°	Number of Metaphases Scored	Per Cent CBA/HT6T6 Type Metaphases †
Yolk sac (10–13-day embryo)	450	12.3
Liver (15–19-day embryo)	1000	13.4
Blood (15–19-day embryo)	376	10.1
Adult bone marrow	550	14.1

° Cell dose was 5×10^5 for yolk sac and blood and 5×10^6 for liver and marrow.
† Per cent CBA/HT6T6 per total number of mitoses scored, 20 days after treatment.

Table 2.—Chromosome Analysis of Lymphoid Tissues From Neonatally Thymectomized CBA/H Mice (45 days old), 40 days after CBA/HT6T6 Yolk Sac Cells With or Without CBA/HT6 Thymus

Experimental Group	Yolk-sac-Type Metaphases Nodes	Marrow
Thymectomy	0/299	6/230 (2.6%)
Thymectomy plus thymus graft°	39/210 (18.5%)	5/180 (2.7%)
Thymectomy plus thymus in DC°	0/237	4/120 (3.3%)
Thymectomy plus thymoma graft	0/306	4/150 (2.6%)

° Thymus graft implanted intraperitoneally. Diffusion chambers (0.1 μ pore) implanted intraperitoneally. All animals received 5×10^5 yolk sac cells from 10–13-day-old CBA/HT6 embryos.

CBA/H hosts, embryonic-type metaphases could be detected in thymus grafts and later in the lymph nodes. Again, the population in lymph nodes was established only if thymus grafts were present. Similarly, when in the experimental model described above the thymus graft was replaced by graft enclosed in a cell impenetrable chamber[3] or by the s.c. graft of a functional thymoma that has only "humoral" function,[3] no lymph-node migrating population derived from the embryonic cells was detected 30–90 days after treatment. Table 2 shows these results with yolk sac cells.

3. *Emigration of embryonic hemopoietic cells from thymus to lymph nodes.* Thymus grafts containing migrating embryonic cells (15 to 20 days after grafting and i.p. cell injection) were retransplanted s.c. or i.p. to 20-day-old neonatally thymectomized CBA/H hosts. Chromosome preparations of lymph nodes from the secondary hosts showed 2–15 per cent embryonic liver and 4–12 per cent yolk-sac-type metaphases, 20 to 40 days after grafting. It has to be stressed that in the secondary host the only source of CBA/HT6 cells, the type of the embryonic tissues injected in the primary host, was the thymus graft itself, indicating emigration of those cells to the lymph nodes.

4. *Emigration of embryonic hemopoietic cells of lymph nodes signifies capacity to respond immunologically.* To test whether this traffic implies a differentiative process towards immune competence, lymph nodes of the secondary hosts described above were tested for immune response in vitro to phytohemagglutinin (PHA) or allogeneic cells. Mitotic arrest was induced in the cultures (after 48 or 72 house for the PHA and after 6 days for the response to C57BL allogeneic cells) and the karyotype of the responding cells was determined. Table 3 indicates the percentage of cells responding to PHA in culture in lymph nodes of the secondary hosts that were originally derived from the hemopoietic cells that migrated to the thymus in the primary host. It can be seen that 10 to 27 per cent of the dividing

Table 3.—Chromosome Analysis of PHA Response of Lymph Nodes Derived From Neonatally Thymectomized CBA/H Secondary Hosts Grafted With CBA/HT6 Thymus Containing CBA/HT6T6 Cells of Various Origins, 60 Days After Intraperitoneal Grafting

Origin of CBA/HT6T6 Cells in Thymus Graft	Number of CBA/HT6T6 Metaphases per Total Scored°
Yolk sac (10–13-day embryo)	39/233 (16%)
Embryonic liver (13–19 days)	664/2466 (27%)
Blood (15–19-day embryo)	20/199 (10%)
Adult bone marrow	130/890 (14%)

° Response measured 48 or 72 hours after culture.

cells are derived from the cells that have migrated from the thymus graft to lymph nodes but that were originally of hemopoietic (yolk sac, embryonic liver, embryonic blood or adult bone marrow) ancestry. The response to allogeneic C57BL lymphoid cells was also studied and it showed that 90 of 899 metaphases studied (11%) were of embryonic liver type and 10 of 130 metaphases (7%) were of yolk sac type.

Embryonic hemopoietic cells (yolk sac, liver or blood) or adult bone marrow cells injected into 45-day-old thymectomized hosts in absence of thymus grafts do not establish a population of cells in lymph nodes capable of response to PHA or allogeneic cells in vitro.

Summary

Embryonic hemopoietic cells (yolk sac, liver or blood) contain prethymic precursors capable of migration to thymus. The migration pattern of these cells is peculiar since they mainly migrate to thymus and bone marrow and not to peripheral lymphoid tissues. After thymus traffic these embryonic precursors develop the capacity to migrate to lymph nodes and this requires a viable intact thymic stroma and represents a true exportation of cells to the periphery. In a sense these cells can be considered thymus-derived, although they did not originate in the thymus itself. The postthymic progeny of the precursors derived from embryonic sources found in the lymph nodes are capable of immune responses (respond to PHA and allogeneic cells in vitro), indicating that the complex traffic pattern is a means of producing cells endowed with immune competence in the peripheral lymphoid tissues. Adult bone marrow exhibits comparable behavior. The presence of the thymus is essential for the development of these immunocompetent cell populations.

REFERENCES

1. Ford, C. E.: *In* Wolstenholme, G. E., and Porter, R. (Eds.): Ciba Foundation Symp. The Thymus. Boston, Little, Brown, 1966, p. 131.
2. Stutman, O., and Good, R. A.: Exp. Hematol. 19:12, 1969.
3. —., Yunis, E. J., and Good, R. A.: Nat. Cancer Inst. 43:499, 1969.

Immunologic and Anatomic Consequences of Calf Thymosin Injection in Rats [1]

J. KRÜGER, A. L. GOLDSTEIN, AND B. H. WAKSMAN

INTRODUCTION

Several lines of evidence have been advanced to support the hypothesis that the thymus secretes a hormone-like substance which may control cell differentiation within the thymus, may govern extrathymic lymphopoiesis, or may stimulate thymus-dependent immune responses (1). Diffusion chamber experiments in thymectomized animals (2–6) and the restoration of immunological reactivity in such animals by processes accompanying pregnancy (7) provided indirect evidence that the thymus operates by a humoral factor capable of inducing immunological competence in lymphoid cells at a distant site. More direct evidence for the production and operation of such a thymic hormone was the fact that injection of different thymic extracts produced lymphocytosis in the peripheral blood (8) and a hyperplastic lymphoid response (9), reduced wasting disease in neonatally thymectomized animals (10), and restored their immunological capacity as determined by a graft-versus-host reaction (11). A lipid fraction of rat thymus was reported to

[1] This work was supported by USPHS Research Grants AI-06112 and AI-06455.

restore the immune potential of thymectomized rats (12). More recently Goldstein et al. (13) prepared from calf thymus a partially purified, protein-rich extract, designated as thymosin, which stimulated lymphopoiesis in normal mice, accelerated regeneration of lymphoid tissue in mice after whole body irradiation, and restored immunological competence to spleen cells from neonatally thymectomized mice (14). The present investigation was undertaken to obtain further insight into the role of thymosin by examing its activity in restoring immunological capacity in thymectomized rats to bovine γ-globulin (BγG).

MATERIALS AND METHODS

Animals. Lewis rats (Microbiological Associates, Bethesda, Md.) were used throughout. Rats 3–4 months old were used both for immunization and as donors of bone marrow cells. For most experiments, animals were irradiated (550 R) at 5–6 weeks of age or were thymectomized at 5–6 weeks, exposed to 900 R of total body X-irradiation 3 weeks later, and within 6 hr of irradiation injected with 2×10^8 nucleated syngeneic bone marrow cells.

Irradiation technique. Rats received 550 or 900 R (central axis dose) whole body X-irradiation in a 12-chamber Lucite cage, at a focus-to-cage distance of 110 cm, beneath a Siemens Stabilipan 250 kV machine at 15 mA using 2 mm aluminum filtration, 0.8 mm copper half-value layer. The measured midline exposure rate was 32.6 R per minute.

Thymosin treatment. Thymosin was prepared in the laboratory of Dr. A. L. Goldstein according to a previously described method (13). A partially purified extract designated as fraction 3 was used for therapeutic injections and for antigenic challenge. One hundred milligrams of the powder was dissolved in 2.5 ml pyrogen-free saline, a small insoluble residue was removed by centrifugation, and the clear supernatant was passed through a 0.45-μ Millipore filter (Millipore Corp., Bedford, Mass.). Calf spleen extracts were prepared in the same manner. Thymosin and spleen extract were injected subcutaneously into different groups of experimental animals. Doses of 5 and 15 mg of protein (determined by the method of Lowry) per 100 g body weight were given on 3 successive days, or three times a week over a period of approximately 6 weeks.

Immunization. BγG (Immunology Inc., Glen Ellyn, Ill., Lot No. 1068) and thymosin were both used for challenge. Rats were given a primary injection of 100 μg BγG or 1 mg thymosin protein in complete Freund's adjuvant (CFA) in one hind footpad and 25 days later were boosted by iv injection of 1 mg BγG or 5 mg thymosin. Skin tests with 30 μg BγG or 50 μg thymosin at 10 and 20 days were read after 3 (Arthus) and 24 hr (delayed). Reaction with less than 6-mm induration was considered negative. Blood specimens from the orbital vein were obtained on day 0, 10, 20, and 32. Antibody determinations were carried out by passive hemagglutination, using the microtitration technique, and by gel diffusion. In two groups of rats a schedule of thymosin injections comparable to that used in treatment was employed (see Table 4). At the end of each experiment, after treatment with thymosin and/or immunization, all rats were sacrificed. Spleen, cervical, mesenteric, and popliteal lymph nodes and thymus (or the tissue of the upper mediastinum) were removed, weighed, and fixed in 10% formalin for staining with hematoxylin and eosin. In some cases the percentages of living nymph node and spleen cells carrying thymus-specific and histocompatibility antigens were determined by dark field and the indirect immunofluorescence technique (15, 16) with absorbed rabbit anti-thymocyte sera and with isoantisera prepared in DA rats. Rats in which thymic remnants were present were discarded from the study.

Endotoxin assay. The assay was conducted in a quiet, temperature-controlled room with trained New Zealand white rabbits, which responded consistently to pyrogen. Animals were restrained in wooden stalls, and their temperatures were recorded every 15 min from an indwelling rectal thermistor (17). Injections were made into the marginal ear vein. Glassware used for all endotoxin experiments was rendered pyrogen-free. Two endotoxins were employed for "tolerance" experiments, a monovalent typhoid vaccine made from *S. typhosa* V-58 (kindly supplied by Dr. E. Atkins) and E Pyrogen from *Proteus vulgaris* (Organon Lab. Ltd., Great Britain).

RESULTS

Response of thymus and peripheral lymphoid organs to thymosin. Groups of four or five female Lewis rats, 5–6 weeks old, were given 550 R whole body X-irradiation, treated from the 4th to the 6th day with two different doses of thymosin or spleen extract, and sacrificed 2 days after the last injection. Normal rats of the same age and X-irradiated, untreated animals (negative controls) were also examined. In Table 1 the organ weights of thymus, spleen, and lymph nodes of experimental animals are expressed as organ indices, which relate them to organ weights in the negative control animals. All treated groups show average indices near 1.0 Thus, under these experimental conditions there was no accelerated regeneration in either the thymus or the peripheral lymphoid organs, nor was there evidence of a feedback inhibition of the thymus during its regenerative phase. Histologically thymus sections showed a similar picture in all irradiated animals. The medulla was markedly shrunken and lymphocytes in the cortex were more loosely packed than in the cortex of the normal thymus. The ratio of small lymphocytes to larger ones was slightly shifted to medium and larger lymphocytic cells. Sections of the lymph nodes and spleens showed moderate numbers of lymphocytes in the para-

TABLE 1

LYMPHOID ORGAN INDICES [a] OF NORMAL AND THYMOSIN-TREATED RATS

Organ	Normal rats	Irradiated rats treated with			
		Thymosin		Spleen extract	
		5 mg/100 g	15 mg/100 g	5 mg/100 g	15 mg/100 g
Spleen	2.22 ± 0.13	1.0 ± 0.15	0.94 ± 0.11	1.03 ± 0.07	0.97 ± 0.05
Lymph node	1.86 ± 0.15	0.95 ± 0.11	0.97 ± 0.12	1.03 ± 0.06	1.08 ± 0.14
Thymus	1.94 ± 0.13	0.95 ± 0.10	0.82 ± 0.05	0.91 ± 0.06	0.91 ± 0.10

[a] Organ index: $\dfrac{\text{Mean organ weight/body weight (experimental)}}{\text{Mean organ weight/body weight (negative control)}} \pm \text{SD}.$

cortical areas and the white pulp, respectively. With the exception of a few minimal foci of small lymphocytes, no follicles or germinal centers could be found. In the lymph node sections there were large numbers of immature and mature plasma cells.

These observations were repeated in groups of male rats thymectomized, given 900 R of whole body irradiation, restored with syngeneic marrow cells, and treated with thymosin or spleen extract at 8–10 days. Again organ indices, 2 days after termination of thymosin treatment, showed no difference between treated and untreated rats. Histologically no repopulation of the splenic white pulp or paracortical areas of lymph nodes could be seen in the treated animals. However in all sections foci of lymphocytes, sometimes with small germinal centers, indicated the recovery of thymus-independent structures by 12 days after irradiation.

Finally in thymectomized, irradiated, bone marrow restored rats immunized with BγG in CFA and autopsied 32 days later (see below), there was no difference between negative controls and animals given 5 mg thymosin per 100 g body weight three times weekly throughout the period of immunization. The reticular structures surrounding the splenic white pulp arterioles and the shrunken paracortical areas of the lymph nodes remained completely lacking small lymphocytes in all animals. In both spleen and lymph nodes, germinal centers appeared to be comparable in number, size, and make-up to those in spleen and lymph node sections from normal controls given BγG and adjuvant. The main cellular element remaining in the lymph nodes were plasma cells and their precursors, which seemed to have occupied the former space of thymus-derived cells.

Thymosin and surface antigens of cells in regenerating lymphoid organs. When bone marrow cells are given to irradiated rodents they repopulate the thymus (18, 19). Within the rat thymus they undergo striking changes in size and rapid replacement of histocompatibility antigen with thymus-specific antigen (16). These alterations are thought to be related to the development of immunocompetence. An attempt was made to find out whether or not treatment with thymosin induces the appearance of thymus-specific surface antigens in cells repopulating the spleen and lymph nodes. Thymectomized, irradiated (900 R) rats restored with syngeneic bone marrow cells were given 5 or 15 mg thymosin or spleen extract per 100 g daily for 3 days 8–10 days after marrow reconstitution. Forty hours after the last injection all rats were sacrificed together with normal rats and untreated negative controls. It could be demonstrated by the indirect fluorescence technique that the histocompatibility antigens of the lymphocytes of spleen and lymph nodes were not replaced by thymus-specific antigen (Table 2). The 2–6% fluorescence among cells tested with the reagents for thymus-specific antigen is within background range.

Effect of thymosin treatment on the immune response to BγG. Thymectomized, irradiated rats reconstituted with marrow cells do not react immunologically on BγG challenge (20). Their failure to develop precipitating or hemagglutinating antibodies and reactions of the delayed type is supposed to be due to a lack of the cooperative effect of thymus-derived lymphocytes with marrow-derived cells. To examine the effect of thymosin or recovery of this immune response rats were thymectomized, 3 weeks later were irradiated and given syngeneic marrow cells, and separate groups were treated with 5 mg thymosin or spleen extract per 100 g or

TABLE 2

Percentage[a] of Spleen and Lymph Node Cells Stained for Thymus-Specific and Lewis Histocompatibility Antigen in Thymectomized, Lethally Irradiated (900 R) Rats Reconstituted with Syngeneic Bone Marrow Cells

Antigen	Cells	Normal rats	Untreated rats	Animals treated with			
				Thymosin		Spleen extract	
				5 mg/100g	15 mg/100g	5 mg/100g	15 mg/100g
Thymus	Spleen	2	5	5	5	5	6
	Lymph node	3	5	4	5	2	3
Histocompatibility	Spleen	99	97	98	100	99	100
	Lymph node	100	100	100	100	99	100

[a] Means for groups of four rats.

kept as negative controls. Five normal rats were positive controls. The extracts were injected subcutaneously three times a week beginning on the eighth day after irradiation and continuing for the duration of the experiment. At 12 days all groups were challenged with BγG in CFA. The skin reactions 10 and 20 days after challenge and serum titers at 32 days show that thymosin-treated rats did not recover immunologic function (Table 3). In similar experiments with thymosin treatment of shorter duration there was also no effect on the response to BγG.

Antigenic properties of thymosin. Rats injected with thymosin subcutaneously, according to the schedule used in treatment, showed only a slight Arthus reaction and failed to develop delayed hypersensitvity or to produce detectable levels of circulating antibody (Table 4). In contrast, rats given a primary thymosin injection in CFA gave good skin reactions of both types and circulating antibodies. Individual sera contained precipitating antibodies for as many as six components present in the thymus extract. Gel diffusion studies showed that thymosin, spleen extract, and calf serum share two identical bands and thymosin and spleen extract a third one. No precipitation line developed against BSA or BγG. Three precipitation bands were found against thymosin alone. By the use of the indirect immunofluorescence technique it could be demonstrated that the 32-day sera contained antibody that was taken up at the surface of calf thymus and lymph node cells (95 and 100%) but not on thymus or lymph node cells of rats and mice. Cytotoxicity assays using the trypan blue exclusion method showed that these sera were cytotoxic for calf thymus and lymph node cells (83 and 70% of these cells were stained after 30-min incubation) but had no measurable effect on the corresponding cells of mice and rats. The thymus glands of all rats immunized with thymosin in CFA were examined histologically for an autoallergic lesion. However, no clear-cut perivascular infiltrates of lymphocytes and histiocytes were found.

Thymosin and endotoxin. Two of the thymosin preparations used in the present study (lots 68102APGFR3 and 681210APJFR3) were examined for possible contamination with bacterial endotoxin. Advantage was taken of the well-known pyrogenic activity of endotoxin. When 10–12 mg thymosin protein in pyrogen-free normal rabbit serum was injected into four rabbits (Fig. 1), a substantial febrile response with a lag period of $\geq$ 30 min was observed. In two rabbits given a large dose of intravenous endotoxin (1 μg E Pyrogen) to produce a refractory state, however, there was no febrile response to a thymosin injection the following day. The refractory state was specific since these animals responded normally to particles of heat-killed *Staphylococcus albus*. In another rabbit with endotoxin tolerance induced by seven daily injections of 6 μg typhoid vaccine, the febrile response following a thymosin injection was reduced to a significant degree. These observations support the inference that the pyrogenic compound found in these batches of thymosin might be endotoxin or a closely similar substance.

DISCUSSION

In attempting to interpret reports from a number of laboratories that injection of crude or partially purified thymus extracts stimulate lymphocyte proliferation in normal or lymphopenic animals and may enhance certain immune responses in such animals, one is confronted with several quite distinct alternatives. First, as sug-

TABLE 3

Effect of Long-Term Thymosin Treatment on the Immune Response of Thymectomized, Lethally Irradiated (900 R) Rats to BγG

Experimental group	No. of rats	Skin reactions (Average diameter mm)					Antibody at 32 days	
		10 days		20 days			Hemagglutination titer (Average log$_2$)	Gel precipitation (No. positive/No. tested)
		Arthus	Delayed		Arthus	Delayed		
5 mg thymosin/100 g	4	0	0		0	0	0	0/4
5 mg spleen extr./100 g	5	0	0		0	0	0	0/5
Negative controls	5	0	0		0	0	0	0/5
Normal positive controls	5	11.0	21.4		14.2	16.2	7.0	5/5

TABLE 4

Immune Response of Rats After Different Forms of Immunization with Calf Thymosin

Experimental group	No. of rats	Skin reactions (Average diameter mm)					Antibody at 32 days	
		10 days		20 days			Hemagglutination titer (Average log$_2$)	Gel precipitation (No. positive/No. tested)
		Arthus	Delayed		Arthus	Delayed		
5 mg thymosin/100 g body weight subcutaneously[a]	3	7.0	0		6.0	0	0	0/3
15 mg thymosin/100 g body weight subcutaneously[a]	3	7.5	0		9.0	0	0	0/3
1 mg thymosin in CFA in hind footpad	7	7.1	17.0		9.5	18.5	5.4	7/7

[a] 5 or 15 mg/100 g were given on 3 successive days sc followed by a single booster injection of 5 or 15 mg sc at day 27.

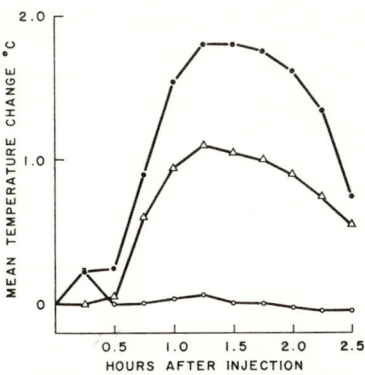

Fig. 1. Comparison of the mean febrile response to thymosin injected into normal (●——●), endotoxin tolerant (△——△), and "endotoxin refractory" (○——○) rabbits.

gested by several authors, the extracts may contain a hormone governing lymphopoiesis. Second, many of the observed effects may be due simply to the antigenicity for the test animals of substances in the heterologous extracts used for treatment. Third, bacterial contamination and the formation of endotoxin during preparation may account for both antigenicity of thymus extracts and their adjuvant effect on immune responses to other antigens such as sheep erythrocytes. A fourth possibility is that certain of the distinctive compounds of the thymus (21) may themselves possess endotoxin-like properties when isolated and injected into a heterologous species. Finally, cross-reactions between components present in thymus extracts (whether derived from the thymus cells themselves or from bacterial contaminants) and antigens later tested in the treated animals might account for accelerated or enhanced responses to the latter.

Thymosin proved, similar to the finding of Hardy *et al.* (22), to be highly immunogenic in rats when injected with CFA, giving rise to delayed sensitization and antibody formation. Two thymosin preparations tested in the present study also proved to contain endotoxin-like activity. With the schedule of treatment used in the present study, thymosin did not stimulate lymphocytopoiesis in sublethally irradiated rats or thymectomized, lethally irradiated rats reconstituted with bone marrow. The striking depletion of lymphocytes in the white pulp of the spleen and paracortical area of the lymph nodes in the thymectomized animals was not influenced by treatment with thymosin or calf spleen extract. In thymectomized, irradiated rats restored with marrow cells, thymosin treatment failed to induce a replacement of histocompatibility antigen with thymus-specific antigen on spleen and lymph node lymphocytes (presumably marrow-derived). Thymus-dependent immune responses to BγG were not restored in similarly treated animals. White and Goldstein were also unable to stimulate humoral antibody responses in adult thymectomized, lethally irradiated (800 R), bone marrow treated mice challenged with sheep erythrocytes (23).

Most reported work with thymus grafts in cell-tight diffusion chambers (2–6) and with thymus extracts (8–13) has ignored the problem of distinguishing thymus-dependent from thymus-independent lymphocytes and their functions. Our histological study confirms and extends morphological evidence that no restoration of thymus-dependent areas of spleen and lymph nodes occurs and that no evidence of thymus characteristics in cells within these organs can be shown. Most reports stress the increase of follicles and germinal centers in treated animals, i.e., the stimulation of nonthymus-dependent areas (5, 6, 24). In the present investigation with thymosin no effect of treatment on these was found, perhaps because our rats were examined too soon after irradiation (8 and 12 days) or after use of CFA. It is also possible that there are species differences in the response to heterologous tissue extracts (Goldstein, Silk, and White, unpublished data). In mice irradiated with 400 or 700 R, thymosin treatment initiated within 2 hr and continued daily thereafter until the mice were sacrificed resulted in extreme proliferation of lymphoid tissue (25). Whenever such immunological functions as the enhancement of antibody production against sheep erythrocytes (4, 6), the accelerated rejection of skin allografts (2, 6, 26), the restoration of immunological competence to spleen cells (11, 14), and the restoration of delayed sensitivity to BSA (2, 12) (which are thymus-dependent or at least partially thymus-dependent) were reported, the experiments were performed with neonatally thymectomized or thymectomized and sublethally irradiated animals which are known to possess residual thymus-derived cells. Therefore it is quite possible that the recovery of thymus-dependent functions reflected a response of these residual cells. Restoration of immunological function in thymectomized, lethally irradiated animals may provide a more incisive experiment because ablation of the thymus-derived pool of lymphocytes is more complete. The partial restoration of delayed sensitization to serum proteins seen in neonatally thymectomized rats (2), for instance, could not be confirmed in thymectomized, lethally irradiated (900 R) animals (20). Similarly, a complete restoration of the 19S antibody response to sheep erythrocytes is seen after administration of thymocytes in neonatally thymectomized mice (27) but not in adult thymectomized, lethally irradiated (800 R), bone marrow treated animals (28).

Abundant evidence that injection of thymus extracts or thymosin, specifically, into normal mice is followed by lymphopoiesis and an increase of peripheral lymphoid tissue weight could simply reflect immunization with foreign antigens, since in almost all cases thymus extracts from heterologous sources have been employed and since the principal response affects nonthymus-dependent components of the tissue. An objection to this argument can be seen in the ineffectiveness of comparable spleen, lymph node, and other organ extracts. However, thymus cells differ strikingly from peripheral lymphocytes in their antigenic makeup (21). The evidence suggests strongly that a thymus-specific substance is responsible for certain of the lymphocytopoietic and immune responses described for thymosin in mice (23).

It is also possible that extracts obtained from isologous or heterologous sources could conceivably be antigenic due to alteration or contamination during extraction and purification procedures. Bacterial endotoxin is one of the most common contaminants in a variety of tissue preparations, and its physiological and immunological effects (29) have always been a source of major errors (30, 31). Dent *et al.*

(30) found that the enhancing effect of extracts prepared from the bursa of Fabricius and of bursal tissue enclosed in cell-tight diffusion chambers on antibody production in bursectomized chickens was due to bacterial products. Endotoxin is itself a good antigen that gives rise to γM-antibody production, and a second injection evokes a "secondary" type of response (32). As an adjuvant, endotoxin enhances markedly the antibody response of normal or sublethally irradiated (400 R) rabbits when given separately or in conjunction with protein antigens (33, 34). A striking splenic germinal center response is correlated with this antibody formation (35). However, animals given a lethal dose of X-ray are unable to make antibodies to BγG alone or to BγG and endotoxin (36). Our experiments are consistent with these findings because thymosin, even with its endotoxin-like activity, failed to restore the capability of thymectomized, lethally irradiated rats to produce antibodies to BγG. Endotoxin also exerts a clear-cut adjuvant effect on first set skin homograft rejection in rabbits (37). The already mentioned hyperplastic lymphoid response after thymosin injection in normal neonatally thymectomized or thymectomized and sublethally or lethally irradiated animals seems to offer further substantiation that thymosin itself causes an antigenic response which may be enhanced by its endotoxin-like component. It cannot be stated with certainty that the endotoxin-like activity of the extracts which we tested was due to bacterial contamination. There exists the possibility that a specific thymus component may exhibit such activity. Characteristic responses are obtained with thymosin preparations which contain less than 0.5% carbohydrate and lack lipid entirely (23).

Immunogenicity and adjuvanticity of thymosin could also explain the restoration of immunological competence to spleen cells from neonatally thymectomized mice as assayed by the graft-versus-host response (14) and may have a bearing on experiments in which thymosin accelerated the rejection of skin allografts in normal mice (24). It seems reasonable to raise the question whether or not the enhanced response, in both cases, may represent the consequence of allograft sensitivity induced by a microbial contaminant of thymosin. Studies on blood group activity of gram-negative bacteria have clearly shown antigenic cross-reactivity in groups as widely separated as bacteria and man (38). Biologically important structural relationships have been demonstrated between streptococcal constituents and mammalian tissue antigens (39), and group A streptococcal membrane antigens have been shown to be capable of inducing allograft sensitivity (40). In contrast, the prolonged survival of skin grafts in mice treated with antiserum to thymosin is clearly reminiscent of the biologic effect of antithymocyte sera as already suggested by Hardy *et al.* (22, 24).

It remains for further studies to attempt to dissect the relative biological contribution of thymosin as an antigen, as a substance with possibly intrinsic endotoxin activity, and as a hormone.

REFERENCES

1. Osoba, D., *In* "Regulation of Antibody Response" (B. Cinader, ed.), p. 232. Thomas, Springfield, Ill., 1968.
2. Aisenberg, A. C., and Wilkes, B., *Nature London* **205,** 716, 1965.
3. Biggart, J. D.,, *Brit. J. Exp. Pathol.* **47,** 586, 1966.
4. Biggart, J. D., *Brit. J. Exp. Pathol.* **47,** 590, 1966.

5. Levey, R. H., Trainin, N., and Law, L. W., *J. Nat. Cancer Inst.* **31**, 199, 1963.
6. Osoba, D., *J. Exp. Med.* **122**, 633, 1965.
7. Osoba, D., *Science* **147**, 298, 1965.
8. Metcalf, D., *Brit. J. Cancer* **10**, 442, 1956.
9. Grégoire, C., and Duchateau, G., *Arch. Biol.* **67**, 269, 1956.
10. De Somer, P., Denys, P., Jr., and Leyten, R., *Life Sci.* **11**, 810, 1963.
11. Law, L. W., and Agnew, H. D., *Proc. Soc. Exp. Biol. Med.* **127**, 953. 1968.
12. Janković, B. D., Isaković. K., and Horvath, J. *Nature London* **208**, 356, 1965.
13. Goldstein, A. L., Slater, F. D., and White, A., *Proc. Nat. Acad. Sci. U.S.* **56**, 1010, 1966.
14. Law, L. W., Goldstein, A. L., and White, A., *Nature London* **219**, 1391, 1968.
15. Möller, G., *J. Exp. Med.* **114**, 415, 1961.
16. Order, S. E., and Waksman, B. H., Transplantation **8**, 783, 1969.
17. Snell, E. S., and Atkins, E., *Amer. J. Physiol.* **212**, 1103, 1967.
18. Gengozian, N., Urso, I. S., Congdon, C. C., Conger, A. D., and Makinodan, T., *Proc. Soc. Exp. Biol. Med.* **96**, 714, 1957.
19. Popp, R. A., *Proc. Soc. Exp. Biol. Med.* **108**, 561, 1962.
20. Isaković, K., Smith, S. B, and Waksman, B H., *J. Exp. Med.* **122**, 1103, 1965.
21. Boyse, E. A., Old, L. J., Stockert, E.. and Shigeno, N., *Cancer Res.* **28**, 1280, 1968.
22. Hardy, M. A., Quint, J., Goldstein, A. L., White, A., State, D., and Battisto, J. R., *Proc. Soc. Exp. Biol. Med.* **130**, 214, 1969.
23. White, A., and Goldstein, A. L., *In* "Control Processes in Multicellular Organisms" (G. E. W. Wolstenholme and J. Knight, eds.). Churchill, London, 1970, pp. 210-237.
24. Hardy, M. A., Quint, J., Goldstein, A. L., State, D., and White, A., *Proc. Nat. Acad. Sci. U.S.* **61**, 875, 1968.
25. Goldstein, A. L., Banerjee, S., Schneebeli, G. L., Dougherty, T. F., and White, A., *Radiat. Res.* **41**, 597, 1970.
26. Buscarini, L., Bedarida, G., and Marandola, P., *Experientia* **20**, 696, 1964.
27. Miller, J. F. A. P., and Mitchell, G. F., *J. Exp. Med.* **128**, 801, 1968.
28. Mitchell, G F, and Miller, J. F. A. P., *J. Exp. Med.* **128**, 821, 1968.
29. Thomas, L., *Ann. Rev. Physiol.* **16**, 467, 1954.
30. Dent, P. B., Perey, D. Y. E., Cooper, M. D., and Good, R. A., *J. Immunol.* **101**, 799, 1968.
31. Merler, E., Perrault, A., Trapani, R. J., Landy, M., and Shear, M. J., *Proc. Soc. Exp. Biol. Med.* **105**, 443, 1960
32. Landy, M., Sanderson, R. P., and Jackson, A. L., *J. Exp. Med.* **122**, 483, 1965.
33. Johnson, A. G., Gaines, S., and Landy, M, *J. Exp. Med.* **103**, 225, 1956.
34. Kind, P., and Johnson, A. G., *J. Immunol.* **82**, 415, 1959.
35. Ward, P. A., Abell, M. R., and Johnson, A. G., *Amer. J. Pathol.* **38**, 189, 1961.
36. Pierce, C. W., *Lab. Invest.* **17**, 380, 1967.
37. Al-Askari, S., Zweiman, B., Lawrence, H. S., and Thomas, L., *J. Immunol.* **93**, 742, 1964.
38. Springer, G. F., Williamson, P., and Brandes, W. C., *J. Exp. Med.* **113**, 1077, 1967.
39. Zabriskie, J. B., *Advan. Immunol.* **7**, 147, 1967.
40. Rapaport, F. T., Markowitz, A. S., and McCluskey, R. T., *J. Exp. Med.* **129**, 623, 1969.

Immunological Studies

The Fate of Thymocytes
A Study of Kinetics of Thymocytes using High Alkaline Phosphatase Activity as an Endogenous Label

OLLI RUUSKANEN, M.D. & KAUKO KOUVALAINEN, M.D.

The kinetics of thymocytes has been studied in several species by using different labels, e. g. isotopes (Diderholm 1961, Mims 1962, Nossal 1964, Fichtelius & Bryant 1964, Murray & Murray 1964, Murray & Woods 1964, Linna & Stillström 1966, Weissman 1967, Iorio et al. 1970), chromosomes (Davies et al. 1968), the number of mitochondria, certain other morphological signs (Fichtelius & Larsson 1961, Ernström & Sandberg 1970, Abe & Ito 1970), and specific antigens (Reif & Allen 1964, Quartey-Papafio 1969, Yata et al. 1970, Miller & Sprent 1971). Indirect observations on thymocyte kinetics have also been made from the quantitative changes of lymphocytes in different lymphoid organs and blood after thymectomy (Waksman et al. 1962). The results of the studies on the kinetics of thymocytes are important for understanding the function of the thymus especially during postnatal life. We know that at least limited numbers of thymocytes leave the organ, and some studies indicate quite a marked release from the thymus to

---

Grant: The National Research Council for Medical Sciences, Finland.

blood and peripheral lymphoid organs, especially to the spleen (Nossal 1964, Ernström et al. 1965, Metcalf & Bromby 1966, Ernström & Sandberg 1970b, Ernström et al. 1971). The cells labelled with isotopes are not quite satisfactory for long-term studies on cell kinetics because the DNA with its label is diluted by cell division and it may also become reutilized by other cells after thymocyte death (see Fichtelius & Bryant 1964). The other methods mentioned before are quite laborious, thus not allowing studies with large numbers of cells to be analyzed. The guinea-pig thymocytes show an extremely high alkaline phosphatase (AP) activity as compared to the main population of lymphocytes in peripheral lymphoid organs and blood (Kouvalainen 1971a). The high content of AP offers a useful label of thymocytes and can easily be used for distinguishing thymocytes from other lymphocytes (Kouvalainen & Ruuskanen 1970, Kouvalainen 1971b). This study was started in order to get further information on the kinetics of thymocytes using the high AP-activity as an endogenous label.

MATERIAL AND METHODS

Young adult guinea pigs and mice of both sexes were used in the study. The suspensions of guinea-pig thymocytes were prepared as follows (Kouvalainen & Ruuskanen 1970): The thymus was gently pressed with anatomic pincers in a small amount of buffered saline in a large Petri dish. Keeping the saline with the free cells and the debris of the thymus at the edge of the dish, it was evenly rotated until the debris and the milky fluid were separated. The milky fluid consisted almost exclusively of thymocytes (Figure 8). HE-stained smear preparations of the thymus-cell suspension, prepared as described, showed that the cell population consisted of small, medium and large thymocytes, the first group being the most frequent cell type. All thymocytes showed AP-activity in the cytoplasm, but it was most marked in the small-cell type (Figure 8). Nigrosine staining showed that about 90 % of the cells were viable after preparation and washing procedures. Chicken red cells (CRC) were used as controls because of their nucleus and characteristic morphology (Figures 6 and 7).

The cells were injected into the tail vein in mice and into the ear lobe vein in guinea pigs. $1.5-18 \times 10^8$ thymocytes in a volume of $0.5-1.0$ ml were injected into guinea pigs and $2-3 \times 10^8$ cells in a volume of $0.3-0.5$ ml into mice. The corresponding number of CRC were $20-30 \times 10^8$ cells in guinea pigs and $8-10 \times 10^8$ cells in mice.

The autologous-thymocyte suspensions were made from the thymuses of the guinea pigs in question by removing both lobes of the thymus in aether anaesthesia 1–2 hrs before the injection. The animals were in good condition when injected. In the group of thymectomized guinea pigs the thymectomy was carried out 1–2 months before the injection of allogeneic thymocytes.

Blood smears for distinguishing the injected thymocytes were obtained after cutting the tail in mice and puncturing the ear lobe vein in guinea pigs. The opposite ear lobe, not the one used for injection of thymocytes, was used for blood sampling.

The AP-activity of cells in smears and sections of the organs was demonstrated by the calcium-cobalt method as described earlier (Kouvalainen 1971a). The following organs were studied: thymus, spleen, lymph node, bone marrow, and liver. In addition intestine, lungs, and kidneys were studied in a number of animals. The staining intensity of guinea-pig granulocytes offered a technical control of the method (Figure 11). For differential counts 300–5000 cells were studied. Quantitative counting of cells was carried out by using Bürger-Türk's chamber. As a background for the occurrence of AP-positive lymphoid cells in the guinea pig and other animal organs, the reader is referred to an earlier paper (Kouvalainen 1971a). The numbers of AP-positive lymphocytes were expressed as percentages of the nucleated cells. Chemical estimation of AP from tissue extracts was also described earlier (Kouvalainen 1971a). In four animals perfusion with 0.9 % saline was carried out 3 hrs after the i.v. injection of thymocytes or CRC: just before the samples were taken for the study.

RESULTS

After the initial rise of the white blood cell count following the i.v. injection of thymocytes their number decreased in all experiments in 10 min to the upper limit of normal values. After 3 hrs, however, there was a significant re-elevation in the number of white blood cells (Figures 1, 3 and 4). This was not directly due to the thymocytes injected but was caused by a marked increase in the number of granulocytes. This phenomenon was found to follow the injection of xenogeneic, allogeneic and autologous thymocytes.

Xenogeneic thymocytes

Guinea-pig thymocytes were injected i.v. into 64 mice. Mouse white blood cells are all AP-negative. Accordingly, the AP-positive guinea-pig thymocytes were very easily discernible in the cell smears. The disappearance rate of the thymocytes from blood is demonstrated in Figure 3. Most thymocytes disappeared from the blood in a few minutes. After 3–5 hrs only very few of them were left (Figure 3, Table I). In a group of animals blood smears were made daily for two weeks following the injection. No guinea-pig thymocytes were observed after the first 24 hrs.

In the sections and smears of organs stained for AP it was seen that a few thymocytes injected were present in the bone marrow, lymph nodes, spleen, and liver (Figure 10). During the first hours after the injection the thymocytes seem to accumulate in the liver and spleen as judged from the quantitative increase in AP-activities of these organs (Figure 2). 10 hrs after the injection there were still occasional thymocytes in the spleen, lymph nodes, and bone marrow. After 24 hrs guinea-pig thymocytes were only found in the mouse organs exceptionally. On no occasion were injected cells found in the mouse thymus. Perfusion with saline in a group sacrificed after 3 hrs did not significantly change the thymocyte counts made from cell smears of the spleen and liver.

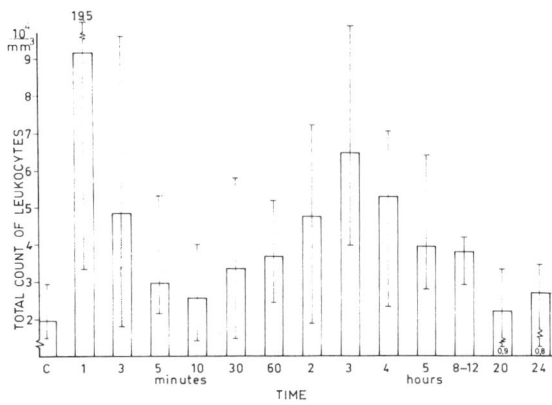

Figure 1. The total number of leucocytes in the blood of mouse after an i.v. injection of guinea-pig thymocytes. The initial rise is due to the enormous number of thymocytes, but the second one at 2 to 4 hrs was observed to be due to the increase of the number of granulocytes.
The range is indicated with the vertical lines.

Allogeneic thymocytes

The spontaneous occurrence of AP-positive lymphocytes, morphologically identical with thymocytes in the guinea pig, is seen in Table I. There was no difference between the frequencies of AP-positive lymphocytes in the thymic and other venous blood (0.44 ± 0.26 and 0.40 ± 0.26 %, respectively). In the arterial blood the frequency of AP-positive lymphocytes was 0.25 ± 0.20 %. In the lymph nodes the frequency of AP-positive cells varied markedly from node to node (1.14 ± 0.68 %). In the spleen the occurrence of AP-positive lymphocytes is quite constant, only 0.13 ± 0.01 %. In the blood the frequency of AP-positive cells varied individually from 0.04 to 0.59 % (mean 0.40 ± 0.26 %) (Table I).

The fate of thymocytes prepared from one guinea pig's thymus was studied in 20 animals. The disappearance rate of the injected cells from blood is seen in Figure 3. The

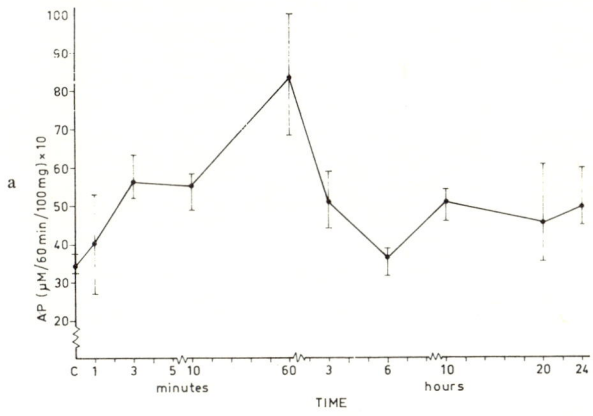

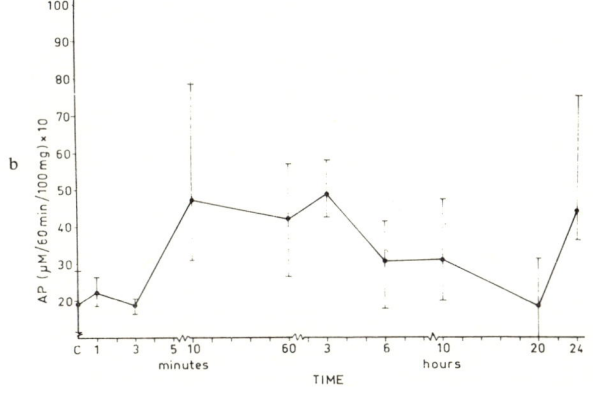

Figure 2. AP-activity in the mouse spleen (a) and liver (b) after an i.v. injection of the guinea-pig thymocytes. Note the rapid increase of AP-activity during the first hr and its decrease during the next 3–10 hrs. There is a re-increase in the liver at 24 hrs.

TABLE I

The percentage of AP-positive lymphocytes (thymocytes) in different organs in controls and after an i.v. injection of AP-positive guinea-pig thymocytes
The figures from different experiments are reduced to correspond to 4×10^8 cells injected
Great individual differences can be seen in high SD-values

Tissues, and the type of cells injected	AP-positive lymphocytes, per cent ± SD			
	Controls	3 hrs	10 hrs	24 hrs
Autologous cells	Guinea pig			
Blood	0.40 ± 0.26	1.75 ± 1.22	0.27 ± 0.36	0.42 ± 0.26
Bone marrow	0.03 ± 0.01	0.36 ± 0.35	0.44 ± 0.52	0.33 ± 0.07
Lymph nodes	1.14 ± 0.68	2.93 ± 1.55	6.30 ± 4.16	2.74 ± 0.74
Liver	0.03 ± 0.03	0.87 ± 1.12	1.40 ± 1.80	0.48 ± 0.56
Spleen	0.13 ± 0.10	3.96 ± 2.67	6.66 ± 2.59	11.34 ± 10.12
Allogeneic cells				
Blood	0.40 ± 0.26	2.88 ± 2.67	3.36 ± 3.51	0.34 ± 0.39
Bone marrow	0.03 ± 0.01	0.26 ± 0.29	3.50 ± 4.96	1.01 ± 1.17
Lymph nodes	1.14 ± 0.68	1.72 ± 2.62	7.54 ± 7.63	2.94 ± 1.18
Liver	0.03 ± 0.03	3.11 ± 4.39	7.60 ± 10.99	0.19 ± 0.21
Spleen	0.13 ± 0.01	5.33 ± 5.55	13.96 ± 7.52	9.71 ± 2.68
Xenogeneic cells	Mouse			
Blood	0	1.27 ± 0.76	0.20 ± 0.60	0.13 ± 0.30
Bone marrow	0	2.00 ± 1.49	0.80 ± 0.87	0.13 ± 0.30
Lymph nodes	0	0.20 ± 0.33	0.33 ± 0.33	0.07 ± 0.15
Liver	0	0.40 ± 0.48	0	0.13 ± 0.30
Spleen	0	0.40 ± 0.60	1.27 ± 0.68	0

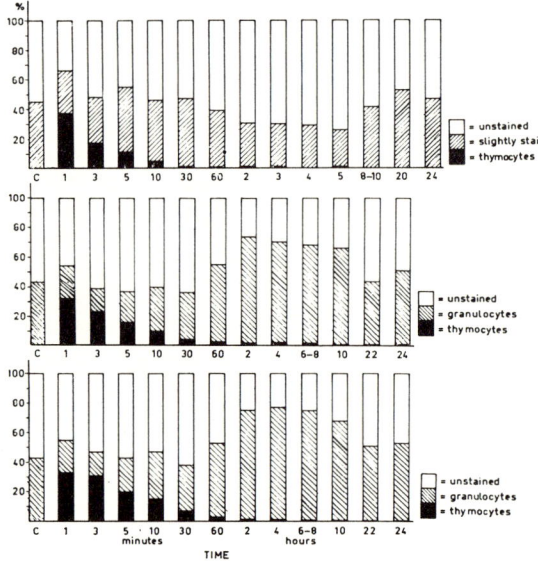

Figure 3. The percentage of xenogeneic and allogeneic thymocytes in blood at different time points after an i.v. injection.
Top: The guinea-pig thymocytes in the mouse.
In the middle: Allogeneic thymocytes in guinea pigs thymectomized 1–2 months before the injection.
Below: Allogeneic thymocytes in intact guinea pigs.
Note the disappearance rates of thymocytes and the marked granulocytosis at 2 to 10 hrs. In mouse the granulocytes are included in the group 'unstained' because they are AP-negative.

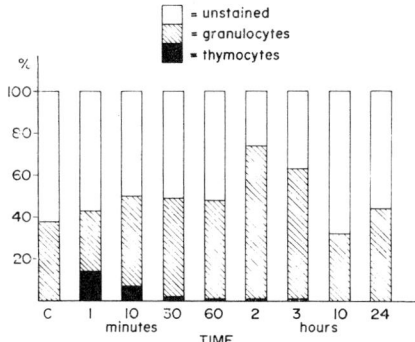

Figure 4. The percentage of autologous thymocytes in blood of the guinea pig after an i.v. injection. Note the disappearance rate and the granulocytosis at 2 to 3 hrs.

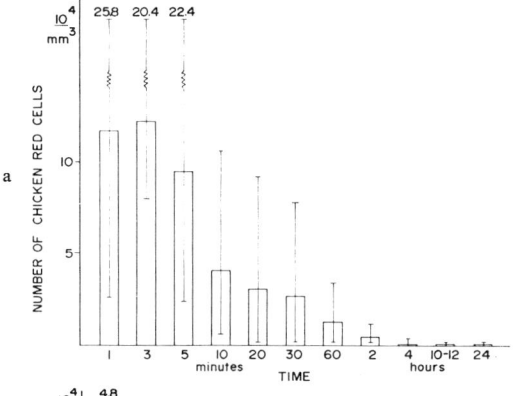

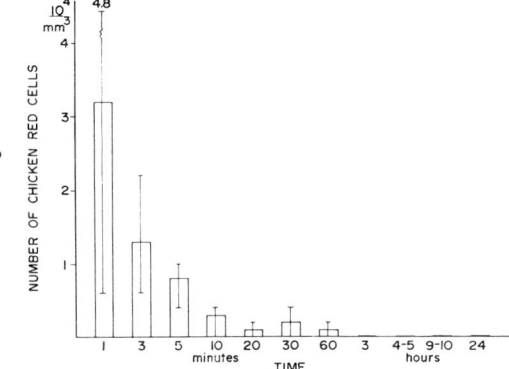

Figure 5

a. The disappearance rate of i.v. injected control cells (chicken red cells, CRC) from the circulation in the mouse. Only occasional cells were seen in blood after 2–4 hrs.

b. The disappearance rate of CRC from blood in the guinea pig. Compare the rapidity of the disappearance with that seen in the mouse.

TABLE II
The percentage of CRS in different organs after an i.v. injection

Species	Time (hrs)	CRS, per cent of nucleated cells ± SD			
		Bone marrow	Lymph nodes	Spleen	Liver
Guinea pig	3	0	0	0	0.4 ± 0.2
	10	0	0	0	0
	24	0	0	0	0
Mouse	3	10.9 ± 9.8	0.3 ± 0.3	30.4 ± 15.3	27.3 ± 3.3
	10	0.2 ± 0.1	0	10.6 ± 7.1	11.0 ± 6.0
	24	0	0	0	0

main population of the thymocytes disappeared from the blood in 2 to 4 hrs. They did not reappear in the circulation during an observation period of 30 days. The occurrence of AP-positive lymphocytes (thymocytes) in different (lymphoid) organs following an i.v. injection of thymocytes is given in Table I. It was seen that the main destination of allogeneic thymocytes in the guinea pig was the spleen, but in addition they were also seen in the peripheral lymph nodes and bone marrow. In two animals a significant accumulation of thymocytes was seen in the liver, but in the remaining animals the thymocytes did not significantly gather in the liver. Thymectomy of the recipients 1–2 months before the injection of allogeneic thymocytes did not change their disappearance rate from blood (Figure 3).

Autologous thymocytes
The disappearance rate of autologous thymocytes injected i.v. into 12 guinea pigs did not significantly differ from that of allogeneic cells (Figure 4). The distribution of the autologous cells in lymphoid organs also corresponded to the one observed when allogeneic cells were used (Table I, Figures 9 and 11).

Xenogeneic control cells
CRC were injected into 13 guinea pigs and 17 mice. Their disappearance from blood and accumulation in different organs were studied.

In guinea pigs CRC disappeared totally from blood in 3 hrs (Figure 5 b). Signs of the destruction of the cells were already seen 5 min after the injection. At 3, 10, and 24 hrs following the injection no CRC were found in the spleen, liver, bone marrow, lymph nodes, and lung (Table II).

In mice the disappearance rate of CRC from circulation was slower than in guinea pigs (Figure 5 a). At 4 hrs and thereafter only occasional CRC were seen in blood. After 3 hrs injected cells were seen in lung, spleen, bone marrow, and liver and, to a lesser extent, in lymph nodes (Figure 7, Table II). After 10 hrs a significant number of cells was still present in the spleen and the liver, and in 2 animals in the lung. After 24 hrs no CRC were found in any organs. Slight degenerative signs of the injected cells were seen in the cell smears in the mouse (Figure 7).

DISCUSSION

The high activity of AP in the guinea pig thymocytes made it possible to follow their fate in the body after an i.v. injection. The disappearance rates of xenogeneic, allogeneic and autologous cells from blood surprisingly resembled each other and were extremely rapid (Figures 3 and 4). The disappearance of control cells, i.e. CRC, resembled that of thymocytes, but was even more rapid, especially in guinea pigs, in which all the CRC were destroyed in 3 hrs. Our study confirms some earlier findings on the development of primary antibodies to CRC in the guinea pig (Litt 1967). The results are in accordance with studies (Halpern et al. 1957, Appelgren & Schildt 1970) showing that foreign red cells are eliminated mainly in the spleen and liver. Xenogeneic thymocytes also seem to be quite rapidly destroyed in the liver and spleen (Figure 2, Table I). The stay of CRC in the body of the guinea pig and the mouse was in general signifiantly shorter than that of thymocytes. This was true despite the fact that much larger amounts of CRC were injected as compared to the amounts of thymocytes. The granulocytosis following the i.v. injection of thymocytes is probably an unspecific reaction resembling the situation described by Jyväsjärvi et al. (1970).

The rapid disappearance rate of thymocytes, including the autologous ones, makes it probable that the thymocytes, or at least the main part of them, are not regular constituents of the blood white cell population. Otherwise it will be hard to find an explanation for the extremely rapid elemination of the injected thymocytes from blood. A quantity of two to twenty-five times the actual total number of blood lymphocytes (Kotani et al. 1966) and an amount equal to the daily output of thoracic duct lymphocytes (Yoffey et al. 1958) were injected into the circulation in the course of 30 sec. The cells injected disappeared from the blood in a few hours and never returned, at least in numbers measurable by the method of this study. Our results accord in this respect with most of the earlier studies on the kinetics of thymocytes in different species (Diderholm 1961, Mims 1962, Murray & Murray 1964). The organism might recognize its own cells as 'foreign' if the cells are damaged by the preparation procedures. The nigrosin test (Kaltenbach et al. 1958) showed, however, that the large majority of cells used in our study was intact. We can conclude that following an i.v. challenge thymocytes leave the circulation with exceptional rapidity. If in the guinea pig about 12.1×10^6 thymocytes leave the thymus in a day, as estimated by Kotani et al. (1966), one could only occasionally find these cells in blood samples. Our findings of the disappearance rates of thymocytes and of the spontaneous occurrence of about 0.4% AP-positive cells (possibly thymocytes) in blood are in fairly good accordance with the number estimated by Ernström & Sandberg (1970b). They also roughly resemble Nossal's calculations (Nossal 1964). If the AP-positive lymphocytes occurring spontaneously in the guinea-pig blood really were thymocytes, their total amount in circulation every moment was about 12×10^5, supposing that the blood volume of a guinea pig weighing 400 g is about 30 ml and the white cell count $10^4/\mu l$. Supposing further that the disappearance rate of the thymocytes from blood corresponds to that seen in the present study, the daily output of thymocytes would be about 8.6×10^7 cells. The relative stability of the frequency of the AP-positive lymphocytes in blood would presuppose a constant release from the thymus. Because no significant differences were found between the frequencies of AP-positive lymphocytes in the thymic and other venous blood, the thymocyte release could probably not be of a very large magnitude. However, there are facts supporting the idea that medullary thymocytes alone or with cortical thymocytes leave the thymus (Borum 1968). There is evidence that the medullary thymocytes are immunologically more competent and may form the main population of long-living cortisone-resistant circulating lymphocytes (Warner 1964, Dougherty et al. 1964, Abe & Ito 1970, Blomgren 1971). In the guinea pig most medullary thymocytes are AP-negative or show only weak AP-activity (Kouvalainen 1971a). Accordingly, our method is not satisfactory for counting medullary thymocytes. That might explain the discrepancy between our results and those of some others showing higher lymphocyte counts in the thymic venous blood than in the blood of the carotid artery (Ernström et al. 1965). On the basis of the very low frequency of AP-positive lymphocytes in the guinea-pig blood and peripheral lymphoid organs, and supposing that they are traceable to the thymus, it seems evident that the so-called T-cells (thymus-derived or thymus-dependent lymphocytes), or at least the main population of them, are not identical with (cortical) thymocytes. It is, however, not excluded that AP-positive cortical thymocytes after leaving the thymus are sooner or later transformed into AP-negative cells. According to our present knowledge, such a transformation does not occur in vitro during an observation period of a few days, but the process might be more active in vivo. After an i.v. injection of thymocytes blast transformed cells seem to derive from cortisone-resistant medullary thymocytes (Blomgren 1971).

The results of this study confirm some earlier findings that the main destination of (cortical) thymocytes in the spleen and to a lesser extent the lymph nodes and other lymphoid and haemopoietic organs (Murray & Murray 1964, Parrot et al. 1964, Goldschneider & McGregor 1968, Iorio et al. 1970, Ernström & Sandberg 1970b, Ernström et al. 1971, Table I). The frequency of AP-positive cells in peripheral lymphoid organs increased during the first 10 hrs after the injection of both allogeneic

---

Figure 6. CRC are demonstrable on the basis of the characteristic morphology. Among the mouse red cells in the middle of the picture there are three CRC (arrows). Note the characteristic oval morphology of these cells. Unstained cells in Bürker-Türk's chamber, × 400.

Figure 7. Nucleated slightly swollen CRC are easily demonstrable among the spleen cells of the mouse. HE × 400.

Figure 8. Smear of the guinea pig thymocytes. AP-activity is demonstrated by the intensity of the dark colour. AP-staining, × 400.

Figure 9. Smear from the spleen of a guinea pig into which autologous thymocytes were injected i.v. 3 hrs earlier. Thymocytes are shown by arrows. Strongly stained granulocytes and AP-negative lymphocytes of the spleen are seen as a background. AP-staining, × 400.

Figure 10. Two guinea-pig thymocytes (arrows) in the mouse spleen smear. All the white cells of the mouse are AP-negative, which makes the distinguishing of injected thymocytes very easy. AP-staining, × 400.

Figure 11. Injected autologous thymocytes in blood smear of the guinea pig (arrows). The granulocytes are intensively stained. Normal AP-negative blood lymphocytes are seen in the middle and to the right. AP-staining, × 400.

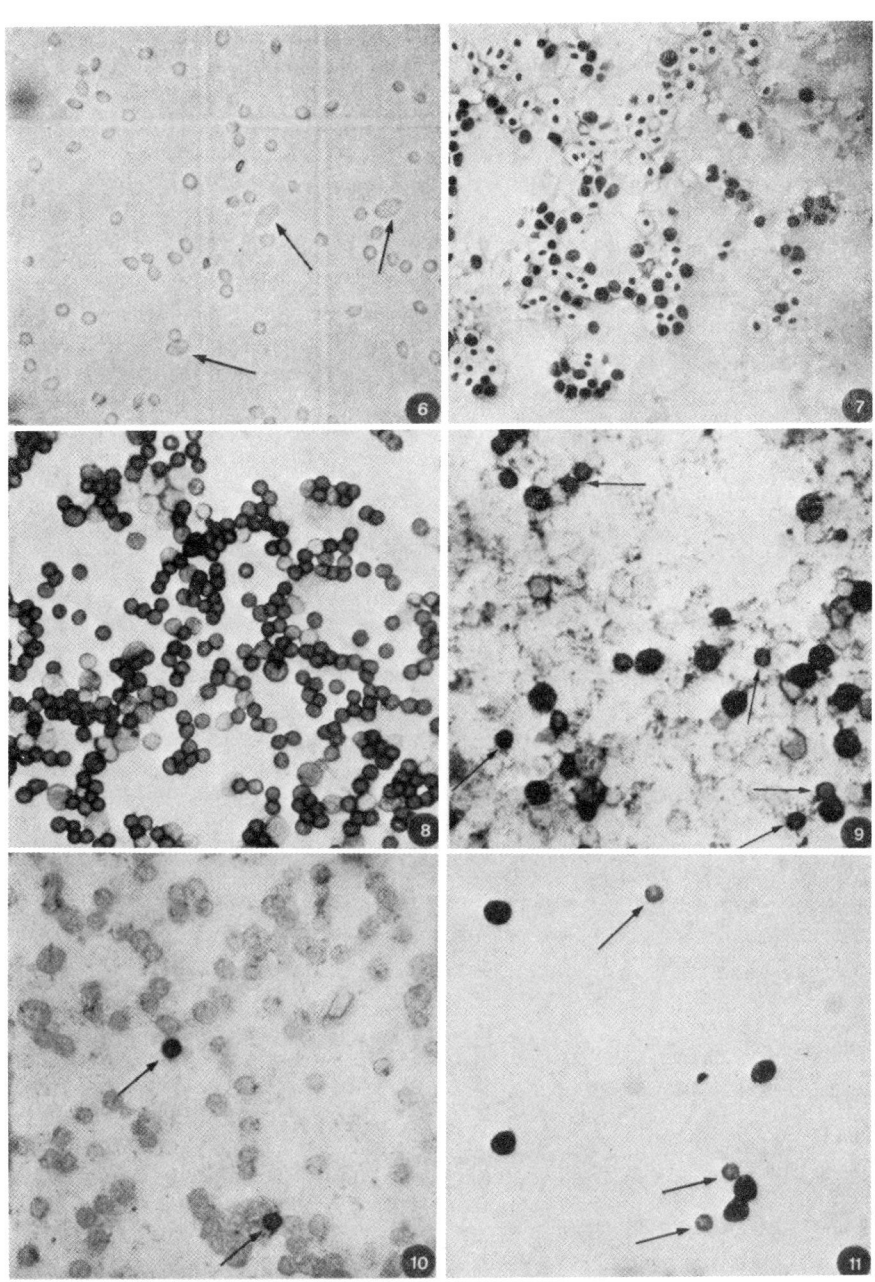

and autologous thymocytes (Table I). The increase seemed to be more marked in the former group. Individual variations were, however, of an extreme magnitude. Whether the autologous and allogeneic thymocytes really behave differently in this respect remains to be clarified. A detailed study on the behaviour of autologous thymocytes in the guinea-pig spleen is in progress. We emphasize the low spontaneous presence of AP-positive lymphocytes in the spleen as seen in this study. Guinea-pig thymocytes were not imported to the thymus in the mouse, in which species observations in this respect were possible. Import has been seen in the guinea pig during the regenerative stage of thymic involution (Larsson 1967).

The AP-positive lymphocytes of blood and peripheral lymphoid organs may derive from the thymus. It is, however, not excluded that lymphocyte clones with high AP-activity also arise in the peripheral lymphoid organs either that they represent a special stage of lymphocytic maturation, or phylogenetic mutative clones without any further biological significance (Kouvalainen 1971a).

REFERENCES

Abe, K. & Ito, T. (1970) 'Fine structure of small lymphocytes in the thymus of mouse: Qualitative and quantitative analysis by electron microscopy.' *Z. Zellforsch.* **110**, 321–35.

Appelgren, L.-E. & Schildt, B. E. (1970) 'Autoradiographic localization of rabbit red cells injected into the mouse.' *Acta path. microbiol. scand.* **78**, 215–18.

Blomgren, H. (1971) 'Studies on the proliferation of thymus cells injected into syngeneic or allogeneic irradiated mice.' *Clin. exp. Immunol.* **8**, 279–89.

Borum, K. (1968) 'Pattern of cell production and cell migration in mouse thymus studied by autoradiography.' *Scand. J. Haemat.* **5**, 339–52.

Davies, A. J. S., Festenstein, H., Leuchars, E., Wallis, V. J. & Doenhoff, M. J. (1968) 'A thymic origin for some peripheral-blood lymphocytes.' *Lancet* **I**, 183–84.

Diderholm, H. (1961) 'Studies on the migration and transformation of lymphocytes in immunized and non-immunized animals.' *Acta path. microbiol. scand.* **51**, Suppl. 146.

Dougherty, T. F., Berliner, M. L., Schneebeli, G. L. & Berliner, D. L. (1964) 'Hormonal control of lymphatic structure and function.' *Ann. N. Y. Acad. Sci.* **113**, 825–43.

Ernström, U., Gyllensten, L. & Larsson, B. (1965) 'Venous output of lymphocytes from the thymus.' *Nature* (Lond.) **207**, 540–41.

Ernström, U., Larsson, B. & Linna, J. (1971) 'Thymus-derived lymphocytes in blood, lymph and lymphoid organs after intrathymic labelling with ^{3}H-thymidine.' *Scand. J. Haemat.* **8**, 141–50.

Ernström, U. & Sandberg, G. (1970a) 'Influence of splenectomy on thymic release of lymphocytes into blood.' *Scand. J. Haemat.* **7**, 342–48.

Ernström, U. & Sandberg, G. (1970b) 'Quantitative relationship between release and intrathymic death of lymphocytes.' *Acta path. microbiol. scand.* **78**, Section A, 362–63.

Fichtelius, K. E. & Bryant, B. J. (1964) 'On the fate of thymocytes.' *In* R. A. Good & A. E. Gabrielsen (eds.) *The Thymus in Immunobiology*, pp. 274–86. Harper & Row, New York/Evanston/London.

Fichtelius, K. E. & Larsson, S. E. (1961) 'Blood lymphocytes in supravital and dried smear preparations studied with mitochondrial stain.' *Acta anat.* (Basel) **44**, 60–69.

Goldschneider, I. & McGregor, D. D. (1968) 'Migration of lymphocytes and thymocytes in the rat. I. The route of migration from blood to spleen and lymph nodes.' *J. exp. Med.* **127**, 155–68.

Halpern, B. N., Biozzi, G., Benacerraf, B. & Stiffel, C. (1957) 'Phagocytosis of foreign red blood cells by the reticuloendothelial system.' *Amer. J. Physiol.* **189**, 520–26.

Iorio, R. J., Chanana, A. D., Cronkite, E. P. & Joel, D. D. (1970) 'Studies on lymphocytes. XVI. Distribution of bovine thymic lymphocytes in the spleen and lymph nodes.' *Cell Tissue Kinet.* **3**, 161–73.

Jyväsjärvi, S., Keinänen, S. & Ruuskanen, O. (1971) 'Leucocytosis in the mouse induced by serial blood sampling from the tail.' *Nature* (Lond.) **230**, 122.

Kaltenbach, J. P., Kaltenbach, M. H. & Lyons, W. B. (1958) 'Nigrosin as a dye for differentiating live and dead ascites cells.' *Exp. Cell Res.* **15**, 112–17.

Kotani, M., Seiki, K., Yamashita, A. & Horii, I. (1966) 'Lymphatic drainage of thymocytes to circulation in the guinea pig.' *Blood* **27**, 511–20.

Kouvalainen, K. (1971a) 'Species and organ dependence of alkaline phosphatase activity in lymphatic tissues. A histochemical, biochemical and electrophoretic study.' *Histochem. J.* **3**, 55–69.

Kouvalainen, K. (1971b) 'The use of alkaline phosphatase for distinguishing thymocytes in the guinea pig.' *In* O. Mäkelä, Anne Cross & T. U. Kosunen (eds.) *Cell Interactions and Receptor Antibodies in Immune Responses.* (Proceed. Third Sigrid Juselius Symposium), pp. 70–74. Academic Press, London/New York.

Kouvalainen, K. & Ruuskanen, O. (1970) 'An easy method for studies on kinetics of thymocytes.' *Scand. J. clin. Lab. Invest.* **25** (Suppl. 113), 68.

Larsson, B. (1967) 'Export and import of ^{3}H-thymidine-labelled lymphocytes in the thymus of normal and steroid-treated guinea-pigs.' *Acta path. microbiol. scand.* **70**, 390–97.

Linna, J. & Stillström, J. (1966) 'Migration of cells from the thymus to the spleen in young guinea pigs.' *Acta path. microbiol. scand.* **68**, 465–75.

Litt, M. (1967) 'Studies on the latent period. I. Primary antibody in guinea pig lymph nodes 7½ minutes after introduction of chicken erythrocytes.' *Cold Spr. Harb. Symp. quant. Biol.* **32**, 477–92.

Metcalf, D. & Brumby, M. (1966) 'The role of thymus in the ontogeny of immune system.' *J. cell. Physiol.* **67** (Suppl. 1), 149–68.

Miller, J. F. A. P. & Sprent, J. (1971) 'Thymus-derived cells in mouse thoracic duct lymph.' *Nature New Biol.* (Lond.) **230**, 267–70.

Mims, C. A. (1962) 'Experiments on the origin and fate of lymphocytes.' *Brit. J. exp. Path.* **43**, 639–49.

Murray, R. G. & Murray, A. (1964) 'Studies on the fate of lymphocytes. II. Intravenous injection of labelled thymic lymphocytes into homologous rats and isologous mice.' *Anat. Rec.* **150**, 95–111.

Murray, R. G. & Woods, P. A. (1964) 'Studies on the fate of lymphocytes. III. The migration and metamorhposis of in situ labelled thymic lymphocytes.' *Anat. Rec.* **150**, 113–28.

Nossal, G. J. V. (1964) 'Studies on rate of seeding of lymphocytes from the intact guinea pig thymus.' *Ann. N. Y. Acad. Sci.* **120**, 171–81.

Parrot, D. M. V., de Sousa, M. A. B. & East, J. (1966) 'Thymus-dependent areas in the lymphoid organs of neonatally thymectomized mice.' *J. exp. Med.* **123**, 191–201.

Quartey-Papafio, J. B. (1969) 'A fluorescent antibody technique for studying thymocyte migration in the rat.' *J. Physiol.* (Lond.) **203**, 2 P.

Reif, A. E. & Allen, J. M. V. (1964) 'The AKR thymic antigen and its distribution in leukemias and nervous tissues.' *J. exp. Med.* **120**, 413–33.

Waksman, B. H., Arnason, B. G. & Jankovic, B. D. (1962) 'Role of the thymus in immune reactions in rats. III. Changes in the lymphoid organs of thymectomized rats.' *J. exp. Med.* **116**, 187–206.

Warner, N. L. (1964) 'Immunological role of different lymphoid organs in chicken. II. The immunological competence of thymic cell suspensions.' *Austr. J. exp. Biol. med. Sci.* **42**, 401–16.

Weissman, I. L. (1967) 'Thymus cell migration.' *J. exp. Med.* **126**, 291–304.

Yata, J., Klein, G., Kobayashi, N., Furukawa, M. & Yanagisawa, M. (1970) 'Human thymus-lymphoid tissue antigen and its presence in leukaemia and lymphoma.' *Clin. exp. Immunol.* **7**, 781–92.

Yoffey, J. M., Hanks, G. A. & Kelly, L. (1958) 'Some problems of lymphocyte production.' *Ann. N. Y. Acad. Sci.* **73**, 47–78.

THE UROPOD-BEARING LYMPHOCYTE OF THE GUINEA PIG

Evidence for Thymic Origin

By DAVID L. ROSENSTREICH, ETHAN SHEVACH, IRA GREEN, and ALAN S. ROSENTHAL

Lymphocytes bearing the highly characteristic foot appendage, or uropod, have been described in small numbers in several different lymphoid populations from a variety of sources and species (1–4). Although lymphocytes with uropods remain a minor component of the total lymphoid population, their frequency can apparently be increased or "stimulated" in vitro by the mixed lymphocyte reaction (2) or by the mitogen, phytohemagglutinin (3, 4). Thus the possibility is raised that the uropod is a marker for "activated" lymphocytes. Alternatively the uropod may represent a region of membrane structural specificity limited to a distinct subset of lymphocytes.

Lymphocytes may be classified in a variety of ways. Lymphoid cells are divided into at least two functional subpopulations based upon their sites of differentiation. Thus the thymus-derived or "T" lymphocytes[1] appear to be responsible for cell-mediated immunity, and the bone marrow–derived or "B" lymphocytes are the apparent precursors of antibody-forming cells. These two populations of cells can be distinguished by the presence of easily detectable membrane immunoglobulin on the B lymphocyte (5), and by the presence of surface differentiation antigens on the T lymphocyte (6). T lymphocytes may be further subdivided by their ability to respond to antigen in vitro, and in the immunized guinea pig, there is clearly a hierarchy of antigen reactivity among different lymphoid subpopulations. Thus, peritoneal exudate lymphocytes are much more reactive to a variety of soluble protein antigens than those derived from draining lymph nodes (7), and thymocytes respond poorly to these antigens, if at all (8).

In order to study the relationship between immunocompetence and uropod formation, lymphocytes from the thymus, draining lymph node, and peritoneal exudate of immunized guinea pigs were obtained and the number of uropod-bearing lymphocytes determined with both light and electron microscope techniques immediately after isolation and before any in vitro antigenic

---

[1] *Abbreviations used in this paper:* B lymphocytes, bone marrow–derived lymphocytes; BSA, bovine serum albumin; FCS, fetal calf serum; MEM, Eagle's minimal essential medium; PELS, peritoneal exudate lymphocytes; PPD, purified protein derivative; TdR-^{3}H, tritiated thymidine; T lymphocytes, thymus-derived lymphocytes.

stimulation. Antigen reactivity was then subsequently determined in each population using the in vitro lymphocyte proliferation assay. Finally, to determine if uropods were found on B cells, T cells, or on both types of lymphocytes, lymphocyte populations containing both B and T cells were studied using an anti-immunoglobulin reagent as a marker for B cells and were simultaneously observed for uropod formation.

We have found that in the lymphoid populations studied there exists a general correlation between the ability to respond to antigen in vitro and uropod formation. Furthermore, in the guinea pig, all those lymphocytes that are spontaneously forming uropods do not bear easily detectable surface membrane immunoglobulin and thus appear to be thymus-dependent or T cells.

Materials and Methods

Strain 2 female guinea pigs were immunized in the four footpads with complete Freund's adjuvant containing 2 mg/ml of *Mycobacterium tuberculosis* H37Ra. 2–4 wk later, 25 ml of sterile mineral oil (Marcol 52, Humble Oil & Refining, Co., Houston, Tex.) was injected intraperitoneally, and 3 days later thymus, draining lymph nodes, and the peritoneal exudate were harvested. Peritoneal exudate lymphocytes were separated from contaminating neutrophiles and macrophages by using an adherence column of nylon fiber (Fenwal Labs., Morton Grove, Ill.) combined with fine glass beads (type 100–5005, Minnesota Mining & Manufacturing Co., St. Paul, Minn.), as previously described (10). The resulting cell population contained more than 95% lymphocytes with a viability of greater than 98% as determined by trypan blue exclusion. Thymus and lymph nodes were trimmed of fat, and single cell suspensions were prepared by teasing with needle and forceps. When indicated in the protocol, thymus and lymph node cells were also purified by passage over columns of nylon and glass beads. Techniques of immunization, cell preparation, and column purification have been described in detail elsewhere (7, 9, 10). After isolation, the cell populations were suspended in Eagle's minimal essential media (MEM, Spinner modification) with 10% fetal calf serum (FCS) and incubated at 37°C for 30 min. Living cell suspensions were examined using Nomarski interference contrast optics on a Zeiss microscope (Carl Zeiss, Oberkochen, West Germany), and uropod-bearing lymphocytes were quantitated. Since uropod formation is temperature dependent, all preparations were allowed to equilibrate to 37°C for 15 min before counting, and during the period of microscope examination, the cells were maintained at 37°C with a Sage air-curtain incubator (Sage Equipment Co., Div. of Orion Research Inc., Cambridge, Mass.). For electron microscope studies, cell suspensions were incubated at either 4° or 37°C for 30 min, fixed in 1% glutaraldehyde for 30 min, processed, and embedded in Maraglas (Polysciences, Inc. Warrington, Pa.) for examination in a Philips 300 electron microscope (Philips Electronic Instruments, Mount Vernon, N. Y.).

For simultaneous evaluation of immunoglobulin-bearing cells and the presence or absence of uropods, whole unfractionated lymph node cells, which contain both B and T cells (9), were incubated in serum-free media, at 4°C for 30 min with a fluoresceinated rabbit anti–guinea pig Fab antiserum (obtained from Dr. Victor Nussenzweig, New York University School of Medicine) (23). This procedure reproducibly stains approximately 30% of lymph node cells with a characteristic "speckled" pattern (25). The cell suspensions were washed twice, resuspended in media with 10% FCS, allowed to equilibrate to 37°C for 15 min, and then maintained at 37°C with the air-curtain incubator. Using a Leitz Ortholux microscope (E. Leitz, Inc., Rockleigh, N. J.), uropod-bearing lymphocytes were first identified with tungsten illumination, then the ultraviolet light was switched on and the presence or absence of fluorescence of these uropod-bearing lymphocytes was determined.

To determine the degree of antigen-mediated in vitro lymphocyte proliferation in different lymphoid populations, cells from different sources were suspended in Spinner's MEM containing 10% strain 2 guinea pig serum plus added glutamine, sodium pyruvate, nonessential amino acids, and penicillin (7). Triplicate tubes of 3×10^6 cells/tube were cultured for 72 hr, with or without 10 µg/ml purified protein derivative (PPD) (Connaught Medical Research Labs, Willowdale, Ontario, Canada), and then were pulsed with 3.0 µCi of tritiated thymidine (TdR-^{3}H, 6.7 Ci/mM, New England Nuclear Corp., Boston, Mass.) for 4 hr and trichloroacetic acid–precipitable radioactivity was determined, as previously described (7). Stimulation is expressed as the ratio of total incorporated counts in antigen-stimulated cultures compared with total incorporated counts in control cultures.

RESULTS

Morphological Observations of Uropod-Bearing Lymphocytes of the Guinea Pig: Ultrastructural Features.—A thin section profile of a typical uropod-bearing lymphocyte is shown in Fig. 1. The uropod is most easily recognized and clearly identified by electron microscopy. Its most characteristic features are the numerous terminal finger-like projections, the microspikes (11). The uropod itself contains occasional mitochondria and more typically, numerous vacuoles of various sizes and a well-developed system of microtubules and microfilaments. Its location on the cell is usually opposite the nuclear hof, and the cytoplasmic region with which it is immediately contiguous typically contains a multitude of cell organelles, including mitochondria, microtubules, a centriole, numerous vacuoles, and the Golgi apparatus. In contrast, pseudopods, which are the means by which the cell moves, generally contain few cell organelles. The small pseudopod-like structure seen in Fig. 1 contains only cytoplasm and numerous free ribosomes. The uropod ultrastructure described here in freshly isolated guinea pig lymphocytes is similar to that described previously in human lymphocytes stimulated by phytohemagglutinin (4) and by the mixed lymphocyte reaction in humans (11, 12).

Light Microscope Observations using the Nomarski Interference Optical System.—Immediately after transfer to the slides, uropod formation in the cell suspensions was minimal. However, after 15 min under the warm stage, the lymphocytes were actively motile and forming uropods. Once equilibrated, (10–15 min) the percentage of uropod-bearing lymphocytes in individual populations remained stable for up to 180 min.

Uropod formation was a rapid and dynamic process. Lymphocytes were observed to extend or retract their uropods, in as little as 60 sec. Many uropod-forming lymphocytes were also actively motile and had a highly irregular shape which was accentuated by pseudopod formation (Fig. 2 c). Nevertheless, some lymphocytes formed uropods although they did not appear to be actively motile, did not have pseudopods, and had the round configuration of resting cells.

The advantage of the Nomarski system over conventional phase-contrast microscopy for observations of living cells is that it clearly delineates both

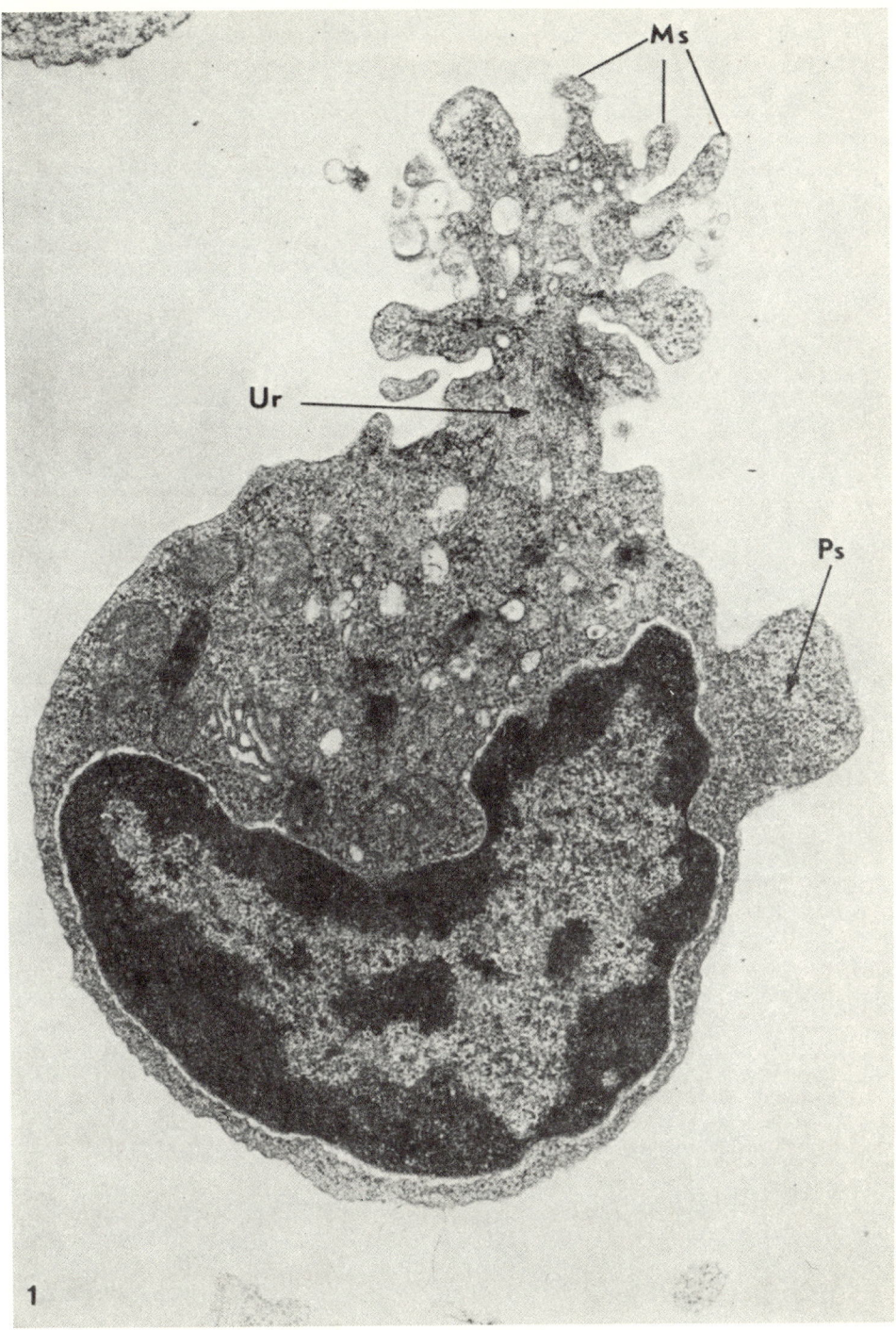

FIG. 1. Electron micrograph of a peritoneal exudate lymphocyte after equilibration at 37°C for 30 min. The cell uropod (Ur) is characterized by terminal microspikes (Ms) and content of vesicles. The small pseudopod (Ps) contains only ribosomes. × 28,000.

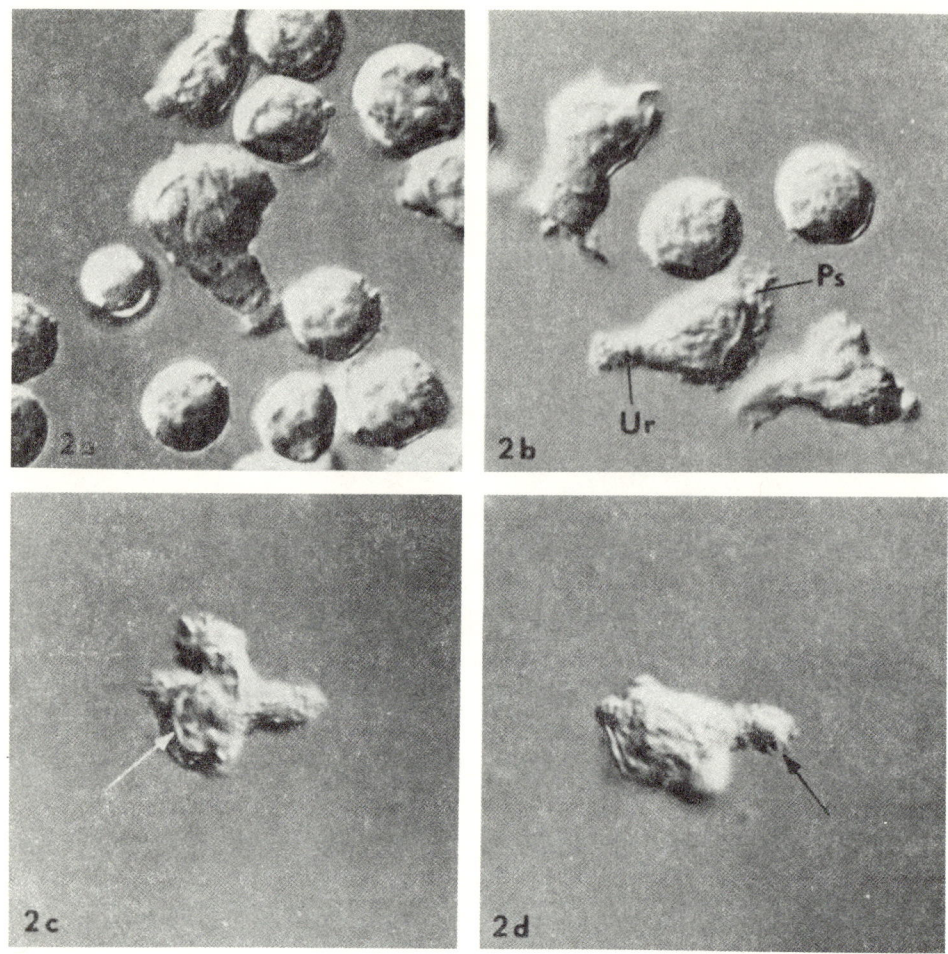

Fig. 2. Lymphocytes derived from either peritoneal exudate or lymph node, fixed after equilibration at 37°C for 30 min, and photographed using Nomarski interference contrast optics. × 1650. (a) Lymph node cell suspension with a large uropod-bearing lymphocyte in the center. (b) Peritoneal exudate lymphocytes. Note the fine-veil like pseudopod (*Ps*) and the thicker uropod (*Ur*). (c) Uropod-bearing lymphocyte with a typical highly irregular shape. The *arrow* points to the clearly visible nuclear rim. (d) Uropod-bearing lymphocyte illustrating the terminal microspikes (*arrow*).

surface structures as well as intracellular elements with good resolution. However, photographic resolution is poor because of the extremely shallow depth of focus, cell motion, and the greatly diminished transmitted light inherent in this optical system. To abolish the variable of cell motility, cells were fixed in 1% glutaraldehyde before photographing.

Several uropod-bearing lymphocytes as photographed using Nomarski optics are illustrated in Fig. 2. Terminal microspikes appear here as either small bumps or fine filaments covering the end of the uropod (Fig. 2 *d*). The uropod itself has a thickness equal to that of the cell body. In contrast, the cell pseudopod presents a thin, more veil-like appearance (Fig. 2 *b*). The outline of the nuclear rim is also visible by this technique, and the small nuclear indentation that is characteristic of many of these cells can also be seen (Fig. 2 *c*). Monocytes are distinguishable from lymphocytes by their large size, numerous long surface microvilli, and a characteristic heavily cratered surface that we have not observed with any other cell type. The intracellular granules and multilobed nuclei of neutrophiles make this cell type also easy to identify.

Quantitation of Uropod-Bearing Lymphocytes in Thymus, Lymph Node, and Peritoneal Exudate Populations.—After incubation at 37°C for 30 min, cell suspensions were mounted on warm cover slips and slides and allowed to equilibrate for 15 min on the warm stage before counting. Thus, the maximum time in culture after isolation and before counting was less than 120 min. Each cell was focused on individually in order to check for uropods that were out of the plane of focus, however, the total time of observation of each cell was generally less than 30 sec, and no attempt was made to observe uropod-negative lymphocytes for longer periods to see if they would become motile and form uropods. At least 300 cells were examined per slide.

Peritoneal exudate lymphocytes clearly contain the highest percentage of uropods (Table I). In counting lymph node cells, only viable cells were counted since up to 30% of these cells may be dead or damaged (7). Nevertheless, there was significantly less uropod formation in lymph node cells than in peritoneal exudate lymphocytes (PELS). Thymus cells had the fewest uropod-bearing lymphocytes.

Since PELS are prepared by a column adherence procedure, both the thymus and lymph node cell preparations were also column purified and the percentage of uropods determined. Column purification of lymph node cells more than doubles the percentage of uropod-bearing lymphocytes (Table I). However, similar column treatment of thymus cells has no effect at all on uropod formation suggesting that the increase in frequency of uropod-bearing cells seen with lymph node cells is the result of the removal of a nonuropod-bearing cell (see below) and is not the result of nonspecific artifacts introduced by the column-purification procedure.

In our observations on these living cell preparations, we have not observed uropod formation by monocytes or macrophages confirming the work of other investigators (13). Monocytes exhibit extensive pseudopod formation, especially as the cells begin to adhere to the glass, but these pseudopods can be differentiated from uropods by the absence of microspikes and their thin veil-like appearance. Polymorphonuclear leukocytes, on the other hand, have been occasionally seen to form what appear to be uropod-like structures. However, neutrophiles are a significant contaminant only in the PEL preparation and can be identified by their typical granules and nuclear structure.

Comparison of PPD-Induced Lymphocyte Proliferation of Thymus, Lymph Node, and Peritoneal Exudate Lymphocytes.—In order to determine if there was any correlation between the percentage of uropod-bearing lymphocytes in a given population, and its subsequent ability to respond to antigen in vitro, the

TABLE I

Quantitation of Uropod-Bearing Lymphocytes from Guinea Pig Lymph Node, Peritoneal Exudate, and Thymus

Column purification	% Uropod-bearing lymphocytes*		
	Thymus	Lymph node	PEL
No	3.2 (1–6)	7.3 (3–12)	—
Yes	3.8 (2–6)	15.2 (7–24)	36.7 (15–57)

* Uropod counts were performed on living cells maintained at 37°C and observed using Nomarski interference contrast optics. In each experiment, at least 300 cells were examined from each population. Results are the geometric means of at least four experiments, expressed as the mean and the range.

TABLE II

Comparative In Vitro Lymphocyte Proliferation of Thymus, Lymph Node, and Peritoneal Exudate Lymphocytes Induced by PPD

	Stimulation ratio (S/C)*		
	Thymus	Lymph node	PEL
Immune‡	1.8 ± 0.4	4.7 ± 1.3	36.1 ± 6.3
Nonimmune	1.3 ± 0.4	1.1 ± 0.2§	1.0 ± 0.5

* S/C is the ratio of total incorporated counts of Tdr-^{3}H in antigen-stimulated cultures to the total incorporated counts in control cultures. Results are expressed as the arithmetic mean ± the standard error of the mean of three experiments.

‡ Immune refers to immunization history (complete Freund's adjuvant) of guinea pigs from which cells were derived. Nonimmune animals had no prior immunization.

§ Lymph node cells from nonimmunized animals were derived from the normally large anterior cervical lymph nodes.

relative antigen reactivity of these populations was tested using the antigen-induced lymphocyte proliferation assay.

In confirmation of our previous studies with other antigens, in vitro lymphocyte proliferation induced by PPD is clearly highest in PELS. Lymph node cells exhibit a small but significant proliferative response, but the response of thymus cells to PPD is not significantly greater than that of control cultures (Table II). This preparation of PPD produces no nonspecific stimulation, as is shown by the absence of stimulation when these cell populations are derived from normal nonimmunized animals, or from animals given only incomplete adjuvant and saline.

Simultaneous Observations of Cells Bearing Immunoglobulin and Cells Forming Uropods.—Adherence columns have been found to preferentially remove B cells (9, 10, 14–16). Therefore, the finding of an increased percentage of uropod-bearing cells after passage of lymph node lymphocytes over an adherence

TABLE III
*Surface Immunoglobulin on Uropod-Bearing Lymph Node Lymphocytes**

Experiment number	No. of uropod-positive lymphocytes with surface immunoglobulin present*
1	0/18
2	0/20
3	1/25

* Number of cells with surface immunoglobulin over the total number of uropod-bearing lymphocytes counted. The percentage of uropod-positive lymphocytes in each experiment ranged from 8 to 11%, and the percentage of surface immunoglobulin positive cells ranged from 25 to 30%.

TABLE IV
Lack of Uropod Formation by a B Cell–Enriched Lymph Node Lymphocyte Population

	Original lymph node lymphocytes*	B cell-enriched lymph node lymphocytes‡
Total number of cells positive for surface immunoglobulin	30/112	59/66
Uropod-positive cells with positive surface immunoglobulin	0/17	0/21

* Number of cells positive or negative over total number of cells counted. Results are the arithmetic mean of two separate experiments.

‡ B cell–enriched population was prepared by killing T cells with a heterologous anti-thymus-derived lymphocyte antiserum, then removing dead cells over a BSA gradient (18). The resulting population had a viability of greater than 90% by dye exclusion.

column suggested that the uropod was a structure found mainly on T cells. The direct simultaneous evaluation of lymph node cell populations for those cells bearing easily detectable immunoglobulin and those cells forming uropods demonstrated in three separate experiments that cells which formed uropods did not have immunoglobulin on their surface (Table III). In another series of experiments the percentage of B cells in the lymph node cell population was enriched by killing the majority of T cells with a heterologous antithymus-derived cell antiserum (17) and then removing dead cells by centrifugation over a bovine serum albumin (BSA) gradient (18). Although approximately 90% of the cells in these enriched populations were positive for surface membrane immunoglobulin, all of the uropod-forming cells were negative for surface fluorescence (Table IV). It was sometimes noted, that in those cell preparations that had been over BSA gradients, a tiny speck of fluorescence was present at the end of the uropod. The appearance of this fluorescence was entirely different from the speckled fluorescence or the rare cap-type of fluorescence noted over B lymphocytes. Thus, it appears that in a mixed population of B and T cells, all the lymphocytes that are spontaneously forming uropods are T cells by the criteria of absence of easily detectable surface membrane immunoglobulin.

DISCUSSION

Previous studies pertaining to the lymphocyte uropod have emphasized stimulation of uropod formation in vitro by a variety of techniques, while noting the relatively low frequency of lymphocytes with uropods in unstimulated populations. In this study, we have shown that the rate of spontaneous uropod formation is very high in some guinea pig lymphoid subpopulations before any in vitro stimulation. Furthermore, we have also demonstrated that lymphocyte populations differ greatly in their percentage of uropod-forming cells. Thus, at any given time an average of 36% of PELS bear uropods, while only 3.8% of thymocytes have these structures. Also, we have found that there is a general correlation between the frequency of uropod formation and the ability of a given population to respond in vitro to antigen.

Peritoneal exudate lymphocytes, which have been found to have both the highest percentage of uropod-bearing cells and the greatest response to antigen, have been shown to possess several unusual features. It has been found that these cells are a highly selected population of lymphocytes that have been generated in response to a new antigenic challenge and preferentially sequestered in the inflammatory exudate (19, 20). It is very possible then, that the uropod-bearing lymphocyte of the guinea pig, both in the peritoneal exudate and in the lymph node, is that cell that has been recently activated by antigen in vivo.

The low percentage of uropod-bearing cells observed in the thymus may be due to a general unresponsiveness of thymus cells to antigenic stimuli (8), or to the fact that there is little antigenic stimulation in vivo of the thymus since antigens do not easily reach this organ when administered at distant sites (21). Alternatively, uropod formation may be a property restricted to differentiated or mature lymphocytes, and the low frequency of uropod formation of thymocytes may be related to their immaturity. Finally, it appears that uropod formation is not merely the general response of lymphocytes that are rapidly dividing, since the mitotic index in the thymus is very high although the frequency of uropod formation is low (22).

Our findings indicate that only thymus-derived or T lymphocytes spontaneously form uropods. First, PELS are greater than 98% pure T cells by the criteria of absent surface immunoglobulin, the absence of antibody-producing cells, and lack of antigen-binding cells, and by the same criteria, 90% of column-purified lymph node lymphocytes are also T cells (9, 10). Both these cell populations are rich in uropod-bearing cells. Second, we have found that passage of lymph node lymphocytes over an adherence column, which removes B cells, significantly increases the percentage of uropod-bearing cells. If both B and T cells were uropod forming, no such increase in frequency after column purification would have been anticipated. Finally, since easily detectable surface membrane immunoglobulin is the hallmark of the B cell, the simultaneously made observation that no uropod-bearing cell had surface immunoglobulin supports the conclusion that in the guinea pig, only T cells spontaneously form uropods.

Recently, Taylor and his coworkers have shown that in the mouse, reaction of "B" cells with a specific anti-immunoglobulin reagent resulted in redistribution of the surface immunoglobulin so that it was concentrated over one pole of the cell forming a fluorescent "cap" (24). Furthermore, they noted that after several hours at 37°C, surface immunoglobulin could no longer be detected on cells that had previously borne this marker. However, we do not feel that the uropod-bearing lymphocytes that we have observed in the guinea pig are merely B cells that have lost their surface immunoglobulin due to treatment with the anti-Fab reagent. In our system, less than 5% of B cells have an immunoglobulin cap, and even after incubation at 37°C for periods as long as 3 hr, we have not detected an increased frequency of cells with caps (25). Furthermore, it is not likely that B cell uropod formation was inhibited by the presence of the fluoresceinated anti-Fab antibody on the cell surface. Work with amebae has shown that membrane motility and uropod formation proceed normally in the presence of large amounts of fluoresceinated antibody on the cell membrane (26). In addition, in lymphocytes that have been stained with a fluoresceinated anti-histocompatibility antibody which binds to both T and B cells, uropod formation is normal (Rosenstreich, D., and E. Shevach, unpublished observation).

The uropod-bearing lymphocyte and the uropod structure itself have been found to possess several properties of possible significance in immunological reactions. It has been shown that the uropod is the structure most intimately involved in lymphocyte-to-lymphocyte and lymphocyte-to-macrophage interactions (2, 11–13). Cytotoxicity mediated by immune lymphocytes has also been found to involve direct contact between a lymphocyte and target cell, often in the region of the uropod (3). Since thymus-dependent lymphocytes appear to lack easily detectable surface antigen receptors, it may be that another mechanism of interaction with antigen exists in these cells. Indeed Biberfeld demonstrated that antigen molecules such as ferritin are taken up by the lymphocyte uropod (4). It is therefore possible that antigen binding and recognition by T cells is mediated through the uptake and concentration of antigen in their uropod region. Further characterization of the nature of the uropod-bearing lymphocyte may help to elucidate the mechanisms of cellular cooperation and the relationship between cell structure and function in immunological reactions.

REFERENCES

1. Lewis, W. H. 1931. Locomotion of lymphocytes. *Bull. Johns Hopkins Hosp.* **49**:29.
2. McFarland, W., D. H. Heilman, and J. F. Moorhead. 1967. Functional anatomy of the lymphocyte in immunological reactions *in vitro*. *J. Exp. Med.* **124**:851.
3. Ax, W., H. Malchow, I. Zeiss, and H. Fischer. 1968. The behaviour of lymphocytes in the process of target cell destruction *in vitro*. *Exp. Cell Res.* **53**:108.
4. Biberfeld, P. 1971. Uropod formation in phytohemagglutinin (PHA) stimulated lymphocytes. *Exp. Cell Res.* **66**:433.
5. Kincade, P. W., A. R. Lawton, and M. D. Cooper. 1971. Restriction of surface immunoglobulin determinants to lymphocytes of the plasma cell line. *J. Immunol.* **106**:1418.
6. Raff, M. C. 1970. Two distinct populations of peripheral lymphocytes in mice distinguishable by immunofluorescence. *Immunology.* **19**:637.
7. Rosenstreich, D. L., J. T. Blake, and A. S. Rosenthal. 1971. The peritoneal exudate lymphocyte. I. Differences in antigen responsiveness between peritoneal exudate and lymph node lymphocytes from immunized guinea pigs. *J. Exp. Med.* **134**:1170.
8. Oppenheim, J. J., R. A. Wolstencroft, and P. G. H. Gell. 1967. Delayed hypersensitivity in the guinea pig to a protein-hapten conjugate and its relationship to *in vitro* transformation of lymph node, spleen, thymus and peripheral blood lymphocytes. *Immunology.* **12**:89.
9. Rosenthal, A. S., J. Davie, D. L. Rosenstreich, and J. T. Blake. 1972. Depletion of antibody-forming cells and their precursors from complex lymphoid cell populations. *J. Immunol.* **108**:279.
10. Rosenthal, A. S., D. L. Rosenstreich, J. Davie, and J. T. Blake. 1971. Isolation and characterization of cellular immune effector cells: evidence for the hetero-

geneity of such cells in the guinea pig. *In* Proceedings of the 6th Leukocyte Culture Conference. M. Roy Schwarz, editor. Academic Press, Nev York. 433.
11. McFarland, W. 1969. Microspikes on the lymphocyte uropod. *Science (Washington*. **163**:818.
12. McFarland, W., and G. P. Schechter. 1970. The lymphocyte in immunological reactions *in vitro*: ultrastructural studies. *Blood.* **35**:683.
13. Salvin, S. B., S. Sell, and J. Nishio. 1971. Activity *in vitro* of lymphocytes and macrophages in delayed hypersensitivity. *J. Immunol.* **107**:655.
14. Plotz, P. H., and N. Talal. 1967. Fractionation of splenic antibody forming cells on glass bead columns. *J. Immunol.* **99**:1236.
15. Shortman, K., N. Williams, H. Jackson, P. Russell, P. Byrt, and E. Diener. 1971. The separation of different cell classes from lymphoid organs. IV. The separation of lymphocytes from phagocytes and antibody-forming cells. *J. Cell Biol.* **48**:566.
16. Bianco, C., R. Patrick, and V. Nussenzweig. 1970. A population of lymphocytes bearing a membrane receptor for antigen-antibody-complement complexes. I. Separation and characterization. *J. Exp. Med.* **132**:702.
17. Shevach, E., I. Green, L. Ellman, and J. Maillard. Heterologous antiserum to thymus derived cells in the guinea pig. *Nature (New Biol.) (London).* **235**:19.
18. Bianco, C., and V. Nussenzweig. 1971. Theta-bearing and complement-receptor lymphocytes are distinct populations of cells. *Science (Washington).* **173**:154.
19. McGregor, D. D., F. T. Koster, and G. B. Mackaness. 1971. The mediator of cellular immunity. I. The life-span and circulation dynamics of the immunologically committed lymphocyte. *J. Exp. Med.* **133**:389.
20. Koster, F. T., D. D. McGregor, and G. B. Mackaness. 1971. The mediator of cellular immunity. II. Migration of immunologically committed lymphocytes into inflammatory exudates. *J. Exp. Med.* **133**:400.
21. Marshall, A. H. E., and R. G. White. 1961. The immunological reactivity of the thymus. *Brit. J. Exp. Pathol.* **42**:379.
22. Metcalf, D. 1964. *In* The Thymus in Immunobiology. Harper and Row, Publishers, New York. 154.
23. Moller, G. 1961. Demonstration of mouse isoantigens at the cellular level by the fluorescent antibody technique. *J. Exp. Med.* **114**:415.
24. Taylor, R. B., W. P. H. Duffus, M. C. Raff, and S. de Petris. 1971. Redistribution and pinocytosis of lymphocyte surface immunoglobulin molecules induced by anti-immunoglobulin antibody. *Nature (New Biol.) (London).* **233**:225.
25. Shevach, E., L. Ellman, J. Davie, and I. Green. 1972. L_2C guinea pig lymphatic leukemia: a "B" cell leukemia. *Blood.* **39**:1.
26. Wolpert, L., and C. H. O'Neill. 1962. Dynamics of the membrane of *amoeba proteus* studied with labelled specific antibody. *Nature (London).* **196**:1261.

Role of the Thymus in the Recovery of Hemolytic Plaque Formation After X-Irradiation[1]

Yumiko Takada, Akikazu Takada, and Julian L. Ambrus

We have reported that the recovery of thymus function after X-irradiation in mice was under genetic control (1). Lower hemolysin levels in a substrain of CBA mice (CBA/St) compared with the other substrain (CBA/H) may be due to a difference in either the number of hemolytic plaque-forming cells or in the amount of production of hemolysin by an individual antibody-forming cell. Jerne's (4) plaque test was employed to answer this question.

The possibility of delayed recovery in thymus function in CBA/St mice after X-irradiation may be due to the fact that either the injected marrow cells did not repopulate the thymus and spleen as rapidly as in CBA/H mice, or they migrated into the thymus and spleen of CBA/St mice in smaller number. This question can be answered by injecting chromosomally marked bone-marrow cells (CBA/HT$_6$T$_6$) into irradiated CBA/H or CBA/St mice and analyzing the cellular composition of various organs of the hosts at intervals (2, 3). This paper deals with the difference between CBA/H and CBA/St mice in the number of hemolytic plaque-forming cells, thymus and spleen weight, and the extent of repopulation of the bone marrow, thymus, and spleen by CBA/HT$_6$T$_6$ marrow cells after X-irradiation and the injection of marrow cells.

Materials and Methods. CBA/H, CBA/St, and CBA/HT$_6$T$_6$ mice were obtained from the inbred colonies in the Springville Laboratories. X-Irradiation, thymectomy, and Jerne's plaque tests were performed as described previously (4, 5), and likewise chromosome analysis (2, 3).

Results. Difference between CBA/H and CBA/St in the number of hemolytic plaque-forming cells. Mice both CBA/H and CBA/St, received 400 R of whole-body X-irradiation, and were injected intraperitoneally with sheep red blood cells (SRBC) at certain intervals. Plaque assays were performed 7 days after SRBC injection. Figure 1 shows the results. Controls were unirradiated CBA/H and CBA/St mice. Statistically there is no difference between these two substrains of mice in the number of plaques per control spleen. CBA/H mice showed a larger number of plaques than CBA/St mice following 22 days after irradiation.

Table I shows the results of two experiments: first, thymectomized and sham-thymectomized CBA/H mice were irradiated with 600 R and injected with 5×10^6 bone-marrow cells obtained from CBA/H mice; second, thymectomized and sham-thymectomized CBA/St mice were irradiated with 600 R and injected with 5×10^6 bone-marrow cells obtained from CBA/St mice. These mice were injected intraperitoneally with SRBC 15 or 22 days after X-irradiation. Spleens were removed for plaque assays 7 days after SRBC injection. Thymectomized mice, both CBA/H and CBA/St, showed very small numbers of hemolytic plaques up to 29 days after X-irradiation. Sham-thymectomized CBA/St mice had smaller numbers of plaques than did sham-thymectomized CBA/H mice.

Percentages of chromosome-marked cells (CBA/HT$_6$T$_6$) in the bone marrow, spleen,

---
[1] This study was supported by General Research Support Grant FR-05648-03 from the National Institutes of Health, U.S. Public Health Service, and American Cancer Society Institutional Grant (K-8).

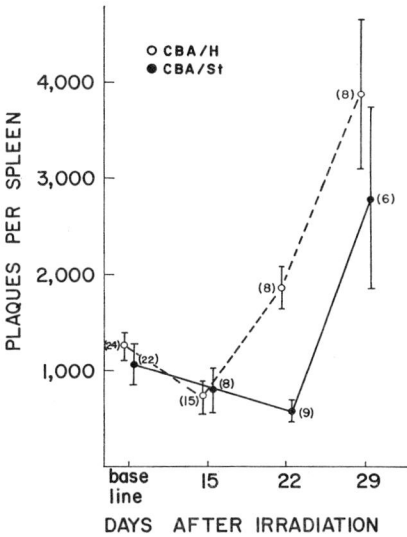

FIG. 1. Recovery of hemolytic plaque formation in CBA/H and CBA/St mice after whole-body irradiation with 400 R. Sheep red blood cells (SRBC) were injected 7 days before mice were sacrificed for plaque assay in the spleens.

and thymus in CBA/H and CBA/St mice. Mice, CBA/H and CBA/St, were irradiated with 600 R, and injected with 5×10^6 CBA/HT$_6$T$_6$ bone-marrow cells in 2 to 4 hr. Mice were sacrificed 22 days after X-irradiation, and the distributions of cell types in the marrow, spleen, and thymus were determined.

Table II shows spleen and thymus weights for normal CBA/H and CBA/St mice and CBA/H and CBA/St mice irradiated and injected with CBA/H and CBA/St marrow cells, respectively. Thymus weights for normal mice were a little larger for CBA/St mice than for CBA/H mice, but thymus weights following irradiation with 600 R and injection of bone-marrow cells were larger for CBA/H mice than for CBA/St mice.

Table III shows the results of chromosome analysis. Although there is a slight histocompatibility difference between CBA/St and CBA/HT$_6$T$_6$, the percentages of T$_6$T$_6$ cells were almost equal in the organs of CBA/St and CBA/H mice. The spleens and thymuses were as fully repopulated with donor marrow cells in CBA/St as in CBA/H mice.

Discussion. We have shown that the recovery of thymus function following X-irradiation is dependent on strains or even substrains of inbred mice (1). CBA/H mice that received 600 R of whole-body irradiation and 5×10^6 bone-marrow cells recovered their antibody-forming ability much more quickly than did CBA/St mice that received the same treatment. Since the same number of bone-marrow cells were injected into each substrain of mice after irradiation, and since thymectomized mice could not produce he-

TABLE I. Plaques per Spleen in Mice Irradiated with 600 R and Injected with 5×10^6 Bone-Marrow Cells.

Strain[a]	Thymectomy	Day[b] of SRBC[c] injection	Day[b] of assay	No. of animals	Hemolytic plaques/spleen[d]
H	No	15	22	13	2811 ± 552
St	No	15	22	13	216 ± 86
H	Yes	15	22	16	34 ± 11
St	Yes	15	22	12	12 ± 3
H	No	22	29	19	4510 ± 526
St	No	22	29	8	1130 ± 184
H	Yes	22	29	9	55 ± 26
St	Yes	22	29	16	50 ± 7

[a] Donors and recipients of marrow cells were of the same strain: H = CBA/H; St = CBA/St.
[b] Days after irradiation.
[c] Sheep red blood cells.
[d] Mean ± standard error.

TABLE II. Weights of Spleens and Thymuses of Normal and Irradiated CBA/H and CBA/St Mice.

Organ	Day of sacrifice[a]	CBA/H		CBA/St	
		No. of animals	Wt of organ (mg)[b]	No. of animals	Wt of organ (mg)[b]
Spleen	(Untreated)	19	68.3 ± 2.0	8	69.3 ± 3.5
	22	9	65.8 ± 9.1	9	87.7 ± 5.6
	29	9	70.9 ± 3.6	7	107.3 ± 7.6
Thymus	(Untreated)	19	33.3 ± 1.6	7	41.0 ± 4.5
	22[c]	9	33.6 ± 2.2	9	23.1 ± 2.8
	29[d]	9	41.9 ± 2.6	6	31.0 ± 4.7

[a] Days after whole-body irradiation with 600 R and injection of 5×10^6 marrow cells.
[b] Mean ± standard error.
[c] The mean of the thymus weight on day 22 was shown by the t test to be larger for CBA/H mice than for CBA/St mice at the 95% level of significance.
[d] The difference between the thymus weights for CBA/H and CBA/St mice on day 29 was shown by the t test to be of borderline significance.

molysin even if marrow cells were injected, it was assumed that the difference between these two substrains in the recovery of hemolysin levels was due to difference in the recovery of thymus function.

However, it is possible that the percentage of immunocyte precursor cells among the injected marrow cells was smaller in CBA/St mice than in CBA/H mice. If this was the case, the lower hemolysin levels in CBA/St mice may have been due not to thymus function, but to the smaller number of precursor cells in the marrow cell population. Precursor cells give rise to antibody-forming cells after interaction with thymus-derived cells (6–9) or under the influence of thymic humoral factors (10).

If marrow precursor cells were fewer or

TABLE III. Percentages of CBA/HT_6T_6 Cells in CBA/H and CBA/St Mice Irradiated with 600 R and Injected with 5×10^6 CBA/HT_6T_6 Bone-Marrow Cells.[a]

Organ	CBA/H				CBA/St			
	Animal	Donor	Host	T_6T_6 (%)	Animal	Donor	Host	T_6T_6 (%)
Spleen	1	50	0	100.0	1	50	4	92.6
	2	50	2	96.1	2	50	6	89.3
	3	50	1	98.0	3	50	0	100.0
	4	50	3	94.3				
	5	50	2	96.1				
Thymus	1	50	1	98.0	1	50	3	94.3
	2	50	4	92.6	2	50	6	89.3
	3	50	2	96.1	3	50	5	90.9
	4	50	7	87.7				
	5	50	5	90.9				
Bone marrow	1	50	0	100.0	1	50	7	87.7
	2	50	0	100.0	2	50	2	96.1
	3	50	1	98.0	3	50	2	96.1
	4	50	0	100.0				
	5	50	0	100.0				

[a] Animals were sacrificed 22 days after irradiation and injection.

proliferated less well after antigen administration in CBA/St mice than in CBA/H mice, the number of hemolytic plaques must be smaller in normal CBA/St mice than in normal CBA/H mice. Figure 1 shows no significant difference between these two substrains in the number of plaques at 7 days.

Table II shows that the weight of the thymus was smaller in CBA/St mice than in CBA/H mice after irradiation. This finding may indicate that functional recovery is related to the speed of cellular repopulation of the thymus, since the thymus could "instruct" immigrating cells.

Table III shows that bone marrows, spleens, and thymuses were almost exclusively repopulated with donor-type cells by day 22 after irradiation. These cells, which participated in antibody production, were of donor origin. Unpublished data indicate that almost all cells in the bone marrow, spleen, and thymus were of donor origin in CBA/H or CBA/St mice that had been thymectomized, irradiated with 600 R, and injected with 5×10^6 CBA/HT$_6$T$_6$ marrow cells. Data in Table I indicate that CBA/H mice could generate larger numbers of hemolytic plaque-forming cells than CBA/St mice at 22 days after irradiation, and that thymectomized and irradiated CBA mice could not generate hemolytic plaque-forming cells.

Although the weight of the thymus was smaller in CBA/St mice than in CBA/H mice at day 22, it was as fully repopulated with bone-marrow cells in the former as in the latter. Accordingly, it is possible that the smaller number of hemolytic plaques in CBA/St mice following irradiation and injection of marrow cells may be due to the fact that these donor-type marrow cells were not well "instructed" in the thymus, so that they could not participate in antibody formation effectively. In fact, almost all of the dividing cells in the spleens of thymectomized and irradiated mice injected with T$_6$T$_6$ marrow cells were of donor origin, but none of them were instructed to react with antigens and with precursors of antibody-forming cells.

On the other hand, some of the donor-type cells in CBA/H mice migrated to the thymus, were instructed, and then emigrated to the spleen, so that they could respond to antigens and precursors. Under the circumstances, recovery of thymus functions following irradiation is influenced by how quickly the thymus is repopulated, how well the ability to instruct is restored, and how quickly the instructed cells seed to peripheral lymphoid organs.

Summary. Relationship between hemolytic plaque formation and repopulation of spleen and thymus after X-irradiation was studied by using two substrains of CBA mice. The CBA/H and CBA/St mice generated almost equal numbers of hemolytic plaques in the spleen at 7 days after intraperitoneal injection of sheep red blood cells (SRBC). The CBA/St mice that received 400 R of whole-body irradiation, or 600 R of irradiation and injection of 5×10^6 marrow cells, generated smaller numbers of plaques at days 22 and 29 than did CBA/H mice that received the same treatment. Bone marrows, thymuses, and spleens of sham-thymectomized and thymectomized CBA/H and CBA/St mice were almost exclusively repopulated with donor-type cells by day 22.

Donor-type cells in the spleens of CBA/H mice had been "instructed" in the thymus, were seeded to the spleen, and responded to antigens, but the spleens of CBA/St mice which were also repopulated with donor marrow cells, had very small numbers of these instructed cells that were capable of responding to antigens.

The excellent technical assistance of Mr. Raymond C. Church is greatly appreciated. Statistical calculations were performed by Mrs. Nina Bates, B.S., of the Department of Biostatistics (Irwin Bross, Ph.D., Director), Roswell Park Memorial Institute.

1. Takada, Y., Takada, A., and Ambrus, J. L., Proc. Soc. Exp. Biol. Med. **135**, 473 (1970).

2. Takada, A., Takada, Y., and Ambrus, J. L., Proc. Soc. Exp. Biol. Med. **136**, 222 (1971).

3. Takada, A., Takada, Y., Kim, U., and Ambrus, J. L., Radiat. Res. **45**, 522 (1971).

4. Jerne, N. K., Nordin, A. A., and Henry, C., *in* "Cell Bound Antibodies" (B. Amos and H. Koprowski, eds.), p. 109. Wistar Inst. Press, Philadelphia (1963).

5. Takada, A., Takada, Y., and Ambrus, J. L., Radiat. Res. **40**, 341 (1969).

6. Claman, H. N., Chaperon, E. A., and Triplett, R. F., J. Immunol. **97**, 828 (1966).

7. Davies, A. J. S., Leuchars, E., Wallis, J., Marchant, R., and Elliot, E. V., Transplantation **5**, 222 (1967).

8. Miller, J. F. A. P., and Mitchell, G. F., Nature (London) **216**, 659 (1967).

9. Taylor, R. B., Nature (London) **220**, 611 (1968).

10. Miller, J. F. A. P., and Osoba, D., Physiol. Rev. **47**, 437 (1967).

Thymus-derived lymphocytes: their distribution and role in the development of peripheral lymphoid tissues of the mouse

M. C. Raff and J.J. T. Owen

1. Introduction

A subpopulation of lymphocytes have recently been demonstrated in peripheral lymphoid tissues of mice which, like thymus lymphocytes, have the Θ alloantigen on their surface [1, 2, 3]. The thymus-dependence of this subpopulation has been shown by the fact that it is markedly depleted in mice which have been treated with anti-lymphocyte serum [1, 2], or which have been thymectomized [3] or are congenitally athymic [3].

There is increasing evidence that "thymus-dependent" lymphocytes in peripheral lymphoid tissues have migrated from the thymus [4, 5, 6] and thus are appropriately termed "thymus-derived". In addition, Θ-bearing lymphocytes have been shown to migrate to peripheral lymphoid tissues from thymus grafts [7, 8]. Although the possibility has not been excluded that a few Θ-bearing cells may mature in peripheral tissues under the influence of the thymus without actually passing through it, it seems reasonable to conclude that the majority, if not all, of those peripheral lymphocytes which carry the Θ alloantigen are not only "thymus-dependent" but also "thymus-derived".

Abbreviations: BBS: Barbital buffered saline   NMS: Normal mouse serum

In this paper we describe the proportions of thymus-derived lymphocytes in adult and developing peripheral lymphoid tissues as demonstrated by dye-exclusion cytotoxic testing to detect Θ-bearing cells.

2. Materials and methods

2.1. Cell suspensions

2.1.1. Adult mice. Cells were obtained from thymus, lymph nodes (pooled mesenteric, inguinal, axillary, brachial and superficial and deep cervical), spleen and Peyer's patches of 3 to 6 months old CBA.H and Balb/c mice of both sexes. Tissues were teased with fine needles in BBS containing 0.1 % bovine serum albumin and each cell suspension was passed through a short column of glass wool prior to cytotoxicity testing.

Peritoneal lymphocytes were obtained by washing the peritoneal cavities of mice with 5 ml of Medium 199 containing 15 % foetal calf serum. The cells were incubated on a glass wool column for 30 min at 37 °C and then eluted with Medium 199.

Blood lymphocytes were obtained using the following procedure: Defibrinated blood was mixed 1 : 1 with Plasmagel (Laboratoire Roger Bellon, Seine France). Erythrocytes were allowed to sediment for 15–30 min at room temperature, after which the supernatant was removed and the cells contained in it were washed in Medium 199 and incubated in a glass wool column for 30 min at 37 °C. Finally the cells were eluted from the column with fresh Medium 199.

2.1.2. Newborn mice. In preparing cell suspensions from newborn mice (up to 17 days old), tissues from several litters were pooled at each stage. Only cells from mesenteric lymph nodes, Peyer's patches and blood were studied. Cell suspensions were prepared as in adult mice, except that mesenteric lymph node cells were not passed through glass wool columns.

More than 90 % of cells in the final suspensions were lymphocytes except in lymph node suspensions of 1 day old mice where 50–80 % of cells were lymphocytes.

Cell counts were made in a haemocytometer chamber and cell smears were made in a cytocentrifuge (Shandon, England). Various developing lymphoid tissues were fixed in

Bouin, embedded in polyester wax and sectioned at 7 microns.

2.2. Cytotoxicity testing to detect Θ alloantigen

Anti-Θ C3H serum was prepared by immunizing AKR mice with CBA thymocytes [9]. The antiserum was heat inactivated at 56°C for 30 min. The cytotoxic activity of the antiserum could be completely absorbed by CBA brain which suggests its anti-Θ specificity [3].

Trypan blue dye-exclusion cytotoxic testing was carried out by the method of Boyse, Old and Chomoulinkov [10], but incorporating the modification described by Schlesinger [11]. In brief, cells at a concentration of 0.5 to 1 x 10^6/ml were first incubated in antiserum at 37 °C, then washed in BBS and finally incubated in complement at 37 °C. Hamster serum, absorbed with mouse liver and spleen to remove its natural toxicity for thymocytes, was used at a final concentration of 1: 21 as a source of complement for tests on thymus cells. Guinea pig serum, absorbed with mouse erythrocytes, was used at a final concentration of 1 : 15 as a source of complement for all other cell types.

After treatment with complement, cells were spun down and the supernatant was discarded. The cells were resuspended in a small quantity of trypan blue in saline and the suspension was examined in a haemocytometer chamber using a thin coverslip and phase contrast optics. In this way not only could stained and unstained cells be clearly distinguished, but red blood cells and lymphocytes could be separately identified.

The anti-ΘC3H serum was titrated with cells of the various tissues and a plateau of maximum cytotoxicity extending over a range of the highest antiserum concentrations was found in each case. An antiserum dilution that was within this range for a particular tissue was selected for use in all subsequent tests on that tissue. A comparable dilution of NMS was used as a control. It was established that for each cell type the level of the plateau of maximum cytotoxicity could not be raised by changing the cell concentration or source or concentration of complement.[12].

A modified cytotoxicity test was developed for lymph nodes and Peyer's patches from mice that were 5 days old or less because cell suspensions from these tissues frequently contained a large proportion of dead cells (mainly cells of the reticular framework). After treatment with antiserum, cells were suspended in 0.2 ml of 0.1 % nigrosin in saline for 10 min at 4 °C so as to stain dead cells present at this stage. The cells were washed with BBS and then incubated at 37 °C in complement. Finally, the cells were examined in saline by phase contrast microscopy. Cells stained with nigrosin (i. e. dead before the addition of complement) were ignored and a number of nuclei stripped of cytoplasm which did not stain but which were present in the original cell suspension were not scored. Among the unstained cells those with a grossly deformed morphology were scored as having been killed by immune lysis [13].

The results obtained when both types of cytotoxicity test were applied to the same population agreed reasonably well (within 10 %).

3. Results

3.1. Adult lymphoid tissues

The results of cytotoxic tests on cell suspensions of adult Balb/c and CBA lymphoid tissues are outlined in Table 1. The results with thymocytes are not included as in all experiments more than 98 % of these cells were killed.

The difficulties in determining percentages of Θ-bearing cells in tissues from cytotoxic data (i. e. how to deal with the proportion of dead cells in control tubes) has been previously discussed [3]. It is clear that only approximate figures can be obtained. In mice of both strains, approximately 70 % of blood lymphocytes, 65–70 % of lymph node lymphocytes, 30–35 % of spleen and peritoneal lymphocytes and 20–25 % of Peyer's patch lymphocytes are Θ-bearing.

3.2. Developing lymphoid tissues

The percentages of Θ-bearing cells in Balb/c mesenteric lymph nodes and blood during the first few days of life are shown in Table 2. Similar figures were obtained in CBA mice, e. g. the proportions of Θ-bearing cells in mesenteric lymph nodes at days 2, 3 and 4 were 10 %, 56 % and 65 % respectively.

Only 50–80 % of cells in suspensions prepared from mesenteric nodes of 1 day old mice were lymphocytes, so the

Table 1. Results of dye exclusion cytotoxic testing on adult Balb/c and CBA lymphoid tissues

	Killed with anti-Θ (%)[a] (A)	Killed with NMS (%)[a] (B)	Cytotoxic Index (%)[b]	Number of experiments
I Balb/c mice				
Blood lymphocytes	73 (72–76)	9 (6–13)	70	4
Lymph node	67 (64–71)	11 (6–14)	63	5
Spleen	40 (37–46)	10 (9–12)	33	4
Peritoneal lymphocytes	37 (32–46)	4 (1–6)	34	3
Peyer's patches	29 (27–30)	11 (5–15)	20	3
II CBA mice				
Blood lymphocytes	71 (61–80)	5 (2–8)	70	15
Lymph node	75 (72–78)	9 (2–13)	72	3
Spleen	38 (35–42)	9 (7–13)	32	3
Peritoneal lymphocytes	36 (25–46)	6 (5–7)	32	3
Peyer's patches	34 (28–38)	11 (9–13)	25	3

a) Expressed as mean (range)
b) This cytotoxic index [(A-B/100-B) x 100] is based on the assumption that both Θ-bearing and non-Θ-bearing cells are proportionally represented among the dead cells in the control (NMS) tubes. (For further discussion, see [3]).

proportion of Θ-bearing cells found at this stage (14 %) is an underestimate of the proportion of Θ-positive cells among lymphocytes of these nodes. However, suspensions prepared from lymph nodes of 2 day old mice and all subsequent ages contained over 90 % lymphocytes. Therefore, the increasing proportion of Θ-bearing cells in suspensions of lymph nodes between 2 day old mice (14 % and 23 %) and 5 day old mice (77 %) shows that there is an increase in percentage of Θ-positive cells among the total lymphocyte population.

Comparison of the histological appearances of mesenteric nodes removed during this period (Fig. 1–2) shows that the number of lymphocytes is greatly expanding as evidenced both by increase in size of nodes and by their greatly increased cellularity. Differential and total cell counts made on cell suspensions from mesenteric nodes at these stages confirmed this conclusion.

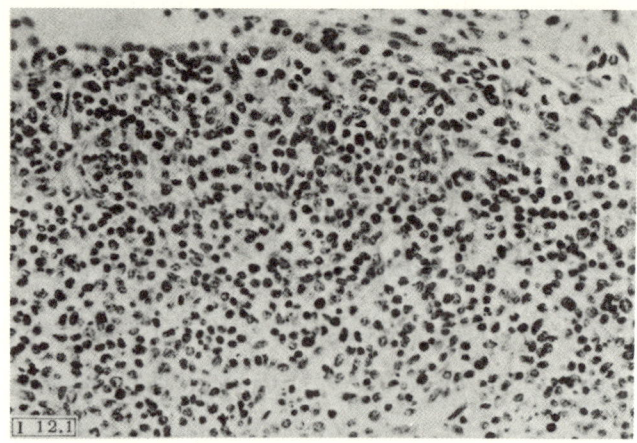

Figure 1. Section of 1-day (within 24 hours of birth) mesenteric lymph node of Balb/c mouse. Cell suspensions from pooled 1-day nodes contained 20–50 % polymorphonuclear leukocytes; the rest of the cells were lymphocytes. Approximately 14 % of cells in these suspensions were Θ-bearing lymphocytes. Gomori trichrome stain x 420.

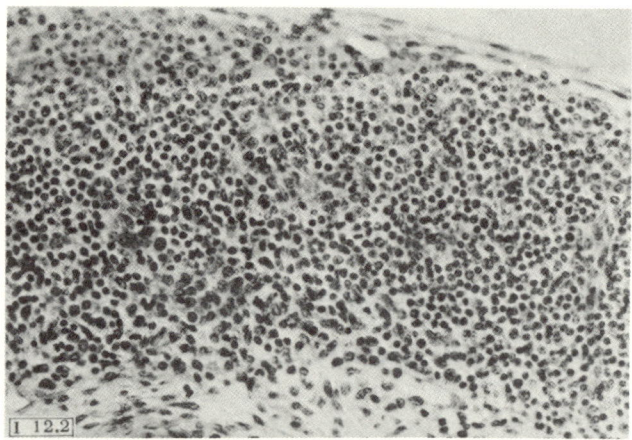

Figure 2. Section of 4-day Balb/c mesenteric lymph node. A greater concentration of lymphocytes can be seen in the node at this stage as compared to day 1. The 4-day lymph node is also of greater overall size. Cell suspensions of 4-day mesenteric nodes contained over 90 % lymphocytes, the majority of which were Θ-bearing. Gomori trichrome stain x 420.

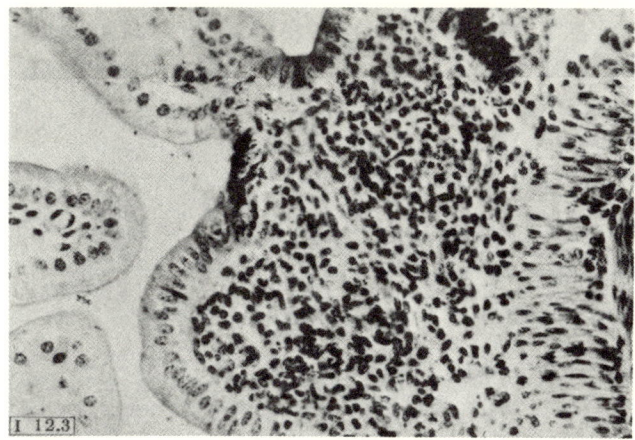

Figure 3. Peyer's patch of 1-day Balb/c mouse. Although Peyer's patches can be dissected out at this stage, too few lymphocytes are obtained in suspension for cytotoxicity testing. Gomori trichrome stain x 420.

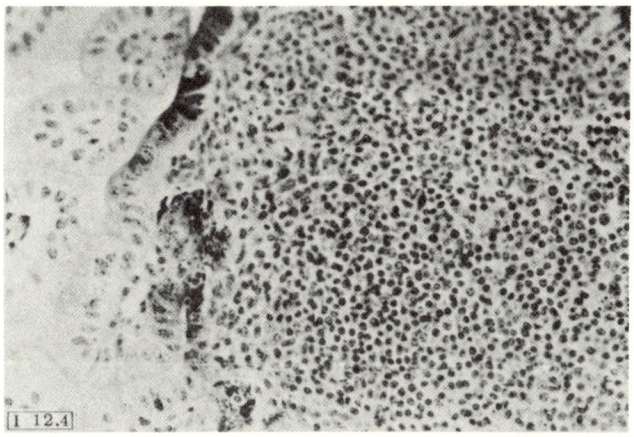

Figure 4. Peyer's patch of 4-day Balb/c mouse showing the rapid increase in size and cellularity which takes place during the first few days after birth. Suspensions of lymphocytes obtained by pooling Payer's patches from a number of animals contained 42−53 % Θ-positive lymphocytes. Gomori trichrome stain x 420.

We were unable to obtain enough cells from Peyer's patches during the first 3 days of life to carry out cytotoxicity tests (see Fig. 3). However, sufficient cells for testing were obtained on day 4 by pooling patches dissected from a number of litters. 40–50 % of lymphocytes present at this stage are Θ-bearing (Table 2 and Fig. 4). At later stages this percentage declines so that by 17 days approximately adult values are obtained (Table 2).

4. Discussion

In studies mainly using ^{51}Cr cytotoxic testing [3] and indirect immunofluorescence [14] the percentages of Θ-bearing cells in adult thymus, lymph nodes, spleen and thoracic duct have been reported. In the results reported here, dye-exclusion cytotoxic testing has been used and the study has been extended to include Peyer's patches, blood and peritoneal lymphocytes. Putting together all the data obtained to date, lymphoid tissues of the adult mouse can be ordered according to their approximate proportions of Θ-bearing lymphocytes: thymus (100 %), thoracic duct lymphocytes (80–85 %), blood lymphocytes (70 %), lymph nodes (65–70 %), spleen (30–35 %), peritoneal lymphocytes (30–35 %) and Peyer's patches (20–25 %). We have been unable to demonstrate Θ-bearing cells in adult CBA bone marrow by either cytotoxic tests or absorption studies.

Although the distribution of Θ-bearing cells found is in broad agreement with the figures for the distribution of cells derived from thymus grafts in lymphoid tissues of thymectomized, irradiated and bone marrow reconstituted mice [6], fewer thymus graft derived cells have been found in lymph nodes, spleen and Peyer's patches of these animals than the figures for Θ-bearing cells reported here. However, thymus graft derived cells were identified by the T 6 chromosome marker and so the figures obtained refer only to dividing cells. The distribution of Θ-bearing cells reported here is also in accord with the figures for the distribution of long-lived [15, 16] and recirculating lymphocytes [17, 18, 19], and there is good evidence that most long-lived and recirculating lymphocytes are thymus-dependent [20].

It is clear from the results obtained on newborn mice that, at birth, a small number of thymus-derived cells are already present in peripheral organs. This provides an explanation for the failure of neonatal thymectomy to eliminate completely cell-mediated immunological functions [21]. The rapid increase in percentage of Θ-bearing lymphocytes in developing

Table 2. Results of dye exclusion cytotoxic testing on developing Balb/c lymphoid tissue

Day of life	Lymph node			Blood			Peyer's patches		
	Killed with Anti-Θ (%) (A)	NMS (%) (B)	Cytotoxic Index (%)c	Killed with Anti-Θ (%) (A)	NMS (%) (B)	Cytotoxic Index (%)c	Killed with Anti-Θ (%) (A)	NMS (%) (B)	Cytotoxic Index (%)c
1a)	21	8	14b)	18 / 15	2 / 2	16b) / 13			
2	27 / 27	15 / 5	14b) / 23b)						
3	49 / 63	9 / 12	44b) / 58b)	55	9	50			
4	80 / 72	9 / 10	78b) / 69				48 / 59	11 / 13	42b) / 53
5	80	12	77	75	15	70	32	7	27b)
6				67	7	65			
8				74	9	71	45	15	35
10	80	13	77						
17	67	10	64	74	6	72	30	14	19
Adult	67	11	63	73	9	70	29	11	20

a) Day 1 = first 24 hours of life
b) Tested by modified cytotoxic test (see section 2.2.)
c) Cytotoxic index: [(A-B/100-B) x 100]

mesenteric lymph nodes at the time when there is a rapidly increasing number of lymphocytes in these organs suggests that their development is largely dependent on thymus-derived cells. The rapidity of this development during the first few days of life explains why thymectomy must be carried out at an early stage to be effective.

Finally, our results showing a definite proportion of Θ-bearing cells in developing Peyer's patches supports the view that lymphoid differentiation in these organs is, in part at least, thymus-dependent.

We thank Misses P. Chivers and F. Rose for excellent technical assistance.

5. References

1. Schlesinger, M. and Yron, I., *Science* 1969. *164*: 1412.
2. Raff, M. C., *Nature* 1969. *224*: 378.
3. Raff, M. C. and Wortis, H. H., *Immunology* 1970. *18*: 929.
4. Miller, J. F. A. P., *Lancet* i 1963. *43*.
5. Weissman, I. L., *J. Exp. Med.* 1967. *126*: 291.
6. Davies, A. J. S., *Transplant. Rev.* 1969. *1*: 43.
7. Schlesinger, M. and Yron, I., *J. Immunol.* 1970. *104*: 798.
8. Owen, J. J. T. and Raff, M. C., *J. Exp. Med.* in press.
9. Reif, A. E. and Allen, J. M. V., *Nature* 1966. *209*: 521.
10. Boyse, E. A., Old, L. J. and Chouroulinkov, I., *Meth. Med. Res.* 1964. *10*: 39.
11. Schlesinger, M., *J. Immunol.* 1965. *94*: 359.
12. Boyse, E. A., Old, L. J. and Stockert, E., *Ann. N. Y. Acad. Sci.* 1962. *99*: 574.
13. Terasaki, P. I. and McClelland, J. D., *Nature* 1964. *204*: 998.
14. Raff, M. C., *Immunology* 1970. *19*: 637.
15. Everett, H. B., Caffrey, R. W. and Rieke, W. O., *Ann. N. Y. Acad. Sci.* 1964. *113*: 887.
16. Denman, A. M., Denman, E. and Embling, P. H., *Lancet* i 1968. *321*.
17. Gowans, J. L. and Knight, E. J., *Proc. Roy. Soc. Lond.* B 1964. *159*: 257.
18. Lance, E. M. and Taub, R. N., *Nature* 1969. *221*: 841.
19. Zalz, M. M. and Lance, E. M., *Cell. Immunol.* 1970. *1*: 3.
20. Mitchell, G. F. and Miller, J. F. A. P., *Nature* 1967. *214*: 992.
21. Miller, J. F. A. P., *Lancet* ii 1961. *748*.

Thymus-Derived Lymphocytes in Blood, Lymph and Lymphoid Organs after Intrathymic Labelling with ^{3}H-Thymidine

ULF ERNSTRÖM, M.D., BENGT LARSSON, M.D. & JUHANI LINNA, M.D.

An intact thymus is necessary for normal development of lymphoid tissue and immunological competence in mammals. Whether this influence of the thymus is primarily mediated by a humoral or a cellular mechanism is much debated.

A flow of lymphocytes from the thymus in rodents is demonstrated in different ways. In guinea-pigs a direct comparison between blood from the thymic vein and the carotid artery is possible; this discloses a difference in number of lymphocytes, indicating a considerable export of small lymphocytes (Ernström et al. 1965, Ernström & Larsson 1967). This technique, combined with administration of ^{3}H-thymidine intraperitoneally has also demonstrated that the emigrating cells are newly formed cells, which have incorporated the thymidine into their DNA within 3 days before leaving the thymus (Ernström & Larsson 1969). A transport of cells from the thymus to peripheral lymphoid tissue has also been demonstrated by local injection of ^{3}H-thymidine into the thymus. The intrathymically injected animals contain more heavily labelled lymphocytes in their spleen and lymph nodes than the intraperitoneally injected controls (Linna & Stillström 1966, Linna 1968). Recent studies emphasize the importance of interaction between cells from the thymus and cells from the bone marrow in the immune response (Mitchell & Miller 1968, Nossal et al. 1968).

The present investigation combines the technique of intrathymic labelling with ^{3}H-thymidine and measurements of the thymic veno-arterial difference in number of lymphocytes.

MATERIAL AND METHODS

A total of 74 young male guinea-pigs (187–415 g) were injected with ^{3}H-thymidine (NEN, Boston, Mass., U.S.A., Spec. act. 6.7 C/mM in a dose of 0.1 μC/g body weight). The isotope was injected either into the thymic parenchyma or intraperitoneally in identical doses.

For intrathymic injection, the cervical skin of the animals was infiltrated with about 0.5 ml, 1 % lidocain (Xylocain®, Astra, Sweden). By an incision in the skin, the thymus was exposed. Both thymic lobes were slowly injected with ^{3}H-TdR using a microsyringe (Hamilton Company, Inc., Whittier, California, U.S.A.). Then the incision was closed with sutures. The control animals were sham-operated and labelled by an intraperitoneal injection with ^{3}H-TdR. The original solution (1 μC/μl) was used for intrathymic injections. This solution, diluted with sterile physiological saline to 0.2 μC/μl, was used for intraperitoneal injections. The intrathymic labelling technique has been described in detail elsewhere (Linna & Stillström 1966).

At 2 days (48 hrs), 4, and 8 days after the administration of ^{3}H-TdR, different groups of guinea-pigs were investigated. They were anaesthetized with sodium mebumal (Nembutal®, Abbot, 0.25–0.50 mg/100 g b.w., i.p.). The thymus was exposed and a thymic vein incised. Blood samples were collected in a heparinized blood pipette (Heparin®, 500 IU/ml, Vitrum, Stockholm, Sweden) for preparation of blood smears and for white cell counts in a Bürker chamber. The right carotid artery was incised close to the origin of the thymic artery and blood samples were taken for the same analysis as mentioned above. The artery was then ligated. Finally, the thoracic duct was exposed at its confluence with the left subclavian and jugular veins, mainly according to the technique of Reinhardt & Yoffey (1957). The duct was incised, and lymph collected for preparation of smears. After that, the animals were killed with an overdose of Nembutal®. Samples of spleen and mesenteric lymph nodes were placed in 4 % carbonate buffered formalin. Samples of thymus, spleen, mesenteric lymph nodes and a 2 cm piece of duodenum were placed in cold 5 % trichloroacetic acid (TCA).

The number of white blood cells was determined in a haemocytometer. The smears of blood and lymph were fixed in methanol and prepared for autoradiography according to the dipping technique (Rogers 1967) with slight modifications (see Ernström & Larsson 1969). After an exposure of one month the slides were developed (Kodak D19), fixed and stained in Giemsa solution.

Altogether 200 cells were counted in each smear (magnification 1000 x). The background labelling was scanty and a minimum load of 3 grains per cell was required for the cell to be regarded as labelled and a minimum load of 11 grains per cell for the cell to be regarded as heavily labelled. The number of heavily labelled, labelled and unlabelled lymphocytes, monocytes and granulocytes was registered. The absolute number of labelled lymphocytes per μl of blood was calculated from the total number of white cells and the percentage of labelled lymphocytes.

The tissue samples in TCA were used for quantitation of tritiated DNA. They were kept at $-20°$ C until extraction of nucleic acids was performed. The extraction was carried out according to a modified Schneider procedure (Schneider 1945). The DNA measurements were made according to Burton's modification (Burton 1956) of the diphenylamine reaction. The radioactivity was measured in a liquid scintillation counting system (Packard Tri-Carb 314 ex) using Bray's solution (Bray 1960) as scintillator. These procedures have been described in detail elsewhere (Linna 1967).

The specific activity (spec. act.) of each sample was calculated (counts per min per mg DNA). Spec. act. of spleen, mesenteric lymph nodes and duodenum were used to calculate relative activity (rel. act.). Rel. act. expresses the spec. act. in one organ in per cent of the total spec. act. of the three organs investigated in each animal. Due to the tritiated DNA carried over by migrating thymic cells, traffic of labelled cells from the thymus to a specific organ should be reflected by a higher rel. act. value for this organ in the intra-

TABLE I

Percentage of heavily labelled lymphocytes of total content of lymphocytes in blood from the thymic vein and the carotid artery and in lymph from the thoracic duct of guinea-pigs at different intervals after a single intrathymic or intraperitoneal injection of ^{3}H-TdR
Mean ± S.E.

Source of blood and lymph	Days after intrathymic labelling			Days after intraperitoneal labelling		
	2	4	8	2	4	8
Thymic vein	1.5 ± 0.3 [2]	1.3 ± 0.3 [2]	0.9 ± 0.2 [2]	0.4 ± 0.2	0.4 ± 0.1	0.2 ± 0.1
Carotid artery	1.0 ± 0.2	0.9 ± 0.3	1.1 ± 0.3 [2]	0.7 ± 0.3	0.5 ± 0.2	0.1 ± 0.0
Thoracic duct	1.3 ± 0.3 [3]	0.4 ± 0.1 [1]	0.8 ± 0.1 [3]	0.1 ± 0.1	0.1 ± 0.1	0.2 ± 0.1
No. of animals	13	12	12	12	11	8

[1], [2], [3] indicate a probability of 95, 99 and 99.9 %, respectively, for the difference between the intrathymically and intraperitoneally labelled animals.

thymically labelled group than in the corresponding intraperitoneally labelled group.

The tissue samples in formalin were used for autoradiography. They were dehydrated in ethanol, cleared in xylene and embedded in paraffin wax. 5/μm sections were cut and placed on carefully cleaned slides. The slides were dipped into NTB 2 photographic emulsion (Eastman Kodak, Rochester, N.Y., U.S.A.). The dipping film technique of Rogers (1967) was used. The slides were exposed in the dark for 1 month. After that, they were developed and stained with haemalun according to Mayer (Romeis 1948). The spleen and mesenteric lymph node sections were screened for heavily labelled cells, i.e. cells with a grain count of 11 or more. Fifty view fields (magnification 1000 ×) were screened from each organ of each animal. The grain count and localization of the heavily labelled cells were recorded.

RESULTS

Autoradiographic investigation of blood and lymph samples

The frequency of heavily labelled lymphocytes in blood and lymph was greater after intrathymic labelling than after intraperitoneal labelling (Table I). This demonstrates a release of heavily labelled lymphocytes from the thymus and a distribution of the thymus-derived cells to both blood and lymph.

After intrathymic labelling about the same frequency of heavily labelled lymphocytes was found in blood and lymph (Table I). However, after intraperitoneal labelling, lower frequency of heavily labelled lymphocytes was found in lymph than in blood (Table II). These results demonstrate an equal distribution of thymus-derived lymphocytes to blood and lymph and support the assumption that the lymphocytes, recirculating between blood and lymph, are of thymic origin.

A positive thymic veno-arterial difference in the number of labelled lymphocytes was found in the animals 2 and 4 days after labelling by an intrathymic injection, but not in those labelled by an intraperitoneal injection (Table III). This indicates that the ^{3}H-TdR injected locally into the thymus is incorporated into DNA-synthesizing thymic lymphocytes, which then leave the thymus through the thymic veins. The ^{3}H-TdR injected intraperitoneally apparently does not reach the thymus in amounts sufficient to cause an emigration of labelled lymphocytes.

A veno-arterial difference in the number of heavily labelled lymphocytes was found 2 and 4 days after the intrathymic injection of ^{3}H-TdR, but not after 8 days (Table IV).

TABLE II

Total number of lymphocytes per μl of blood from the thymic vein and the carotid artery of guinea-pigs at different intervals after a single intrathymic or intraperitoneal injection of ^3H-TdR
Mean ± S.E.

Source of blood	Days after intrathymic labelling			Days after intraperitoneal labelling		
	8	4	2	2	4	8
Thymic vein	2465 ± 271	2017 ± 255	2008 ± 106	1567 ± 147	2326 ± 213	2306 ± 264
Carotid artery	2066 ± 253	1885 ± 234	1939 ± 120	1464 ± 173	2151 ± 203	2190 ± 268

This finding confirms earlier results indicating a release of lymphocytes from the thymus in the guinea-pig within a limited period (about 4 days) after the cells have synthesized DNA (Larsson 1966, Ernström & Larsson 1969).

No release of labelled thymic lymphocytes was demonstrated 8 days after labelling. Despite this, almost the same frequency and number of labelled lymphocytes per μl of blood were found as after 2 and 4 days, indicating that lymphocytes previously released from the thymus remain recirculating between blood and lymph (Tables III and IV).

Quantitation of ^3H-DNA in tissue samples

The spec. act. of the different organs varied from animal to animal and did not allow any conclusions about a specific transport from the thymus. Thus, the duodenum had a higher spec. act. after intrathymic than after intraperitoneal injection, but the rel. act. proved that this was not due to a specific transport of DNA from the thymus (Table V).

Two days after labelling, the spleen of the intra-thymically labelled animals had a higher relative activity than that of the intra-

TABLE III

Total number of labelled lymphocytes per μl of blood from the thymic vein and the carotid artery of guinea-pigs at different intervals after a single intrathymic or intraperitoneal injection of ^3H-TdR
Mean ± S.E.

Source of blood	Days after intrathymic labelling			Days after intraperitoneal labelling		
	2	4	8	2	4	8
Thymic vein	100 ± 21[2]	94 ± 17	88 ± 8[3]	34 ± 9	62 ± 13	23 ± 11
Carotid artery	89 ± 20	71 ± 11	94 ± 14[1]	54 ± 14	70 ± 29	41 ± 16
Veno-arterial difference	11 ± 29	23 ± 20	−6 ± 16	−20 ± 17	−8 ± 32	−18 ± 19

[1], [2], [3] indicate a probability of 95, 99 and 99.9 %, respectively, for the difference between the intrathymically and intraperitoneally labelled animals.

TABLE IV

Number of heavily labelled lymphocytes per µl of blood from the thymic vein and the carotid artery of guinea-pigs at different intervals after a single intrathymic or intraperitoneal injection of ^3H-TdR
Mean ± S.E.

Source of blood	Days after intrathymic labelling			Days after intraperitoneal labelling		
	2	4	8	2	4	8
Thymic vein	29±7[1]	31±8[1]	19±4[1]	7±3	8±3	4±3
Carotid artery	18±6	12±3[1]	22±7[1]	10±4	11±6	1±1
Veno-arterial difference	11±9	19±8	−3±8	−3±5	−3±7	3±3
p	—	<0.05	—	—	—	—

[1] indicates a probability of 99 % for the difference between the intrathymically and intraperitoneally labelled animals.

peritoneally labelled animals (p < 0.05). After 4 and 8 days the differences in rel. act. values did not reach statistically significant levels (Table V).

As regards the mesenteric lymph nodes, no difference was found between the intrathymically and the intraperitoneally labelled animals.

The findings confirm the earlier observations of a quantitatively significant cell migration from the thymus to the spleen (Linna & Stillström 1966).

TABLE V

Mean values of spec. act. and rel. act. of different organs sampled from guinea-pigs 2, 4 and 8 days after intrathymic (i.t.) or intraperitoneal (i.p.) labelling with ^3H-TdR. The success of the intrathymic labelling is demonstrated by the difference in mean spec. act. of thymus samples between all intrathymically and intraperitoneally labelled groups of animals. Statistically significant differences between rel. act. values of intrathymically and intraperitoneally labelled groups of animals were obtained for spleens sampled 2 days after labelling, demonstrating quantitatively significant thymus cell migration to the spleen by this time.
Mean ± S.E.

	Way of labelling	2 days			4 days			8 days		
		spec.act.	rel.act.[1]	p[2]	spec.act.	rel.act.[1]	p[2]	spec.act.	rel.act.[1]	p[2]
Spleen	i.t.	19,877	22.2±1.7	<0.05	17,867	30.0±0.3	—	12,814	30.9±1.6	—
	i.p.	11,839	17.1±1.7		10,559	28.1±1.7		4,492	29.1±2.2	
Mes. lymph node	i.t.	16,264	18.8±0.8	—	13,025	22.3±0.2	—	12,946	30.8±1.6	—
	i.p.	18,020	23.2±2.1		9,469	23.1±1.0		5,355	33.2±1.7	
Duodenum	i.t.	51,259	59.0±1.9	—	28,790	47.7±1.2	—	16,030	38.3±1.3	—
	i.p.	42,774	59.6±3.2		20,565	48.8±1.4		5,802	37.7±3.0	
Thymus	i.t.	249,497			156,061			98,429		
	i.p.	2,762			3,840			1,730		

[1] Rel. act. = $\dfrac{\text{spec. act. of an organ} \times 100}{\text{spec. act. of spleen} + \text{spec. act. of mes. lymph node} + \text{spec. act. of duodenum of the same animal}}$

[2] Comparison between rel. act. of intrathymically and intraperitoneally labelled animals.

Autoradiographic investigation of lymphoid tissue samples

At all times after labelling, the mesenteric lymph nodes contained more heavily labelled cells (of all grain classes) after intrathymic labelling than after intraperitoneal labelling (Figure 1). This shows that many of the heavily labelled cells must be derived from the thymus. The number of heavily labelled cells in the mesenteric lymph nodes was essentially unchanged during the experimental period after intrathymic labelling, but decreased with time after intraperitoneal labelling.

At 2 days after labelling, the spleen contained more heavily labelled cells (of all grain classes) after intrathymic labelling than after intraperitoneal labelling (Figure 2). As regards the grain class 11–15, this was also the case 4 and 8 days after labelling. This demonstrates that many heavily labelled cells in the spleen were derived from the thymus.

At 4 days after labelling the heavily labelled spleen cells of the grain classes above 15 grains were as frequent or more frequent after intraperitoneal than after intrathymic labelling (Figure 2). Between days 2 and 4 an increase in cell number of all grain classes above 15 grains occurred in the intraperitoneally labelled animals. The data cannot be explained in terms of division of labelled spleen cells, which should

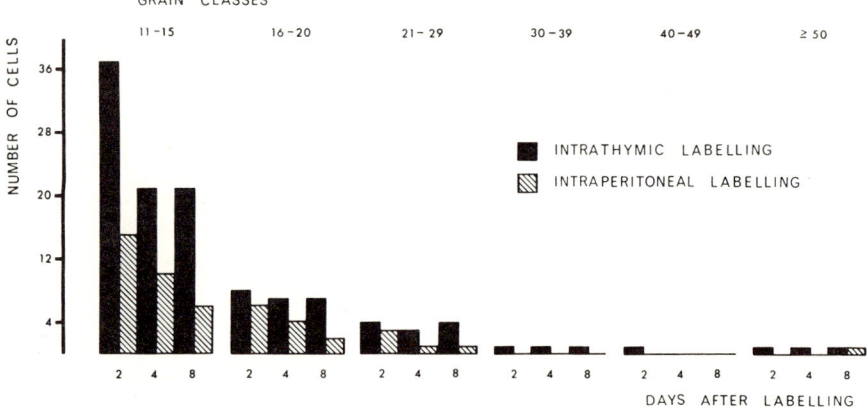

Figure 1. Frequency of heavily labelled lymphocytes of different grain classes in the mesenteric lymph nodes of intrathymically and intraperitoneally labelled animals. The lymph nodes were sampled 2, 4 and 8 days after labelling with ^{3}H-TdR.

Heavily labelled cells of all grain classes were more frequent at all times in the intrathymically labelled animals than in the intraperitoneally labelled ones. Cells with grain count $>$ 30 were very infrequent in the intraperitoneally labelled animals. Thus, many heavily labelled cells are thymus-derived. The number of cells in each grain class remained virtually unchanged in the intrathymically labelled animals during the experimental period, indicating that thymus-derived lymphocytes recirculate between blood, lymph and lymph nodes (see also Table I). An exception was the decrease in cell number in the grain class 11–15 from day 2 to 4.

cause dilution of labelling. Instead the data indicate an immigration to the spleen of heavily labelled cells of extrathymic origin, when 4 days old.

At 8 days after labelling the heavily labelled cells in the spleen were again more frequent in the intrathymically labelled animals. After intrathymic labelling, the heavily labelled cells of the spleen were localized mainly in the white pulp and occasionally also in the germinal centres. In the mesenteric lymph nodes they were found in the outer cortex as well as in the paracortical areas (Turk & Oort 1967) and in the medulla. Occasionally, they were found in germinal centres.

DISCUSSION

The risks with the local labelling procedure are discussed by Linna (1968). A certain traumatic damage at the intrathymic injection can not be prevented. This damage may of course influence the export of living lymphocytes from the thymus. The existence of an export of living cells in the present experiment is obvious from the autoradiographic findings of heavily labelled lymphocytes circulating in blood and lymph and localized to spleen and mesenteric lymph nodes as late as 8 days after the local labelling of the thymus. Furthermore, transfusion experiments by Diderholm (1961)

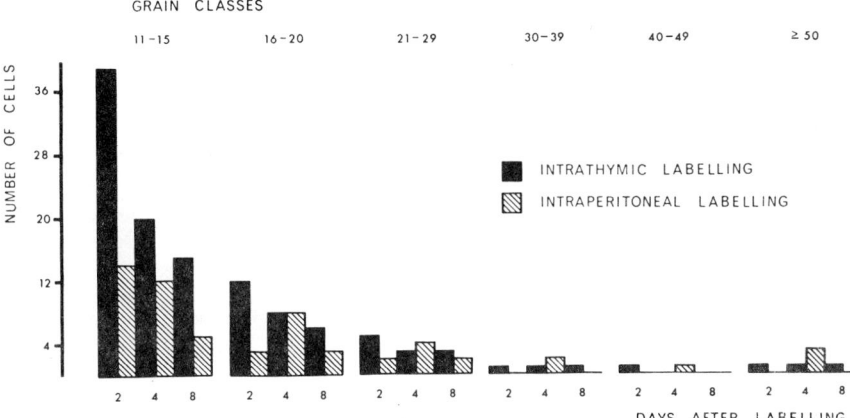

Figure 2. Frequency of heavily labelled lymphocytes of different grain classes in the spleen of intrathymically and intraperitoneally labelled animals. The spleens were sampled 2, 4 and 8 days after labelling with ^{3}H-TdR.
Heavily labelled cells of all grain classes were more frequent in the intrathymically labelled animals 2 and 8 days after labelling, showing that many heavily labelled cells in the spleen are thymus-derived. At 4 days, the results in the intraperitoneally labelled animals indicate an immigration of heavily labelled cells from an extrathymic source.

showed that ³H-thymidine labelled dead thymus cells are not found in spleen and mesenteric lymph nodes like labelled living cells.

The comparison between afferent and efferent thymic blood demonstrates a release of heavily labelled lymphocytes from the thymus 2 and 4 days after labelling but not 8 days afterwards. The result supports the opinion that the thymus contains a rapidly proliferating population of lymphocytes which is exchanged within few days (Craddock et al. 1964, Steel & Lamerton 1965, Everett et al. 1964, Larsson 1966, Metcalf 1966, Ernström & Larsson 1969), and that a great deal of the lymphocytes are leaving the thymus (Murray & Woods 1964, Nossal 1964, Ernström et al. 1965, Linna & Stillström 1966, Weissman 1967, Michalke et al. 1969, Iorio et al. 1970). In the guinea-pig the number of lymphocytes leaving the thymus by the veins have been estimated to 30 % of the lymphocytes produced, the remaining dying within the thymus (Ernström & Sandberg 1970).

The determination of tritiated DNA demonstrated a quantitatively significant migration to the spleen 2 days after labelling, conforming earlier observations (Linna & Stillström 1966). Later on, 4 and 8 days after labelling, the differences in the rel. act. values of the spleen did not reach statistically significant levels. The data thus do not indicate an emigration of thymic cells to the spleen later than 3 days after labelling with ³H-TdR. The results supports the evidence for a rapid traffic of lymphocytes through the splenic tissue (Ford 1969) and a considerable export of lymphocytes from the spleen (Ernström & Sandberg 1968).

The autoradiographic data demonstrate heavily labelled thymus-derived lymphocytes in the spleen and mesenteric lymph nodes 2, 4 and still 8 days after the local thymus labelling with ³H-TdR. The heavily labelled cells after intrathymic labelling were found both in- and outside the so-called thymus-dependent areas (Parrot et al. 1966, Parrot & de Sousa 1969, Turk & Oort 1967), supporting earlier observations of the homing of thymus-derived cells (Linna 1970). Iorio et al. (1970) demonstrated the efflux of thymic lymphocytes to other lymphoid organs after the infusion of ³H-TdR into the thymic artery of calves and traced most of the thymus-derived lymphocytes to the thymus-dependent areas of the spleen and lymph nodes.

The demonstration of an essentially unchanged content of heavily labelled lymphocytes in blood, lymph and lymph nodes 2, 4 and 8 days after intrathymic labelling in contrast to the findings after intraperitoneal labelling, shows that the labelled thymus-derived cells are recirculating for at least 8 days and are more long-lived than those labelled by the intraperitoneal injection.

Four days after labelling, heavily labelled cells of non-thymic origin were found in the spleen. The bone marrow is the most probable source of the immigrants, as the bone marrow like the thymus has an intense DNA-synthesis in its lymphocytes. A migration of cells from the bone marrow to the spleen has also been demonstrated after local labelling of the bone marrow in young guinea-pigs (Linna & Lidén 1969).

REFERENCES

Bray, G. A. (1960) 'A simple efficient liquid scintillator for counting aqueous solutions in a liquid scintillation counter.' *Analyt. Biochem. J.* **1**, 279–85.

Burton, K. (1965) 'A study of the conditions and mechanisms of the diphenylamine reaction for the colorimetric estimation of DNA.' *Biochem. J.* **62**, 315–23.

Craddock, C. G., Nakai, G. S., Fukuta, H. & Vanslager, L. M. (1964) 'Proliferation activity of the lymphatic tissues of rats as studied with tritium-labeled thymidine.' *J. exp. Med.* **120**, 389–412.

Diderholm, H. (1961) 'Studies on the migration and transformation of lymphocytes in immunized and non-immunized animals.' *Acta path. microbiol. scand.*, Suppl. 146 ad vol. 51.

Ernström, U., Gyllensten, L. & Larsson, B. (1965) 'Venous output of lymphocytes from the thymus.' *Nature* (Lond.) **207**, 540–41.

Ernström, U. & Larsson, B. (1967) 'Export and import of lymphocytes in the thymus during steroid-induced involution and regeneration.' *Acta path. microbiol. scand.* **70**, 371–84.

Ernström, U. & Larsson, B. (1969) 'Thymic export of lymphocytes 3 days after labelling with tritiated thymidine.' *Nature* (Lond.) **222**, 279–80.

Ernström, U. & Sandberg, G. (1968) 'Migration of splenic lymphocytes.' *Acta path. microbiol. scand.* **72**, 379–84.

Ernström, U. & Sandberg, G. (1970) 'Quantitative relationship between release and intrathymic death of lymphocytes.' *Acta path. microbiol. scand.*, Sect. A. **78**, 362–63.

Everett, N. B., Rieke, W. O. & Caffrey, R. W. (1964) 'The kinetics of small lymphocytes in the rat, with special reference to those of thymic origin.' *In* R. A. Good & A. E. Gabrielsen (eds.) *The Thymus in Immunobiology*, pp. 291–97. Harper & Row, New York/Evanston/London.

Ford, W. L. (1969) 'The kinetics of lymphocyte recirculation within the rat spleen.' *Cell Tissue Kinetics* **2**, 171–91.

Iorio, R. J., Chanana, A. D., Cronkite, E. P. & Joel, D. D. (1970) 'Studies on lymphocytes. XVI. Distribution of bovine thymic lymphocytes in the spleen and lymph nodes.' *Cell Tissue Kinetics* **3**, 161–73.

Larsson, B. (1966) 'Venous output of ^{3}H-thymidine-labelled lymphocytes from the thymus.' *Acta path. microbiol. scand.* **68**, 622–24.

Lidén, S. & Linna, T. J. (1969) 'Bone marrow cell migration to the spleen in young guinea pigs.' *Int. Arch. Allergy* **35**, 47–57.

Linna, J. (1968) 'Cell migration from the thymus to other lymphoid organs in hamsters of different ages.' *Blood* **21**, 727–46.

Linna, T. J. (1967) 'Transport of tritium-labelled DNA from the thymus to other lymphoid organs in rabbits under normal conditions and after administration of endotoxin.' *Int. Arch. Allergy* **31**, 313–37.

Linna, T. J. (1970) 'Influence of contact allergy on thymus lymphoid cell migration.' *Int. Arch. Allergy* **38**, 230–45.

Linna, T. J. & Stillström, J. (1966) 'Migration of cells from the thymus to the spleen in young guinea pigs.' *Acta path. microbiol. scand.* **68**, 465–75.

Metcalf, D. N. (1966) 'Lymphocyte kinetics in the thymus.' *In* J. M. Yoffey (ed.) *The Lymphocyte in Immunology Haemopoiesis*, pp. 333–41. Edw. Arnold Ltd., London.

Michalke, W. D., Hess, M. W., Riedwyl, H., Stoner, R. D. & Cottier, H. (1969) 'Thymic lymphopoiesis and cell loss in newborn mice.' *Blood* **33**, 541–54.

Mitchell, G. F. & Miller, J. F. A. P. (1968) 'Cell to cell interaction in the immune response. II. The source of hemolysin-forming cells in irradiated mice given bone marrow and thymus or thoracic duct lymphocytes.' *J. exp. Med.* **128**, 821–38.

Murray, R. G. & Woods, P. A. (1964) 'Studies on the fate of lymphocytes. III. The migration and metamorphosis of in situ labeled thymic lymphocytes.' *Anat. Rec.* **150**, 113–28.

Nossal, G. J. V. (1964) 'Studies on the rate of seeding of lymphocytes from the intact guinea pig thymus.' *Ann. N. Y. Acad. Sci.* **120**, 171–81.

Nossal, G. J. V., Cunningham, A., Mitchell, G. F. & Miller, J. F. A. P. (1968) 'Cell to cell interaction in the immune response. III. Chromosomal marker analysis of single antibody-forming cells in reconstituted, irradiated, or thymectomized mice.' *J. exp. Med.* **128**, 839–54.

Parrott, D. M. V. & de Sousa, M. A. B. (1969) 'The source of cells within different areas of lymph nodes draining the site of primary stimulation with a contact sensitizing agent.' *In* L. Fiore-Donati & M. G. Hanna, Jr. (eds.) *Lymphatic Tissue and Germinal Centers in Immune Response*. Plenum Press, New York. *Adv. exp. Med. Biol.* **5**, 293–307.

Parrott, D. M. V., de Sousa, M. A. B. & East, J. (1966) 'Thymus-dependent areas in the lymphoid organs of neonatally thymectomized mice.' *J. exp. Med.* **123**, 191–204.

Reinhardt, W. O. & Yoffey, J. M. (1957) 'Lymphocyte content of lymph from the thoracic and cervical ducts in the guinea pig.' *J. Physiol.* (Lond.) **136**, 227–34.

Rogers, A. W. (1967) *Techniques of Autoradiography*. Elsevier, Amsterdam/London/New York.

Romeis, B. (1948) *Mikroskopische Technik*. 15th ed. Oldenburg, München.

Schneider, W. C. (1945) 'Phosphorus compounds in animal tissue. I. Extraction and estimation of desoxypentose nucleic acid and of pentose nucleic acid.' *J. biol. Chem.* **161**, 293–302.

Steel, G. G. & Lamerton, L. F. (1965) 'The turnover of tritium from thymidine in tissues of the rat.' *Exp. Cell Res.* **37**, 117–31.

Turk, J. L. & Oort, J. (1967) 'Germinal center activity in relation to delayed hypersensitivity.' In H. Cottier, N. Odartchenko, J. Schindler & C. C. Congdon (eds.) *Germinal Centers in Immune Responses*, pp. 311–16. Springer, Berlin/Heidelberg/New York.

Weissman, I. L. (1967) 'Thymus cell migration.' *J. exp. Med.* **126**, 291–304

SURFACE IMMUNOGLOBULINS ON THYMUS AND THYMUS-DERIVED LYMPHOID CELLS*

By ARTHUR D. BANKHURST, M.D., NOEL L. WARNER, Ph.D., AND JOHN SPRENT, M.B.

Materials and Methods

Animals.—CBA and (CBA × C57BL)F_1 mice raised and maintained at the Hall Institute were used throughout. The mice were of either sex and were 50–120 days of age.

Cell Suspensions.—Thymuses were obtained from CBA mice of 50–70 days of age. Cell suspensions were prepared by passing the thymuses gently through a fine stainless steel mesh into cold Eisen's balanced salt solution (EBSS). Thoracic duct lymphocytes (TDL) from 120-day old CBA mice and H2-activated thymus-derived cells in the thoracic duct effluent (TTDL) were obtained by procedures described below. Cells were washed once in EBSS and four additional times through fetal calf serum (FCS) gradients according to the method of Byrt and Ada (14) to remove debris. The cells were finally suspended in 10% FCS in Dulbecco's solution and counted in a hemacytometer. The viability of thymus suspensions and TDL or TTDL suspensions were generally 90–95% and 98–99%, respectively.

Operative Procedures.—Thoracic duct fistulas were prepared using the modification of Miller and Mitchell (15) of the technique described by Boak and Woodruff (16). Generally the mice received an intravenous infusion of isotonic saline during the first 24 hr after cannulation to ensure optimal yield of lymphocytes. The cells were collected in 10% FCS in cold Dulbecco's

---

* This is publication 1554 from the Walter and Eliza Hall Institute of Medical Research. This work was supported by the U.S. Public Health Service Research Grant AM-11234-04.

Abbreviations used in this paper: B, nonthymus-derived; EBSS, Eisen's balanced salt solution; FCS, fetal calf serum; PAPS, polyaminopolystyrene; RFC, rosette-forming cells; T, thymus-derived; TDL, thoracic duct lymphocytes; TTDL, H2-activated, thymus-derived thoracic duct lymphocytes.

solution. Preservative free heparin (Evans Medical Ltd., Liverpool, England) was used to prevent coagulation.

Preparation and Collection of TTDL.—The TTDL were obtained from thoracic duct cannulation of 120-day old (CBA × C57BL)F_1 male mice. These mice had undergone whole body irradiation (800 R) followed by intravenous administration of 100×10^6 CBA thymus cells (50–56-day old female donors). The TTDL were collected starting 4 days after irradiation. The details of these procedures are described elsewhere (17).

Anti-Immunoglobulin Materials.—Antisera against mouse immunoglobulins were prepared in rabbits according to methods described previously by Herzenberg and Warner (18). The antisera with their corresponding immunogens were as follows: anti-light chain (κ) = anti HPC-2 (diethylaminoethyl [DEAE] fraction of Bence Jones kappa protein from BALB/c mouse bearing plasma cell tumor HPC-2); anti-IgM = anti-HPC-76 (starch gel electrophoresis fraction of serum from BALB/c mouse bearing plasma cell tumor HPC-76); anti-polyvalent heavy chain = anti-NZB normal serum globulin. The anti-polyheavy chain serum was shown to have high titers against μ, α, and $\gamma 2$ heavy chains.

The gamma globulin fraction of the rabbit antiserum was then separated by starch gel electrophoresis in Veronal buffer, pH 8.2. This globulin fraction (IgG) was then tested for anti-immunoglobulin activity by precipitation with ^{125}I-labeled purified myeloma proteins (18). In the case of the monospecific anti-μ serum, all absorptions to remove other antibody activities were made with immunoglobulins conjugated to polyaminopolystyrene (PAPS) (18), and the light chain activity of the anti-polyvalent heavy chain serum was removed by absorption with soluble purified HPC-4 (DEAE fraction of Bence Jones protein from [NZB × BALB/c]F_1 mouse bearing plasma cell tumor HPC-4).

In some cases where indicated, thymus absorptions of the anti-immunoglobulin protein were performed. This was done by two successive incubations for 1 hr at 0°C with thymus suspensions from young BALB/c or (CBA × C57BL)F_1 mice. (The equivalent of 5 thymuses/ml of protein solution containing 2–6 mg/ml)

Blocking of Anti-Immunoglobulin Protein.—The specific anti-immunoglobulin activity of the various rabbit globulin fractions was removed (blocked) by purified myelomas coupled to PAPS with the exception of the light chain (HPC-4) which was in solution. The absorptions were performed as follows: anti-κ absorbed with HPC-4 (κ) or HPC-1 (IgA-κ) and MPC-86 (IgG2b-κ); anti-polyheavy chain absorbed with HPC-1 (IgA-κ), MPC-25 (IgG1-κ), MPC-86 (IgG2b-κ), MOPC-104 (IgM-λ), GPC-7 (IgG2a-κ).

Iodination of Anti-Immunoglobulin Protein.—The globulin fractions of anti-immunoglobulin sera were iodinated with ^{125}I according to the method of Klinman and Taylor (19) with minor modifications in that 10% FCS in Dulbecco's solution was used to wash through the ion exchange column. The specific activity of the preparations varied between 4–6 μCi/μg protein.

Cell Labeling.—The cell suspensions were labeled with radioiodinated anti-immunoglobulins according to the method described by Bankhurst and Warner (10). 5 million viable cells were incubated for 1 hr at 0°C with labeled protein (2000–4000 ng in 0.25 ml total incubation volume) and subsequently washed four times through FCS gradients (14) before radioautography.

Radioautography.—The procedures for radioautography have been described by Byrt and Ada (14). The cells were stained with Giemsa, and only lymphoid-like cells of definitive morphology were scored. Positive cells had at least 15 grains on their surface or immediately adjacent to the surface. Clumped cells were excluded. 300 cells were counted on each slide to obtain the percentage of labeled cells.

RESULTS

Per Cent Labeling of Thymus, TDL, and TTDL Cell Suspensions.—TDL cell suspensions labeled on short exposure (4–6 days) with anti-light chain and anti-heavy chain radioiodinated IgG (Table I). The percentage of labeled cells in the TDL preparation remained essentially unchanged between the short (4–7 days) and prolonged (30–60 days) exposure times (19.0 and 17.9% average, respectively, with anti-light chain) even though the number of grains per cell increased. The TDL labeling with the anti-polyheavy chain IgG (20.2% with prolonged exposure) was approximately equal to the anti-light chain labeling. Of interest is the experiment performed with anti-μ which showed a percentage of labeled cells (17.6% on prolonged exposure) approaching the percentage

TABLE I

Labeling of TDL, TTDL, and Thymus Cell Suspensions by Unblocked and Blocked Anti-Immunoglobulin IgG

Experiment	Cell source	Percentage of labeled cells											
		Anti-κ*		Anti-κ blocked*		Anti-poly-heavy chain‡		Anti-poly-heavy chain blocked‡		Anti-μ		NRG§	
		S‖	L‖	S	L	S	L	S	L	S	L	S	L
1	TDL	18.6	16.6	0.3	—	20.0	32.0	0	4.0				
	TTDL	0.6	50.0	0	0	0	1.6	0	0				
	Thymus	2.6	14.3	0.3	3.0	0	1.3	0	0.3				
2	TDL	15.3	17.0	0	0	—	11.3	0.3	3.0				
	TTDL	1.3	42.0	0.3	1.6	0	0	0	0.3				
	Thymus	1.6	19.0	0.3	2.0	0	0	0	0.3				
3	TDL	23.0	20.0	0	1.0	17.0	17.3	0	1.0	12.0	17.6	0	0
	TTDL	0	19.0	0	2.6	0	0.3	0	0	0	0	0	0.3
	Thymus	1.0	10.0	0	2.6	0.1	1.0	0	0	0	0.3	0	0
Average	TDL	19.0	17.9	0.1	0.5	18.5	20.2	0.1	2.7				
	TTDL	0.6	37.0	0.1	1.4	0	0.6	0	0.1				
	Thymus	1.7	14.4	0.2	2.5	0.03	0.8	0	0.2				

* These proteins in experiments 1 and 2 were thymus absorbed. The proteins in experiment 3 were not.
‡ These proteins in 1 and 3 were thymus absorbed.
§ Normal rabbit globulin.
‖ S = 4–7 day exposure; L = 30–60 day exposure.

labeled with anti-polyheavy chain IgG. In all cases binding activity on the TDL, TTDL, or thymus could be selectively removed by preabsorption of the anti-immunoglobulin IgG with purified myeloma. On the average only 0.5 and 2.7% of TDL labeled, respectively, with blocked anti-light chain and blocked anti-polyheavy chain IgG.

The thymus and TTDL suspensions labeled in a different manner (Table I). There was essentially no labeling on short exposures with any radioiodinated anti-immunoglobulin IgG. On prolonged exposure, however, labeling was observed with anti-light chain IgG but not with the anti-heavy chain IgG. The percentage of TTDL labeled with anti-light chain IgG was greater than the percentage of thymus cells labeled (37.0% average *versus* 14.4% average).

Each experiment in Table I was performed as a unit with the simultaneous incubation of thymus, TDL, and TTDL suspensions with the identical freshly radioiodinated IgG. The binding of the anti-heavy chain IgG (and the lack of binding with the blocked IgG) could therefore be observed on TDL even though under identical conditions no labeling was observed on TTDL and thymus cells.

Grain Counts on Labeled Cells.—The grain counts of cells with either unblocked or blocked radioiodinated IgG were compared. The thymus cell suspensions in experiment 2 were tabulated according to the number of grains per labeled cell (Fig. 1). With the unblocked anti-light chain IgG, a total of 302 cells had to be observed to find 100 labeled cells. Accordingly, 302 were observed with the blocked IgG-treated thymus cell suspension. The difference in grain distribution was marked. There were many cells (19%) with greater than 15 grains/cell in the unblocked IgG suspension but very few with a similar grain count (2.0%) with the blocked IgG. Similarly the TTDL suspension from experiment 2 was examined (Fig. 1). In this case only 145 cells had to be observed to tabulate 100 labaled cells. The grain distribution of thymus and TTDL were similar. Again it was apparent that the difference between cell suspensions labeled with unblocked and blocked materials was in the cells bearing 15 or more grains/cell (44.7% *versus* 1%, respectively). The anti-heavy chain IgG produced no significant labeling of TTDL or thymus cells (less than 10% had 1–6 grains/cell) and there was no difference between blocked and unblocked anti-heavy chain preparations.

Size Distribution of Labeled Thymus and TTDL.—It was observed that the labeled cells in the thymus suspension were predominantly large cells. Therefore, the thymus cells were divided into two groups; one group comprised those cells greater than 10 μ in diameter and the other group those less than 10 μ (Fig. 2). Whereas only 25% of all thymus cells were greater than 10 mm, 79% of the labeled cells were in this category.

The TTDL cells were evaluated in the same manner (Fig. 2). The total suspension was mainly comprised of larger cells (76% greater than 10 μ) and the label was distributed equally between the larger and smaller cells.

DISCUSSION

The results of the above experiments directly demonstrate the presence of immunoglobulin light chains on the surface of thymus and thymus-derived lymphoid cells. Previous studies on the question of the presence of surface immunoglobulins have been performed mainly on mixed B cell and T cell populations or have reported negative results for thymus cells. These studies have used a variety of techniques to investigate surface immunoglobulins. Some workers have used blast transformation by anti-allotype sera (20) or anti-immunoglobulin sera (21). Other approaches have included the inhibition of rosette-forming cells (RFC) by anti-immunoglobulin sera (22, 23), the inhibition of the binding of radioiodinated antigen on the antigen-sensitive cell by anti-immunoglobulin sera (5), and the formation of rosettes with mouse lymphocytes and heterologous erythrocytes coated with mouse immunoglobulin in a

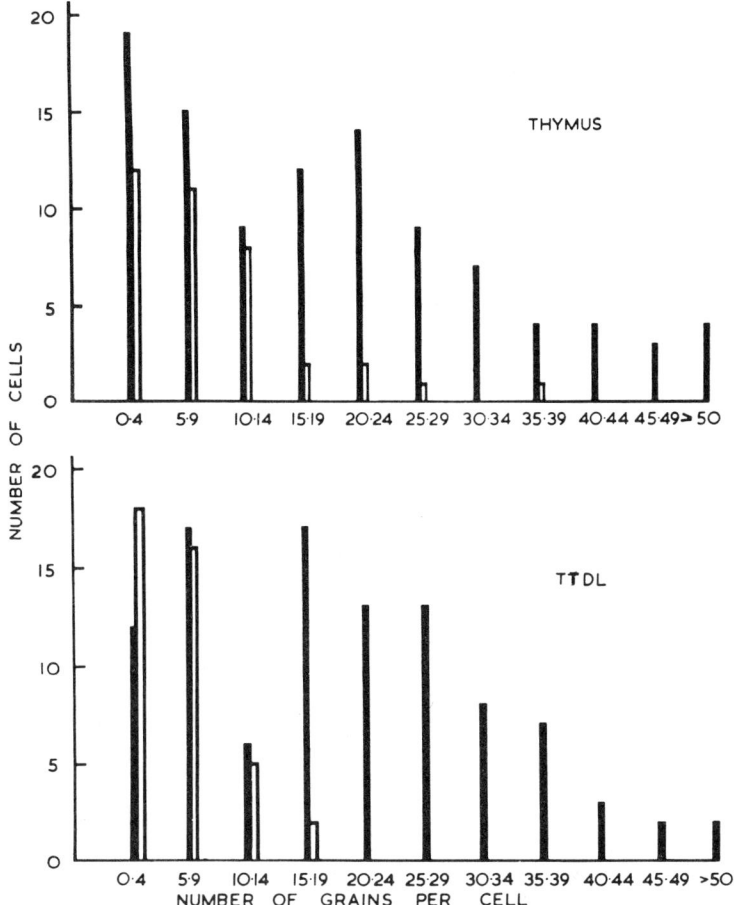

FIG. 1. Distribution of grain counts on labeled cells from thymus and TTDL. Solid bar represents grain counts with anti-light chain protein and open bar represents grain counts with the same protein absorbed (blocked) with purified light chain. 302 and 145 cells from experiment 2 after long exposures were counted, respectively, for thymus and TTDL.

Coombs'-type reaction (24). Functional approaches have included the inhibition of responses to a variety of antigens in irradiated mice reconstituted with spleen cells treated with anti-μ sera (5),[2] and the inhibition of a similar response

---

[2] Herrod, H., and N. L. Warner. Inhibition by anti-μ chain sera of the cellular transfer of antibody and immunoglobulin synthesis in mice. Manuscript in preparation.

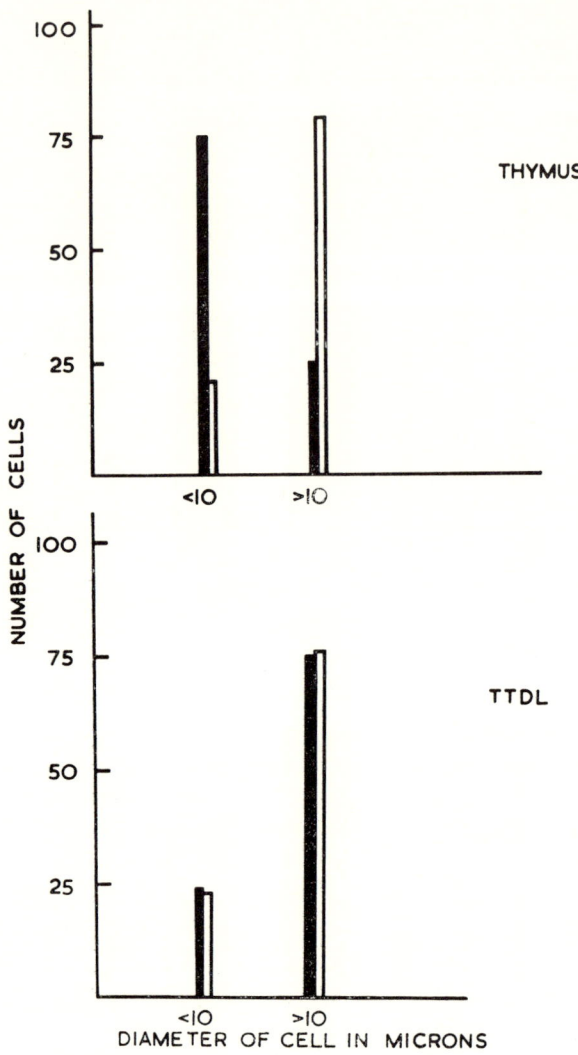

Fig. 2. Distribution of cell diameters on cells from thymus and TTDL. Open bar represents cells labeled with anti-light chain protein (greater than 15 grains/cell) while solid bar represents all cells regardless of label. 100 cells from experiments 1 and 2 after long exposures were averaged to obtain these distributions.

in vitro with anti-light chain sera (25). Experiments on the direct verification of the presence of surface immunoglobulin have used anti-immunoglobulin proteins labeled with radioactive iodine (10, 13) or fluorescein (11, 12).

The above studies have all verified the presence of surface immunoglobulins on B cells and its presumptive role as an antigen receptor. Heretofore direct evidence of the presence of immunoglobulin on thymus or thymus-derived cells by the binding of anti-immunoglobulin proteins has been lacking. Several investigators have suggested immunoglobulins are present on T cells by the use of indirect techniques such as the inhibition of RFC by anti-μ and anti-light chain sera in a population which was enriched to 85% with theta-positive cells (22). T cell-mediated immune reactions have also been blocked with anti-immunoglobulin sera such as in the inhibition of graft-*versus*-host reactions by anti-light chain sera in neonatal mice (6) and chickens,[3] and the inhibition of graft-*versus*-host reactions in adult, irradiated mice receiving parenteral spleen or bone marrow cells (7). Only anti-light chain sera were observed to block the reaction in the neonatal mice or chickens, whereas only anti-globulin sera with broad specificity was used in the other experiments (7). Anti-light chain serum has also been reported to block the antigen-^{125}I–induced suicide of T cells (4).

The experiments described in this present paper report on two lymphoid cell populations, thymus and TTDL, which are exclusively composed of T cells as shown by the presence of the theta marker on greater than 95% of the cells (17) and the absence of a B cell receptor for antigen-antibody complexes (26). With these cell suspensions a maximum of 19 and 50%, respectively, of thymus and TTDL were labeled with radioiodinated anti-light chain IgG. Such results could not be explained by the presence of B cell contamination. It might be speculated that the true number of T cells with surface light chains might approach 100% with even more prolonged exposures, or alternatively, it may be that only antigen-activated cells or cells which have recently achieved immunocompetence (antigen-sensitive cells) are expressing surface immunoglobulin. This possibility of a young population of antigen-activated cells bearing surface immunoglobulin is reinforced by the finding that 79% of the lymphoid cells labeling in the thymus were large cells greater than 10 μ in diameter. It is well known that such a population of larger cells is correlated with recent mitotic activity (27). Furthermore the TTDL population was comprised mostly of large, blast-like cells which predictably had a larger number of labeled cells than was present in the thymus (average of 37% *versus* 14.4% for TTDL and thymus, respectively). Since the medulla of the thymus has a higher percentage of large lymphocytes than the cortex (28), it is interesting to speculate that the labeled thymus cells might correspond to the medullary steroid-resistant population which are particularly active against allogenic cells (29) and are the cells which eventually appear as TTDL.

---

[3] Rouse, B. T., and N. L. Warner. Suppression of graft-*versus*-host reactions in chickens by pretreatment of donor cells with anti-light chain sera. Manuscript in preparation.

On the basis of RFC-blocking studies with specific anti-immunoglobulin sera on primed and unprimed mice, some authors (22) have proposed that T cell antigen activation may involve the progressive exposure of an IgM receptor molecule. The unprimed cell would have only the Fab portion of the molecule exposed while the primed cell would sequentially expose the "hinge region" and, finally, essentially the entire IgM molecule. It should be stressed that the studies reported here do not support this concept, since no labeling by radio-iodinated anti-heavy chain reagents was observed on an antigen-activated population (TTDL). There may, however, be a difference in the nature of surface immunoglobulins on the "collaborative" cells involved in the SRBC response and the "killer cell" population of the TTDL activated against the histocompatability antigen.

No claim is made here concerning the functional role of surface immunoglobulins demonstrated on T cells; however, if one were to speculate that their role is as an antigen receptor, it would perhaps be unlikely that there was not an associated variable part of a heavy chain. Such a statement is based on the poor antigen-binding efficiency of an artificial molecule reconstituted from light chains alone (30) although such an artificial molecule may be a distant approximation of such a configuration in nature. There are several explanations for the absence of at least part of a heavy chain demonstrable with the present techniques. It is possible that the T cell has a heavy chain buried in the surface matrix and unavailable for detection by anti-immunoglobulins; there may be a new, unidentified heavy chain class (IgX); or the antisera prepared against purified myeloma proteins did not possess activities against an exposed hinge region, variable part of a heavy chain, or the monomer of an IgM molecule.

The fact that 19% of TDL label on short exposures correlates well with the data on the incidence of theta-positive lymphocytes (approximately 80%) (31) and suggests that this population labeling rapidly with anti-immunoglobulin IgG is a B cell population. The results of cell labeling with anti-immunoglobulin reagents on TDL from neonatally thymectomized mice (10) and TDL from mice with the congenital absence of a thymus[4] also suggest that the rapid labeling cells are B cells. In contrast to this, the T cell population did not label unless exposed for 1 month or longer and suggests a difference in immunoglobulin surface density between the B and T cell. Although no attempt was made to correlate grain count with surface molecular density, other studies (10, 11) have suggested a difference between the T cell and B cell in the range of 0.1–1.0%. The single experiment performed on TDL with anti-light chain IgG, anti-polyheavy chain IgG, and anti-μ IgG (17.9, 20.2, and 17.6%, respectively) suggests that there are multiple heavy chains present on lymphoid cells at some stage of their development. This has been suggested in several studies

---

[4] Bankhurst, A. D., and N. L. Warner. Unpublished observations.

(10, 20, 23). It is not clear why there is not a subpopulation in TDL representing the T cells which will become labeled after prolonged exposure like thymus or TTDL. It is conceivable that the small lymphocytes comprising such a T cell population have a much denser surface matrix of unrelated materials that would submerge the surface immunoglobulins and make them inaccessible for detection. Some support for this concept comes from work done on the greater density of histocompatability antigens on mouse lymphocytes from lymph nodes or spleen *versus* thymus (32).

The possibility that cytophilic immunoglobulin accounts for the observed results cannot be rigorously excluded despite extensive efforts at cell washing. This is not likely since heavy chain labeling would also be expected if this were the case. In addition there could conceivably be other surface antigens which cross-react with the anti-immunoglobulin IgG.

SUMMARY

Lymphoid cells from thymus, thoracic duct lymph (TDL), and thoracic duct lymph in irradiated animals reconstituted with allogeneic thymus cells (TTDL) were labeled with radioiodinated anti-immunoglobulins using radioautographic techniques. Thymus and TTDL were labeled (14.4 and 37.0%, respectively) with anti-light chain protein after prolonged exposures (30–60 days). No labeling was observed on thymus and TTDL with anti-polyheavy chain globulin. In contrast 18.5–19.0% of TDL labeled on short exposure (6 days) with anti-polyheavy chain and anti-light chain materials. It is proposed that the difference between the labeling observed on short exposures *versus* long exposures can be related to the difference in surface density of immunoglobulins between nonthymus-derived (B) and thymus-derived (T) cells.

The distribution of labeled cells in the thymus was preferentially among the larger cells (greater than 10 μ diameter). The TTDL population was mostly composed of a larger, blast-like population and the distribution of label was independent of size.

As the thymus and TTDL preparations contain almost exclusively T cells, this represents a direct demonstration of surface immunoglobulin light chains on T lymphoid cells.

BIBLIOGRAPHY

1. Wigzell, H., and O. Mäkelä. 1970. Separation of normal and immune lymphoid cells by antigen-coated columns. Antigen-binding characteristics of membrane antibodies as analyzed by hapten-protein antigens. *J. Exp. Med.* **132**:110.
2. Miller, J. F. A. P., and J. Sprent. 1971. Cell-to-cell interaction in the immune response. VI. Contribution of thymus-derived cells and antibody-forming cell precursors to immunological memory. *J. Exp. Med.* **134**:66.
3. Chiller, J. H., G. S. Habicht, and W. O. Weigle. 1970. Cellular sites of immunologic unresponsiveness. *Proc. Nat. Acad. Sci. U.S.A.* **65**:551.

4. Basten, A., J. F. A. P. Miller, N. L. Warner, and J. Pye. 1971. Specific inactivation of thymus-derived (T) and nonthymus-derived (B) lymphocytes by ^{125}I-labeled antigen. *Nature (London).* In press.
5. Warner, N. L., P. Byrt, and G. L. Ada. 1970. Blocking of the lymphocyte antigen receptor site with anti-immunoglobulin sera *in vitro*. *Nature (London).* **226:**942.
6. Mason, S., and N. L. Warner. 1970. The immunoglobulin nature of the antigen recognition site on cells mediating transplantation immunity and delayed hypersensitivity. *J. Immunol.* **104:**762.
7. Tyan, M. L. 1971. Modification of bone marrow induced GVH disease with heterologous antisera to gamma globulin or whole serum. *J. Immunol.* **106:**586.
8. Greaves, M. F. 1970. Biological effects of anti-immunoglobulins. Evidence for immunoglobulin receptors on "T" and "B" lymphocytes. *Transplant. Rev.* **5:**45.
9. Warner, N. L. 1971. Surface immunoglobulins on lymphoid cells. *In* Contemporary Topics in Immunobiology. M. G. Hanna, editor. Plenum Publishing Corp., New York. In press.
10. Bankhurst, A. D., and N. L. Warner. 1971. Surface immunoglobulins on mouse lymphoid cells. *J. Immunol.* In press.
11. Rabellino, E., S. Colon, H. M. Gray, and E. R. Unanue. 1971. Immunoglobulins on the surface of lymphocytes. I. Distribution and quantitation. *J. Exp. Med.* **133:**156.
12. Pernis, B., L. Forni, and L. Amante. 1970. Immunoglobulin spots on the surface of rabbit lymphocytes. *J. Exp. Med.* **132:**1001.
13. Raff, M. C. 1970. Two distinct populations of peripheral lymphocytes in mice distinguishable by immunofluorescence. *Immunology.* **19:**637.
14. Byrt, P., and G. L. Ada. 1969. An *in vitro* reaction between labeled flagellin or haemocyanin and lymphocyte-like cells from normal animals. *Immunology.* **17:** 503.
15. Miller, J. F. A. P., and G. Mitchell. 1968. Cell to cell interaction in the immune response. I. Hemolysin-forming cells in neonatally thymectomized mice reconstituted with thymus or thoracic duct lymphocytes. *J. Exp. Med.* **128:**801.
16. Boak, J. L., and M. F. A. Woodruff. 1965. A modified technique for collecting mouse thoracic duct lymph. *Nature (London).* **205:**396.
17. Sprent, J., and J. F. A. P. Miller. 1971. Interaction of thymus lymphocytes with histoincompatible cells. II. Recirculating lymphocytes derived from antigen-activated thymus cells. *J. Cell. Immunol.* In press.
18. Herzenberg, L. A., and N. L. Warner. 1968. Genetic control of mouse immunoglobulins. *In* Regulation of the Antibody Response. B. Cinader, editor. Charles C Thomas, Publisher, Springfield, Ill.
19. Klinman, N. R., and R. B. Taylor. 1969. General methods for the study of cells and serum during the immune response: the response to dinitrophenyl in mice. *Clin. Exp. Immunol.* **4:**473.
20. Sell, S., J. A. Lowe, and P. G. H. Gell. 1970. Studies on rabbit lymphocytes *in vitro*. XI. Superaddition of anti-allotypic lymphocytes transformation: evidence for multipotent lymphoid cells. *J. Immunol.* **104:**103.
21. Sell, S. 1967. Studies on rabbit lymphocytes *in vitro*. VI. The induction of blast

transformation with sheep antisera to rabbit IgA and IgM. *J. Exp. Med.* **125:** 393.
22. Greaves, M. F., and N. M. Hogg. 1970. Antigen binding sites on mouse lymphoid cells. *In* Proceedings of the 3rd Sigrid Julius Symposium on Cell Collaboration in the Immune Response. A. Cross, T. Kosunen, and O. Mäkelä, editors. Academic Press Inc., New York.
23. Biozzi, G., R. A. Binaghi, C. Stiffel, and D. Mouton. 1969. Production of different classes of immunoglobulins by individual cells in the guineapig. *Immunology.* **16:**349.
24. Coombs, R. R. A., B. W. Gurner, I. McConnell, and A. Munro. 1970. Immunoglobulin determinants on mouse lymphocytes from blood, lymph nodes, bone marrow and thymus. *Int. Arch. Allergy Appl. Immunol.* **39:**280.
25. Lesley, J., and R. W. Dutton. 1970. Antigen receptor molecules: inhibition by antiserum against kappa light chains. *Science (Washington).* **169:**487.
26. Basten, A., J. Sprent, and J. F. A. P. Miller. 1971. A receptor for antibody-antigen complexes on B cells: its value in separating T cells from lymphocyte populations. *Nature (London).* In press.
27. Terasima, T., and L. J. Tolmach. 1963. Growth and nucleic acid synthesis in synchronously dividing populations of HeLa cells. *Exp. Cell Res.* **30:**344.
28. Smith, C. 1964. The microscopic anatomy of the thymus. *In* The Thymus in Immunobiology. R. A. Good and A. E. Gabrielsen, editors. Harper and Row, Publishers, New York.
29. Blomgren, H. 1971. Studies on the proliferation of thymus cells injected into syngeneic or allogeneic irradiated mice. *Clin. Exp. Immunol.* **8:**279.
30. Edelman, G. M., D. E. Olins, J. A. Gally, and N. D. Zinder. 1963. Reconstitution of immunologic activity by interaction of polypeptide chains of antibodies. *Proc. Nat. Acad. Sci. U.S.A.* **50:**573.
31. Miller, J. F. A. P., and J. Sprent. 1971. Thymus-derived cells in mouse thoracic duct lymph. *Nature (London).* **230:**267.
32. Aoki, T., U. Hammerling, E. deHarven, E. A. Boyse, and L. J. Old. 1969. Antigenic structure of cell surfaces. An immunoferritin study of the occurrence and topography of H-2,θ, and TL alloantigens on mouse cells. *J. Exp. Med.* **130:**979.

DECREASED LONGEVITY OF MICE FOLLOWING THYMECTOMY IN ADULT LIFE[1]

H. F. JEEJEEBHOY

It has been shown that an animal which has been thymectomized in adult life gradually develops a decreased ability to produce a normal immune response to sheep red blood cells and to reject allografts (*3, 5, 6, 8*). Hence, it is tempting to think that the results obtained in clinical transplantation might be improved if the recipient of a renal allograft was thymectomized in addition to receiving the various therapeutic agents in current use. Heterologous antilymphocyte serum is frequently administered at the present time (for reviews see references *1* and *4*); its immunosuppressive properties are significantly potentiated by prior thymectomy of the recipient (*2, 7*). Unfortunately, the present study shows that thymectomy performed in adult life significantly decreases the life span of a mouse. Hence, our findings would suggest that the routine use of thymectomy in clinical transplantation is probably undesirable. This last statement

[1] Supported by grants from the Medical Research Council of Canada, the National Cancer Institute of Canada, and the John A. Hartford Foundation, Inc.

TABLE 1. Life span of thymectomized and sham thymectomized mice[a]

Procedure	No. of mice	Survival after operation (days)	P[b]
Thymectomy	14	133, 189, 259, 280, 309, 350, 358, 361, 369, 430, 465, 472, 538, 542	<0.01
Sham thymectomy	9	458, 476, 500, 503, 523, 541, 550, 553, 553	

[a] Male C57BL/6J mice paired for weight and age (14-week-old and weighing 22-24 g) and either thymectomized or sham thymectomized.
[b] Determined by Mann-Whitney U test.

is based on the assumption, which may not be valid, that thymectomized human subjects would show a decrease in their life spans similar to that found in mice.

A group of male C57BL/6J mice (14-week-old and weighing 22-24 g) were thymectomized. On the same day a sham operation (3) was performed on another group of male C57BL/6J mice which had been paired for weight and age with the first group. The two groups of animals were kept under identical laboratory conditions and fed similar diets (Purina chow and water ad libitum). In order to avoid the possibility of introducing infections, no investigations were performed on these animals during their lifetimes. In particular, they were never bled for determination of peripheral blood counts. Only the day of death was recorded and an autopsy was performed if the carcass had not been destroyed by cannibalism. Animals which died in the immediate postoperative period were excluded from the study.

The results presented in Table 1 show that the life span of a mouse is significantly decreased if it has been thymectomized in adult life. The body weights of the thymectomized and sham thymectomized animals were at all times comparable. Ten of the 14 thymectomized mice and 7 of the 9 sham thymectomized mice were autopsied. The first thymectomized animal which died succumbed to pneumonia. No obvious cause of death was found in any of the other animals. However, the earlier death of mice in the thymectomized group of animals was probably attributable to undetected infections. There is a gradual decrease in the ability to produce a normal immune response if an animal has been thymectomized in adult life. This decrease might render the animal susceptible to infections which could normally be quite adequately dealt with by a nonthymectomized animal with an intact immune response.

Acknowledgments. I thank Mr. R. White and Mr. L. Elder for their expert technical assistance.

REFERENCES

1. James, K. 1969. Progr. Surg. 7: 140.
2. Jeejeebhoy, H. F. 1965. Lancet 2: 106.
3. Jeejeebhoy, H. F. 1965. Immunology 9: 417.
4. Jeejeebhoy, H. F. 1971. Canad. J. Surg. 14: 5.
5. Metcalf, D. 1965. Nature 208: 1337.
6. Miller, J. F. A. P. 1965. Nature 208: 1337.
7. Monaco, A. P.; Wood, M. L.; Russell, P. S. 1965. Science 149: 432.
8. Taylor, R. B. 1965. Nature 208: 1334.

Isogeneic Lymphocyte Interaction: Recognition of Self Antigens by Cells of the Neonatal Thymus*

Michael L. Howe , Allan L. Goldstein , and Jack R. Battisto

In most mammals the thymus is essential for normal development and expression of cellular immunity.[1] Considerable interest is currently focused on the mechanism by which the thymus endows primitive lymphoid elements with the capacity to function as mature immunologically competent cells.[2,3] Recently, it has been demonstrated by both *in vivo*[4,5] and *in vitro*[6] methods that the neonatal thymus contains a population of cells capable of recognizing foreign histocompatibility antigens. The studies reported here demonstrate by means of *in vitro* isogeneic lymphocyte interaction (ILI) that the thymus of the neonate also contains, for a limited period of time, a population of cells capable of self-recognition.

Materials and Methods. Animals: Mice used in this study were of strains CBA/J and Balb/c (Jackson Laboratories, Bar Harbor, Me.) and CBA/Wh (obtained from the colony of Dr. A. White). Male and female animals were used in each experiment. Animals designated as "neonatal" were 1-4 days of age; those termed "adult" were 2-6 months old.

Preparation of lymphoid cells for culture: Animals were exsanguinated by decapitation; their lymphoid organs were removed aseptically and teased with small forceps into a cell suspension in RPMI Medium 1640[7] supplemented with 5% fetal calf serum, 100 units/ml penicillin, and 100 μg/ml streptomycin. Larger particles were allowed to settle and the suspension of single cells was removed. Cell suspensions were centrifuged at $150 \times g$ for 20 min, then resuspended in culture medium to a final concentration of 1 or 2×10^6 cells/ml. All cell cultures were established in 12×75 mm disposable polystyrene tubes and incubated at 37°C in an atmosphere of 5% CO_2 in air. The final volume of all cultures was 1.0 ml. Each value in the text represents the mean of triplicate cultures.

Determination of cellular proliferation: Twenty hr. before termination of culture, 0.25 μCi of [^{14}C]thymidine (50 mCi/mmol, Schwarz Bioresearch, Orangeburg, N.Y.) was added to each tube. Cells were collected by Millipore filtration[8] and incorporation of labeled thymidine was estimated by standard scintillation techniques.

Mitomycin treatment: In some of the experiments it was necessary to prevent cellular division. Cells were incubated at a concentration of 2×10^6 cells/ml at 37°C for 20 min in the presence of 25 μg/ml of mitomycin C.[9] The cells were then washed twice with 20-ml volumes of complete medium and resuspended to the final concentration desired.

Results. During the course of some experiments involving the mixed lymphocyte interaction, control studies were conducted in which thymus cells from neonatal CBA/Wh mice were cultured with spleen cells from the same mouse strain.[10] When instead of control values we observed stimulation of the cells, our attention was directed to the phenomenon itself. A typical experiment (Fig. 1) shows the proliferative response observed over a period of time in mixtures containing 1×10^6 CBA/J neonatal thymus (T^n) cells and an equal number of CBA/J adult spleen (S^a) cells. The response within this isogeneic mixture of cells was first apparent at 48 hr, reached a maximum at 96 hr, and declined thereafter. During the same time interval the proliferative activity of the cultures

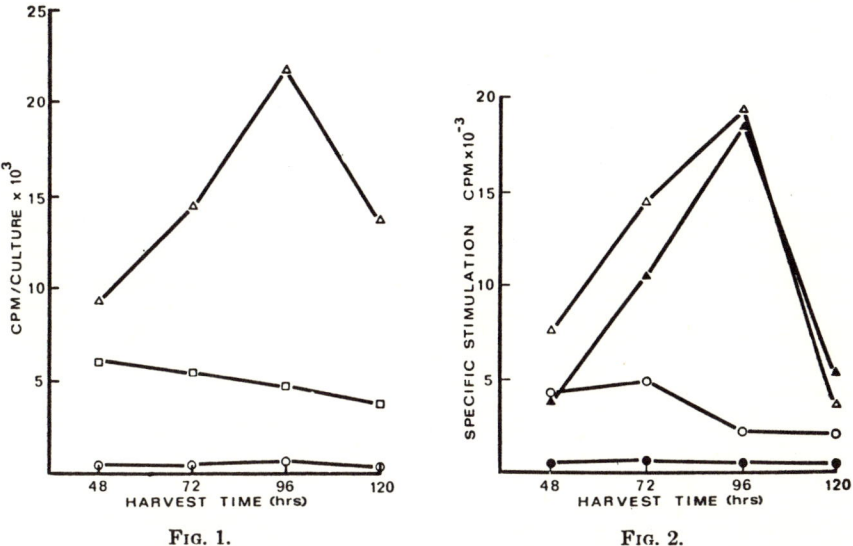

FIG. 1. FIG. 2.

FIG. 1. Proliferative response in mixtures of isogeneic spleen and thymus cells from CBA/Wh mice. O, 2×10^6 neonatal thymus cells (cpm/2); □, 2×10^6 adult spleen cells (cpm/2); △, 1×10^6 neonatal thymus cells cultured with 1×10^6 adult spleen cells.

FIG. 2. Relative contribution of each cell type to the ILI. Cells were rendered incapable of division by treatment with mitomycin C. The response of appropriate control cultures was subtracted from the response of the mixtures. Each mixture contained 1×10^6 adult CBA/J spleen cells and 1×10^6 neonatal CBA/J thymus cells. ●, mitomycin C-treated thymus cells + mitomycin C-treated spleen cells; O, mitomycin C-treated thymus cells + normal spleen cells; ▲, normal thymus cells + mitomycin C-treated spleen cells; △, normal thymus cells + normal spleen cells.

containing S^a cells alone declined steadily while the T^n cells cultured separately remained relatively nonresponsive throughout the experiment. Thus, despite the fact that both populations of lymphoid cells originated from the same inbred strain of mice, when they were mixed *in vitro* a proliferative response was observed that was similar to that seen when lymphoid cells from allogeneic strains of mice were cultured together.

We determined the relative contribution of each cell type to the total proliferative response by rendering the cultures one-way reactive, i.e., by prior incubation of one of the cell types with mitomycin C. The quantity of thymidine incorporated in mixtures of cells containing untreated T^n and mitomycin-treated S^a cells was approximately equal to that in mixtures of untreated T^n and S^a cells (Fig. 2). On the other hand, proliferation was almost entirely abolished when mitomycin-treated T^n cells were cultured with untreated S^a cells. As expected, mitomycin treatment of both sets of cells destroyed the proliferative activity. Thus, the activity seen in $T^n \times S^a$ cell mixtures was almost entirely due to the proliferation of T^n cells.

That the peak of proliferative activity in $T^n \times S^a$ cultures actually fluctuated between 72 and 96 hr is demonstrated in Table 1. It can also be seen that although the specific stimulation was somewhat variable, it usually exceeded 15,000 cpm at the response peak.

Having established that T^n cells were capable of undergoing proliferation in the presence of isogeneic S^a cells, we next sought to determine whether isogeneic cells from other tissues were capable of provoking thymus cells to respond. Accordingly, CBA/Wh neonatal thymic cells were cultured separately with CBA/Wh adult bone marrow, lymph node cells, and newborn liver cells. These results, presented elsewhere,[10] indicate that a small degree of proliferative activity occurred in mixtures of thymic cells with bone marrow cells (1000 cpm above controls), less in mixtures containing lymph node cells, and least in those with newborn liver cells. None of these cells provoked thymic cell proliferation in the mixtures to the extent seen in cultures containing spleen cells.

TABLE 1. *Summary of ILI experiments: interaction of isogeneic neonatal thymus cells (T^n) and adult spleen cells (S^a).* *

| Experiment number | Peak of response (hr) | Proliferation (cpm) in control and mixed cultures | | | Specific stimulation† |
		$\frac{S^a}{2}$	$\frac{T^n}{2}$	$S^a + T^n$	
70	96	3030	284	12,281	8,967
71	72	7476	217	19,302	11,609
72	96	9009	984	33,608	23,615
73	72	6942	210	31,937	24,785
74	96	7602	184	27,325	19,539
76	96	6354	3157	28,552	19,041
78	72	11349	587	41,978	30,042
81	96	7192	215	24,881	17,474

* Each mixed culture contained 1×10^6 T^n cells and 0.5×10^6 S^a cells. Control cultures contained 2×10^6 T^n cells or 1×10^6 S^a cells.

† Mean cpm of mixed culture minus mean cpm/2 of each control culture.

Comparison of the mean values of mixed and control cultures using the Student's *t* test indicates that the differences are all significant at the 2% level.

To ascertain whether neonatal thymic cells possess the capacity to proliferate in the presence of allogeneic cells, T^n cells from CBA/J mice were mixed with mitomycin-treated adult thymus and spleen cells from Balb/c and CBA/J mice. Fig. 3 shows that T^n cells were stimulated to proliferate to the same extent by mitomycin-treated Balb/c and CBA/J spleen cells. In addition, T^n cells responded to mitomycin-treated T^a cells from Balb/c donors but not to those from isogeneic donors. Thus, neonatal CBA/J thymic cells respond well to allogeneic cells of splenic or thymic origin, but will respond to isogeneic cells only if the latter are derived from the spleen.

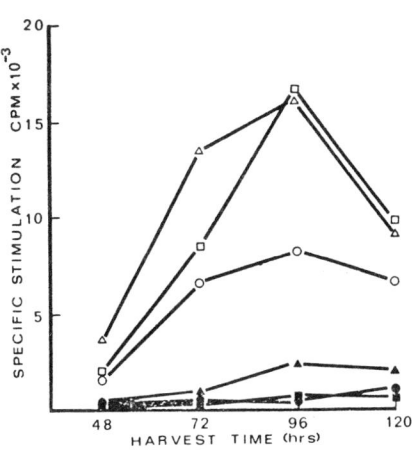

FIG. 3. The ability of CBA/Wh thymocytes to respond to allogeneic cells and the effect of age of thymus cell donor on this response. Each culture contained 1×10^6 cells of each type. The response of appropriate control cultures was subtracted from the response of the mixtures. ■, normal CBA/Wh neonatal thymocytes + mitomycin C-treated CBA/Wh adult thymocytes; ●, normal CBA/Wh adult thymocytes + mitomycin C-treated Balb/c adult thymocytes; ▲, normal CBA/Wh adult thymocytes + mitomycin C-treated Balb/c adult spleen cells; ○, normal CBA/Wh neonatal thymocytes + mitomycin C-treated Balb/c adult thymocytes; △, normal CBA/Wh neonatal thymocytes + mitomycin C-treated Balb/c adult spleen cells; □, normal CBA/Wh neonatal thymocytes + mitomycin C-treated CBA/Wh adult spleen cells.

In the same experiment (Fig. 3) the capacity of CBA/J adult thymus (T^a) cells to respond to an allogeneic stimulus was also examined. Whereas T^n cells responded well to the Balb/c spleen cells and gave a lesser, though positive, response to Balb/c thymic cells, the T^a cells did not respond well to either allogeneic cell type. Thus it is apparent that the capacity of the neonatal thymus to recognize alloantigens is significantly reduced in the thymus of the adult animal.

In view of the latter observation, it became necessary to know at precisely what age thymic cells acquire and lose the capacity to respond to isogeneic cells. Adult CBA/J spleen cells were cultured with isogeneic thymic cells from donors of different ages. The data in Fig. 4 indicate that proliferative activity was greatest in cultures containing cells from 1- to 2-day-old donors and only slightly reduced in those containing cells from 3- to 4-day-old donors. Significantly reduced, though positive, responses were observed in the cultures containing older (35 days) or younger (1-day-old and embryonic) cells. Thymocytes from 70-day-old animals produced only minimal responses. Thus, the ability of neonatal thymus cells to respond in the presence of isogeneic spleen cells is low in the embryo, increases sharply just after birth, declines after 4 days of age, and almost falls to background levels by adulthood.

Discussion. Cells capable of recognizing self and non-self have long been postulated to co-exist within an individual for a short time during immunological

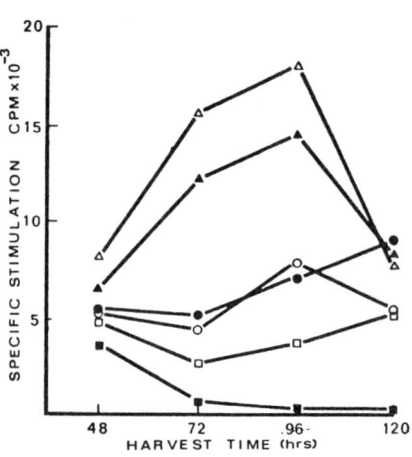

FIG. 4. Effect of age of cell donor on the response of CBA/J thymocytes to isogeneic adult spleen cells. 1×10^6 CBA/J spleen cells were mixed with 1×10^6 CBA/J thymocytes from donors of different ages. The response of appropriate control cultures was subtracted from the response of the mixtures. None of the cells were treated with mitomycin C. ■, thymocytes from 70-day-old donors; □, thymocytes from 1-day-old donors; ○, thymocytes from embryonic (18–19 days gestation) donors; ●, thymocytes from 35-day-old donors; ▲, thymocytes from 3- to 4-day-old donors; △, thymocytes from 2- to 3-day-old donors.

development.[11] Presumably, cells capable of recognizing non-self are maintained in small numbers throughout life unless stimulated by the appropriate antigen, while cells recognizing self are rendered tolerant by early exposure to self antigens. Although this theory of the existence and neonatal "tolerance" of self-recognition cells has been widely accepted, its support has rested mainly upon indirect evidence. The ILI described in this communication clearly suggests the existence of the postulated self-recognition cells within the neonatal thymus and offers an *in vitro* system for their study.

This interpretation is dependent upon the assumption that the proliferative activity of thymocytes in the ILI is triggered by thymocyte recognition of spleen cell antigen(s) (Fig. 2). The possibility also exists that spleen cells recognize thymic cell antigens and synthesize specific immunoglobulins and these, in turn, stimulate thymus cells to divide. Although our data do not permit a definitive choice between these two possibilities, we are inclined to assume that thymocytes recognize spleen cell antigens since proliferation in allogeneic cell mixtures is always due to proliferation of the recognizing cells. A third possibility is that spleen cells produce a mitogenic factor which stimulates thymic cell division. This possibility appears unlikely since it would require that thymus cells be sensitive to a mitogenic factor for only a few days after birth. Further, in preliminary experiments, supernatants from either $S^a \times T^n$ cultures or S^a cultures alone have failed to stimulate T^n proliferation (unpublished observations).

The theory that proliferation in the ILI is due to thymic-cell recognition of surface antigens of spleen cells would be considerably strengthened if thymic cells would proliferate, as well, in the presence of lymphoid cells with known antigenic differences. This was actually observed when CBA thymic cells were mixed with allogeneic thymus or spleen cells of Balb/c origin (Fig. 3). Indeed, the kinetics and magnitude of the response in the allogeneic mixtures so closely resemble those seen in the ILI as to lend support to the view that, in the ILI, T^n cells are responding to splenic antigen(s).

Mixtures of T^n cells with isogeneic cells from sources other than the spleen results in a marked decrease in proliferative activity.[10] This disparity in the stimulatory activity of spleen cells as compared to other types of isogeneic cells may reflect quantitative or qualitative variations of the cellular antigens that elicit the ILI.

Presumably, the loss of ability to recognize self antigens in the aging thymus (Fig. 4) reflects an acquisition of immunological tolerance; loss of responsiveness to foreign antigens (Fig. 3) may be due to relocation of the responsible cells in peripheral lymphoid organs.[5]

Several explanations could account for the marked increase in reactivity of thymic cells to self antigens that occurs just after birth. The influence of thymic hormones upon immature cells, the antigenic effects of newly established intestinal flora, and the influence of maternal antigens or hormones present in the colostrum are all possibilities. Our data do not allow a selection from among these possibilities.

A number of recent studies have alluded to the capacity of thymocytes to recognize self antigens *in vitro* and *in vivo*. Llacer and Uyeki[12] reported that proliferation occurred in mixtures of authochthonous spleen and thymus cells from adult rats. Although their observation may be analogous to the ILI, this is not certain since they could not render the mixtures one-way reactive by irradiation. In addition, although proliferative activity at 44 hr was reported in their preliminary communication, no extended time study of the response was reported. Finally, the fact that these authors observed proliferation in mixtures of adult rat cells while we were unable to do so with adult mouse cells (Fig. 4) may reflect a species difference. This possibility is supported by the fact that adult rat thymus cells are also capable of recognizing allogeneic cellular antigens[13] whereas those of the CBA mouse cannot (Fig. 3).

Other instances have been reported of lymphoid cells being reactive when transferred into isogeneic hosts. For example, Playfair and Krsiakova[14] found that significant graft-versus-host reactions resulted when spleen cells from 2-month-old donors or thymus cells from 3-month-old donors were injected into isogeneic Balb/c or NZB recipients. In addition, Van Bekkum[15] has reported "isologous secondary disease" in irradiated mice receiving isogeneic bone marrow cells.

Although the specific antigen(s) responsible for the ILI has not yet been identified it is most likely that it belongs to the differentiation antigen category.[16] These antigens, which occur only on certain lymphoid cells within an individual, may also exhibit allelic variation and thus qualify as alloantigens. Indeed, the extent to which they contribute to allogeneic lymphocyte interactions is unknown.

Currently, we are attempting to define the antigenic basis of the ILI, identify the cause and function of the sudden burst of ILI activity in the post-natal thymus, and to demonstrate this self-recognition phenomenon in other *in vitro* and *in vivo* systems.

Abbreviations: ILI, Isogeneic lymphocyte interaction; S^a or T^a, adult spleen or thymus cells; S^n or T^n, neonatal spleen or thymus cells.

* Supported by Grants AI-04131 and AI-00307 from the National Institute of Allergy and Infectious Diseases, U.S. Public Health Service.

[1] Miller, J. F. A. P., and D. Osoba, *Physiol. Rev.*, **47,** 1 (1967).
[2] Davies, A. J. S., *Transplant. Rev.*, **1,** 92 (1969).
[3] White, A., and A. L. Goldstein, in CIBA Foundation Study Section: *Hormones and the Immune Response* (London: J. & A. Churchill, Ltd., 1970), in press.
[4] Sosin, H., H. Hilgard, and C. Martinez, *J. Immunol.*, **96,** 189 (1966).
[5] Goldstein, A., A. Guha, M. L. Howe, and A. White, in preparation.
[6] Knight, S. C., and G. J. Thorbecke, *Fed. Proc.*, **29,** 301 (1970).
[7] Moore, G. E., A. A. Sandberg, and K. Ulrich, *J. Nat. Can. Inst.*, **36,** 405 (1966).
[8] Robbins, J. H., P. G. Burk, and W. R. Levis, *Fed. Proc.*, **28,** 363 (1969).
[9] Bach, F. H., and N. K. Voynow, *Science*, **153,** 545 (1966).
[10] Howe, M. L., A. L. Goldstein, and J. R. Battisto, in *Proceedings of the 5th Annual Leukocyte Culture Conference*, 1970, in press.
[11] Burnet, F. M., *The Clonal Selection Theory of Acquired Immunity* (Cambridge University Press, 1959).
[12] Llacer, V., and E. M. Uyeki, *Intl. Arch. Allergy*, **35,** 88 (1969).
[13] Schwarz, M. R., *Immunology*, **10,** 281 (1966).
[14] Playfair, J. H. L., and M. Krsiakova, *Transplant.*, **7,** 443 (1969).
[15] Van Bekkum, D. W., *Brookhaven Symp. in Biology*, **20,** 190 (1967).
[16] Boyse, E. A. and L. J. Old, *Ann. Rev. Genetics*, **3,** 269 (1970).

Thymus Derived Lymphocytes and Their Function in Immunity

THYMUS ORIGIN OF LYMPHOCYTES REACTING AND STIMULATING REACTION IN MIXED LYMPHOCYTE CULTURES—STUDIES IN THE RAT

B. P. MACLAURIN

INTRODUCTION

Since the original description of blastic transformation in cultures of peripheral blood lymphocytes derived from genetically different human donors (Bain, Vas & Lowenstein, 1964), this reaction has been intensively investigated. It is now established that the mixed lymphocyte reaction (MLR) is a valid indicator of difference at one or more major histocompatibility loci between human lymphocyte donors (Amos, & Bach, 1968; Schellekens *et al.*, 1970). Silvers, Wilson & Palm (1967) have presented evidence which strongly suggests that in the rat, response in the MLR is similarly dependent upon difference between responding inbred rat strains determined by the major histocompatibility locus AgB.

Schwarz (1967, 1968) has reported several studies of the MLR in rats, using thymus spleen or lymph nodes as the source of the participating lymphocytes, but without assessment of reactivity between lymphocytes of different tissue origin. Wilson (1967), Wilson, Silvers & Nowell (1967) and Wilson, Blyth & Nowell (1968) have described similar and additional experiments, with extensive assessments of the optimal conditions necessary for rat lymphocyte culture, and evidence that lymphocytes responding in the MLR are thymus derived.

There is evidence in mice of antigenic difference between thymus derived and non-thymus-derived lymphocytes (Reif & Allen, 1964; Raff 1969) and Iversen (1970) has recently reported a similar conclusion from work on inbred rats using different techniques. It seemed possible that the extra antigen found upon the surface of thymus-derived lymphocytes might be relevant in the MLR, both for reaction to allogeneic cells and also for stimulation of this response.

The present report describes studies on the MLR in inbred rat strains using interstrain mixtures of thymocytes and thymocytes mixed with lymphocytes derived from different lymphoid organs. The evidence indicates a descending gradient of reactivity from thymus, to lymph node, to spleen, to bone marrow. Lymphocytes of mature animals previously subjected to neonatal thymectomy, show diminished or absent capacity to *stimulate* allogeneic thymocytes, thus suggesting a thymus origin for lymphocytes capable of stimulating as well as reacting in the mixed lymphocyte reaction.

METHODS

Inbred rats of the AS_2 and HS strains were used throughout. These strains are known to show histocompatibility differences determined by the major AgB histocompatibility locus (Heslop 1968). Lymphocyte suspensions were prepared from animals after complete exsanguination under ether anaesthesia, using the technique of needle aspiration of the abdominal aorta. Blood from both strains was pooled and the serum obtained was stored at $-20°C$.

The thymus, lymph nodes and spleen were removed aseptically, washed in Hanks' balanced salt solution to remove any adherent blood, and dissected free of fat and other tissue. The thymus and lymph nodes were separately minced with fine scissors in fresh Hanks' solution. The resulting cell suspensions were passed through fine nylon-gauze mesh and then centrifuged for 5 min at 1000 rev/min. After one further wash in Hanks' solution, cell viability was checked by the trypan blue method and the lymphocyte deposit was resuspended in culture medium at a concentration of 2×10^6 viable cells/ml. Cell suspensions from the spleen were prepared by gentle homogenization in Hanks' solution, using a simple pestle in a sterile glass tube. The cell suspension was then passed through nylon-gauze mesh and handled as for the thymus and lymph node preparations.

Bone marrow cell suspensions were obtained by washing out with Hanks' solution, the marrow space of the shaft of the femur on both sides. The bones were first dissected out asceptically. The marrow particles were gently homogenized as with the spleen and the resulting cell suspension was passed through two layers of nylon-gauze mesh prior to washing and resuspension in culture medium. Approximately one third of the marrow cells obtained in this way were small lymphocytes.

The culture medium used throughout was RPMI, supplemented with 10% foetal-calf serum and 10% pooled rat serum (used fresh or within 2–3 weeks of collection). For all experiments, white cell suspensions were cultured at a concentration of 2×10^6 per ml. They were grown in $3 \times \frac{1}{2}''$ capped glass tubes and were maintained for 4 days at 37°C in an atmosphere of 5% CO_2 95% air. Preliminary assessment had indicated that with these methods, response in mixed cultures was maximal at the 3rd and 4th day and fell off markedly by the sixth day of culture. Contrary to previous findings with medium 199, survival of unstimulated rat lymphocytes in RPMI supplemented as described, was found to be satisfactory at 4 days.

After preliminary morphological assessment of rat mixed lymphocyte cultures, all subsequent analysis of transformation potential was made on the basis of comparisons of tritiated thymidine incorporation into DNA for unmixed and mixed lymphocyte populations. All cultures received tritiated thymidine (0·5 μCi/ml—specific activity 150 mCi/mM) after 72 hr and were harvested 24 hr later. The method of processing and counting thymidine treated cultures was that described by Knight & Ling (1969).

Thymocytes from one strain were mixed in culture in equal numbers with lymphocytes from the other incompatible strain, these latter cells being derived either from thymus, lymph nodes, spleen or bone marrow. Control cultures of each lymphocyte suspension separately were set up for each experiment. All cultures were performed in triplicate and the results recorded are the means of triplicate counts. Syngeneic mixtures of lymphocytes of different tissue origin were also set up as additional controls for each experiment.

Where indicated in the text, neonatal thymectomy was performed on AS_2 animals within 24 hr of birth by a sternal split procedure under deep hypothermia, and application of suction for removal of the thymus. Histological assessment for completeness of removal was carried out at the time of killing. In sham thymectomized animals, the sternum was split under hypothermia but the thymus was left intact.

Rabbit anti-rat thymocyte serum was produced by five-weekly intravenous injections of 3×10^7 thymocytes. Serum was obtained 1 week later and after heat inactivation for 30 min at 56°C, it was repeatedly absorbed with washed rat red cells in the cold. The serum was administered to newborn AS_2 strain rats twice weekly by intraperitoneal injection in a dose of 1 ml for a total of seven injections. Lymphocyte suspensions were prepared from the treated animals 1 week later.

RESULTS

These are set out in Tables 1–3 and summarized in Fig. 1. In all experiments, maximal stimulation of ^{3}H tdr. incorporation was observed in mixed cultures of incompatible thymocytes, and least stimulation was found in cultures with bone-marrow lymphocytes. Thymocytes versus lymph node or spleen lymphocytes produced intermediate levels of stimulation. The same pattern and gradient of response was observed when cultures were made 'one way' by X-irradiation (1500 r) of the stimulating cell suspensions. As expected the stimulation factor after irradiation was more than halved for thymocyte-versus-thymocyte cultures but reduction was very much less in mixtures with other cell suspensions, possibly indicating that most of the increase in thymidine incorporation in the latter mixed cultures is a function of the thymocyte rather than the tissue lymphocytes; or that intact lymph node and spleen lymphocytes may have an inhibitory influence on thymocytes.

Interpretation of mixed cultures, with stimulation by lymphocytes of non-thymic origin was complicated by the fact that in autologous mixtures of tissue lymphocytes with thymocytes, mild but definite stimulations of ^{3}H tdr. incorporation was observed (Table 2). The net stimulation results shown in the Tables were obtained by subtraction of the autologous from the homologous stimulation values. Following X-irradiation of the stimulating cell suspensions, this non-allogeneic increased stimulation was largely eliminated but autologous mixtures then showed some reduction of observed as compared with expected counts, presumably as a consequence of cell death. Accordingly, it has still seemed desirable

TABLE 1. Stimulation of ^{3}H-thymidine incorporation by mixing thymocytes and allogeneic tissue lymphocytes

	Two-way (without irradiation)				One-way—by irradiation—1500 r— of *stimulating* lymphocytes from thymus, lymph node, spleen or bone marrow			
Mean DPM cultured separately	DPM in mixed culture	*Net DPM in mixed culture	Stimulation index (S.I.)	Mean S.I.	Mean DPM cultured separately	DPM in mixed culture	*Net DPM in mixed culture	Stimulation index (S.I.)	Mean S.I.

Mean DPM cultured separately	DPM in mixed culture	*Net DPM in mixed culture	Stimulation index (S.I.)	Mean S.I.	Mean DPM cultured separately	DPM in mixed culture	*Net DPM in mixed culture	Stimulation index (S.I.)	Mean S.I.
Thymus-versus-thymus									
162	4250	—	26		57	557	—	9·7	
423	6311	—	15		17	128	—	7·5	8·0
320	4480	—	13·4		91	610	—	6·7	
170	8430	—	47						
399	5696	—	14·2	24					
250	4787	—	20						
236	4021	—	18						
77	2060	—	28						
75	2732	—	38						

			Net S.I.	Mean Net S.I.				† Net S.I.	Mean Net S.I.
Thymus-versus-lymph node									
30	174	156	5·2		14	95	106	7·6	
157	1057	939	5·1	5·2	51	140	162	3·2	6·9
113	870	714	6·3		37	335	300	8·1	
142	715	610	4·3		92	829	796	8·6	
Thymus-versus-spleen									
162	655	621	3·8		14	62	42	3·0	
40	185	110	2·7	3·1	46	52	87	1·9	3·8
96	301	163	1·8		37	124	135	6·6	
55	331	253	4·6						
125	358	338	2·7						
Thymus-versus-bone marrow									
159	331	245	1·5		52	72	124	2·4	
104	213	197	1·9	1·6	73	34	119	1·6	1·6
107	458	171	1·5		20	50	49	2·4	
					45	47	0	0	

* Net DPM = count obtained—DPM increment in the corresponding *autologous* mixed culture (see Table 2)

† Net S.I. = stimulation index, i.e. $\frac{\text{net DPM in mixed culture}}{\text{mean DPM from same lymphocytes cultured separately}}$.

to subtract the autologous from the homologous stimulation values obtained to correct for this.

The stimulation indices for one way and two way mixed lymphocyte reactions are compared in Fig. 1. The gradient in stimulation capacity of lymphocytes from various sources is well seen. The low response by thymocytes to intact or irradiated spleen and bone marrow lymphocytes might be explained in part as due to contaminating red cells, polymorphs etc., but this objection does not apply to the lymph-node cell suspensions which were virtually free of non-lymphocytic elements.

TABLE 2. Stimulation of ^{3}H-thymidine incorporation by mixing thymocytes and **autologous** tissue lymphocytes

	Two-way (without irradiation)			One-way (after irradiation of lymph node, spleen or bone marrow lymphocytes)			
Mean DPM cultured separately	DPM in mixed culture	Stimulation index (S.I.)	Mean S.I.	Mean DPM cultured separately	DPM in mixed culture	Stimulation index (S.I)	Mean S.I.
Thymus-versus-lymph node							
9	12	1·3		42	20	0·5	
104	302	2·9		19	9	0·5	0·8
164	363	2·2	1·9	18	22	1·2	
100	138	1·4		52	54	1·0	
Thymus-versus-spleen							
122	133	1·1		45	10	0·2	
116	283	2·4		40	15	0·4	0·4
19	54	2·8	1·9	18	8	0·4	
60	125	2·1		49	34	0·7	
84	86	1·0					
Thymus-versus-bone marrow							
283	396	1·4		119	25	0·2	
83	123	1·5	2·1	70	14	0·2	0·6
153	538	3·5		51	55	1·1	
				13	14	1·1	

In an attempt to overcome this objection and to demonstrate in a different and more conclusive manner the role of thymus-derived lymphocytes in *stimulating* the mixed-lymphocyte reaction, experiments with anti-thymocyte serum treated animals and with neonatally-thymectomized animals were carried out.

The results of treatment with antithymocyte serum (ATS) proved rather inconclusive because the serum appeared to stimulate thymidine incorporation by lymphocytes from treated animals, independently of any allogeneic-lymphocyte stimulation. By subtraction of the values obtained with isogeneic-lymphocyte mixtures, it does appear that the stimulation index for intact thymocytes, versus lymphocytes from ATS treated animals has been moderately reduced. The results of one such experiment are shown in Table 3.

The results after neonatal thymectomy provide more definite evidence that thymus-derived lymphocytes are required to *stimulate* the mixed lymphocyte reaction since, after total thymectomy lymph-node lymphocytes showed diminished or absent capacity to stimulate intact allogeneic thymocytes (Table 3). Lymph-node lymphocytes from the thymectomized animals were not obtained until 5 weeks or more after operation, and at this time immunological maturation, at least in respect of skin-graft rejection times, is

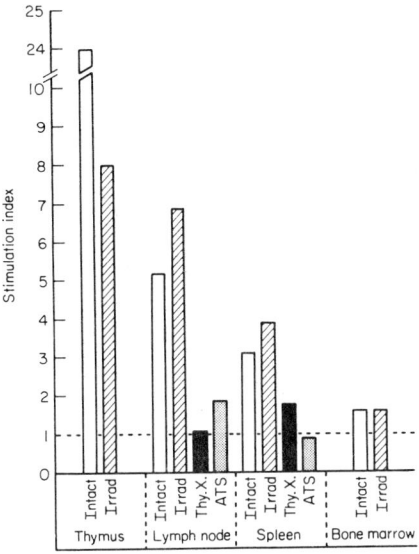

FIG. 1. Mean stimulation indexes: Mixed culture of normal thymocytes with allogeneic stimulating lymphocytes from thymus lymph node, spleen or bone marrow.

For all tissues except thymus, the stimulation index is net (see Tables 1 and 2). Irrad. = lymphocytes X-irradiated at dose of 1500 r. Thy. X. = lymphocytes from mature rats after neonatal thymectomy. ATS = lymphocytes from mature rat, treated with antithymocyte serum from birth.

known to be in the adult range (Heslop, 1969). If thymectomy was incomplete no depression of mixed lymphocyte response was observed.

When the MLR was made one way, by X-irradiation (1500 r) of the stimulating-lymphocytes derived from the complete neonatally-thymectomized group, partial restoration of stimulant capacity by these cells was observed in one experiment but not in a second experiment. No convincing explanation for this change in response can be given. It is similar in kind though different in magnitude to that observed with mixed cultures of thymocytes and X-irradiated lymph-node lymphocytes from intact animals.

DISCUSSION

The frequency with which mouse lymphocytes carrying the θ-thymus antigen marker can be detected in various lymphoid organs shows a gradient, with maximal numbers in thymus and thoracic duct (90–100%) and decreasing numbers in peripheral blood, lymph node, spleen and bone marrow in that order (Raff, 1969). A similar gradient has been demonstrated in rats by Iversen (1970), employing specific antisera against recirculating and non-recirculating lymphocytes.

TABLE 3. ³HTdr Incorporation after stimulation of normal allogeneic thymocytes with lymphocytes (lymph node or spleen) from mature rats after neonatal thymectomy or sham thymectomy, or anti-thymocyte serum from birth

Treatment of animal providing lymphocytes for *stimulation* (from lymph nodes or spleen)	Mean DPM cultured separately	DPM in mixed culture	Net DPM in mixed culture	Net stimulation index (S.I.)	Mean net S.I.
A. Complete Neonatal Thymectomy					
Thymus-versus-lymph node	255	1025	141	0·5	
	* 111	83	102	0·9	1·1
	163	306	327	2·0	
Thymus-versus-spleen	150	271	336	2·2	
	* 104	83	118	1·1	1·8
	105	209	221	2·2	
B. Incomplete neonatal thymectomy					
Thymus-versus-lymph node	190	1397	1427	7·5	
	* 36	287	289	8·0	7·7
Thymus-versus-spleen	158	75	344	2·1	
	* 37	137	148	4·0	3·0
C. Sham neonatal thymectomy					
Thymus-versus-lymph node	142	714	677	4·8	
	91	828	824	9·0	6·9
Thymus-versus-spleen	* 37	124	134	3·6	
	125	358	356	2·9	3·2
D. Anti-thymocyte serum†					
Thymus-versus-lymph node	402	1334	774	1·9	1·9
Thymus-versus-spleen	559	1041	493	0·9	0·9

* Indicates results in which responses made 'one way' by X-irradiaton (1500 r) of *stimulating* lymphocytes from spleen or lymph node.

† 1 ml of anti-thymocyte serum given twice weekly to neonatal recipient for 4 weeks, and lymphocytes obtained 1 week later.

The present paper shows that there is also a gradient from thymus, to lymph node, to spleen, to bone marrow in the degree to which these various lymphocyte populations will stimulate allogeneic rat thymocytes, in a two-way or one-way MLR. However this finding may partly have resulted from contamination of the lymphocyte suspensions from spleen and bone marrow with fairly large numbers of red cells and other cell types. Nonetheless the anti-thymocyte serum experiments described, tend to confirm that the gradient relates to the proportion of thymus-derived lymphocytes. The strongest supportive evidence of stimulation requirement for T cells (terminology of Roitt et al., 1969) is provided by the neonatal-thymectomy studies. Similar results in thymus-deprived dogs have been reported by Kisken & Swenson (1969), but in their study, thymectomy was performed 3 years previously on adult animals of uncertain genetic disparity.

Major histocompatibility antigens appear to be represented upon all lymphocytes and not just T cells and hence the diminished stimulation capacity by B lymphocytes requires explanation. Differences in metabolic activity between B and T cells might account for the diminution shown. In rats Iversen (1969) has shown a higher basal rate of RNA synthesis in the non-recirculating lymphocyte population. Part of the proliferative response of normal human lymphocytes on mixed culture with lymphoma cell line lymphocytes in a 'one way' reaction has been attributed to the state of metabolic activation of the lymphoma cells (Hardy, Ling & Knight, 1969); and a positive response can still be obtained in autochthonous mixtures of normal lymphocytes and cell lines derived a year previously from the same donor (Steel & Hardy, 1970).

Preliminary cultures of thymocytes mixed in equal proportions showed maximal thymidine incorporation between the third and fourth days, but it could be argued that these conditions of culture were not optimal for stimulation by lymphocytes from nodes, spleen or bone marrow. However, neonatal thymectomy drastically reduced their stimulation capacity, and it seems unlikely that alteration in culture conditions would have materially influenced the results.

As an alternative hypothesis, it is suggested that a supplementary, membrane-related antigen system expressed only on thymus passaged lymphocytes could modify the existing histocompatibility antigen display on the T cell surface, by a subtle, spatial, reorientation, significant for cellular recognition but not generating any additional antibody specificities. As a consequence, B cells might present an intact but relatively inactive set of histocompatibility antigens, resulting in diminished stimulation capacity in the MLR.

Bone-marrow-derived lymphocytes of mice and rats also carry an extra surface antigen not shared by T cells (Raff 1970; Iversen 1970). This antigen might additionally have a modifying influence upon the histocompatibility antigen display of B lymphocytes. Expression of the T cell antigen on thymus passaging lymphocytes might involve either deletion or concealment of the B antigen.

The further concept that recirculating lymphocytes may carry a more active histocompatibility antigen display than that possessed by other tissues is supported by the experiments of Guttman, Lindquist & Ochner (1969). They showed that most of the immunogenic properties of rat kidney, transplanted between histoincompatible strains, resided in the contained lymphoid cells rather than the renal tissue itself. A similar conclusion can be drawn from the rat experiments described by Elkins (1964), who reported that local graft-versus-host reactions in the kidney were absent if recipient animals were first depleted of lymphocytes by preliminary lethal irradiation.

Lack of stimulant function by B lymphocytes in the MLR may partly explain the absence of maternal response to foetal lymphocytes and avoidance of host-versus-graft reaction against the foetus. Tissues of non-lymphoid origin appear to have only limited capacity to stimulate allogeneic lymphocytes (Hardy & Ling, 1969).

The increased thymidine incorporation found in autologous mixtures, appears to be a response of B lymphocytes to contact with thymocytes and is eliminated by prior X-irradiation of the non-thymic cells. It may indicate a relative paucity of T compared to

B lymphocytes in the rat bone-marrow environment, and supplementation may enable B lymphocyte response to circulating antigen in the serum used for medium supplementation.

ACKNOWLEDGMENTS

I am greatly indebted to Dr N. R. Ling and Professor P. G. H. Gell of the Department of Experimental Pathology, University of Birmingham for their encouragment and suggestions in this study and for provision of facilities and staff. The inbred rat strains used were generously made available by Mr N. Nisbet, Director of the Salt Research Centre at Oswestry. I am grateful to Mrs Frances Levy for technical assistance. The work was carried out during the tenure of a Nuffield Foundation Travelling Fellowship in Medicine while on sabbatical leave from the University of Otago Medical School.

REFERENCES

AMOS, D.B. & BACH, F.H. (1968) Phenotypic expressions of the major histocompatibility locus in man (HLA): leukocyte antigens and mixed leukocyte culture reactivity. *J. exp. Med.*, **128**, 623.

BAIN, B., VAS. M.R. & LOWENSTEIN, L. (1964) The development of large immature mononuclear cells in mixed leukocyte cultures. *Blood*, **23**, 108.

ELKINS, W.L. (1964) Invasion and destruction of homologous kidney by locally inoculated lymphoid cells. *J. exp. Med.*, **120**, 329.

GUTTMAN, R.D., LINDQUIST, R.R. & OCHNER, S.A. (1969) Renal transplantation in the inbred rat. IX. Hematopoietic origin of an immunogenic stimulus of rejection. *Transplantation*, **8**, 472.

HARDY, D.A. & LING, N.R. (1969) Effects of some cellular antigens on lymphocytes and the nature of the mixed lymphocyte reaction. *Nature (Lond.)*, **221**, 545.

HARDY, D.A., LING, N.R. & KNIGHT, S.C. (1969) Exceptional lymphocyte stimulating capacity of cells from lymphoid cell lines. *Nature (Lond.)*, **223**, 511.

HESLOP, B.F. (1968) Histocompatibility antigens in the rat: the AS2 strain in relation to the AS, BS and HS strains. *Aust. J. exp. Biol. med. Sci.* **46**, 479.

HESLOP, B.F. (1969) Maturation of histocompatibility antigens and host reactivity in the rat. *Transplantation Proceedings*, **1**, 560.

IVERSEN, J.G. (1970) Specific antisera against recirculating and non-recirculating lymphocytes in the rat. *Clin. exp. Immunol.*, **6**, 101.

KISKEN, W.A., SWENSON, N.A. (1969) Unresponsiveness of mixed lymphocyte cultures from thymectomized adult dogs. *Nature (Lond.)*, **224**, 76.

KNIGHT, S. & LING, N.R. (1969) A comparison of the responses of lymphocytes from blood, spleen thymus and appendix of rabbits of different ages to stimulation *in vitro* with staphylococcal filtrate. *Clin. exp. Immunol.* **4**, 667.

RAFF, M.C. (1969) Theta isoantigen as a marker of thymus-derived lymphocytes in mice. *Nature (Lond.)*, **224**, 378.

RAFF, M.C. (1970) Preliminary studies with an anti-lymphocytic serum specific for thymus-independent mouse lymphocytes. Paper read to the October meeting of the British Society for Immunology.

REIF, A.E. & ALLEN, J.M.V. (1964) The AKR thymic antigen and its distribution in leukemias and nervous tissues. *J. exp. Med.* **120**, 413.

ROITT, I.M., GREAVES, M.F., TORRIGIANI, G., BROSTOFF, J. & PLAYFAIR, J.H.L. (1969) The cellular basis of immunological responses. A synthesis of some current views. *Lancet*, **ii**, 367.

SCHELLEKENS, P.TH.A., VRIESENDORP, B., EIJSVOOGEL, V.P., VAN LEENWEN, A., VAN ROOD, J.J., MIGGIANO, V. & CEPELLINI, R. (1970) Lymphocyte transformation *in vitro*. II. Mixed lymphocyte culture in relation to leucocyte antigens. *Clin. exp. Immunol.* **6**, 241.

SCHWARZ, M.R. (1967) Transformation of rat small lymphocytes with allogeneic lymphoid cells. *Amer. J. Anat.* **121**, 559.

SCHARZ, M.R. (1968) The mixed lymphocyte reaction: an *in vitro* rest for tolerance. *J. exp. Med.* **127**, 879.

SILVERS, W.K., WILSON, D.B. & PALM, J. (1967) Mixed leukocyte reactions and histocompatibility in rats. *Science*, **155**, 703.

STEEL, C.M. & HARDY, D.A. (1970) Evidence of altered antigenicity in cultured lymphoid cells from patients with infectious mononucleosis. *Lancet*, i, 1322.

WILSON, D.B. (1967) Quantitative studies on the mixed lymphocyte interaction in rats. I. Conditions and parameters of response. *J. exp. Med.* **126,** 625.

WILSON, D.B., SILVERS, W.K. & NOWELL, P.C. (1967) Quantitative studies on the mixed lymphocyte interaction in rats. II. Relationship of the proliferative response to the immunologic status of the donors. *J. exp. Med.* **126,** 655.

WILSON, D.B., BLYTH, J.L. & NOWELL, P.C. (1968) Quantitative studies on the mixed lymphocyte interaction in rats. III. Kinetics of the response. *J. exp. Med.* **128,** 1157.

Capacity of Thymic Cells to Effect Target Cell Lysis Following Treatment with Concanavalin A [1]

L. STAVY, A. J. TREVES, AND M. FELDMAN

INTRODUCTION

Antibody production to a wide range of antigens was shown to involve cooperation between thymus and bone marrow-derived cells (1–5). Cellular immunity was likewise claimed to be based on a bicellular interaction (6–10). Although the determination of the effector cell in cellular immunity is still unclear, there is mounting evidence that it may be the thymus cell population (11, 12). To analyze certain aspects of cell cooperation in graft reaction, an *in vitro* system for the primary induction of cellular immunity was employed in our laboratory (13, 14). In this system rat lymphocytes were sensitized by mouse fibroblasts. The sensitized cells underwent blast transformation and acquired the capacity to lyse mouse fibroblasts. When rat thymus cells were interacted with mouse fibroblasts, however, blast transformation occurred but the transformed cells were by themselves hardly capable of lysing the mouse fibroblasts. It was necessary to admix these cells with nonsensitized rat spleen cells, or with spleens of animals previously exposed to irradiation and repopulated with bone marrow cells, to obtain a significant lysis. It was shown that the immunological specificity of this lytic reaction is determined by the antigens stimulating the thymic cells (15, 16). Hence, thymus cells do appear to recognize mouse transplantation antigens.

In a parallel study we demonstrated that concanavalin A (con A), a protein possessing two sugar-binding sites per molecule (17–21), confers cytolytic activity to lymph node cells interacting with fibroblasts (22). This cytotoxicity is expressed in a manner which is indistinguishable from the lysis caused by lymphocytes sensi-

---

[1] This work was supported by a grant from the Max and Ida Hillson Foundation, New York, and by the Freudenberg Foundation for Research on Multiple Sclerosis, Weinheim, Germany.

tized on a monolayer (antigenic sensitization). It was deduced from these experiments that the capacity to effect cellular cytotoxicity is an inherent property of lymph node cells, the expression of which is triggered by an antigen as well as by con A. In the present study we test whether thymus cells also possess an inherent capacity to effect lysis of target cells which can be manifested by con A.

MATERIALS AND METHODS

Animals. Inbred Lewis/Mai rats, outbred Wistar rats, and inbred C3H/eb mice were obtained from the Weizmann Institute Animal Breeding Center.

Preparation of fibroblast monolayers. Primary monolayer cultures of embryonic fibroblasts were prepared from 13–15-day-old embryos. The fibroblasts were grown in 100 mm plastic tissue culture dishes (Falcon) in Waymouth's medium supplemented with 5% calf serum. Primary monolayers were trypsinized on day 7–9, collected, suspended in lactalbumin hydrolysate in Earle's saline (LA) and were then replated in new culture dishes. Four to five days later the above procedure was repeated; this time the fibroblasts were suspended in LA at a concentration of 0.75×10^6 cells/ml. Four milliliters of this suspension were plated in 60 mm tissue culture dishes and 1 ml was plated in 35 mm dishes. The plates were then X-irradiated at 2000 R to prevent further cell replication. All cultures were kept at 37° in a humidified incubator with an inflow of 10% CO_2 in air. A detailed description of the procedure is given in previous publications (13, 14, 23).

Preparation of ^{51}Cr-labeled fibroblast monolayers (test monolayers). The medium in the 35 mm dishes was replaced immediately following irradiation with 1 ml of LA containing 1 μCi/ml of ^{51}Cr–Na_2CrO_4 (Radiochemical Center, Amersham). After 24 hr the radioactive medium was in turn replaced with 1.5 ml of unlabeled LA. The monolayers were used 3–5 days after labeling.

Preparation of lymphocytes and thymocytes. The cells were obtained from 2.5–3-month-old female Lewis rats which were ether-anesthetized and bled from the eye. The lymph nodes and the thymus were collected in sterile phosphate-buffered saline (PBS), pH 7.2. Fat and fasciae were trimmed from them and the cells were teased out by forceps, counted, centrifuged and resuspended in Eagle's medium supplemented with 15% horse serum (EM). The horse serum was obtained from Grand Island Biological Co.

Cell suspensions were plated in culture dishes—30×10^6 cells in 4 ml medium in 60 mm dishes and $3-5 \times 10^6$ cells in 1.5 ml in 35 mm dishes. Culture medium in dishes kept for more than 4 days was changed on the third day.

Preparation of bone marrow cells. Bone marrow cells were obtained by washing out the contents of the humerus and the femur with PBS. The rest of the procedure is the same as described for lymph node cells. The numbers of bone marrow cells quoted in this paper represent the number of nucleated cells obtained after treatment with Türk's solution.

Assay of cytolysis. Injury to fibroblasts was determined by the percentage of ^{51}Cr released from the monolayers into the culture medium. The medium was collected in counting tubes after gentle agitation of the plates. The remaining monolayer was washed once with 1.5 ml of PBS and combined with the original medium. The monolayers were then incubated with 1.5 ml 0.6% trypsin for 1 hr at

37° with continuous shaking, after which the plates were washed with 1.5 ml PBS and the wash combined with the original trypsinized monolayer in the counting tubes. The tubes were counted in an Autogamma Spectrometer (Packard). Cytolysis is expressed as the percent of ^{51}Cr released into the test culture medium, as compared to the total amount of ^{51}Cr in the culture (monolayer plus medium). In each experiment the spontaneous release of ^{51}Cr from intact monolayers was determined and these values were subtracted from the experimental results. All measurements were carried out in triplicate. The detailed procedure has been described elsewhere (13, 14, 23).

RESULTS

The capacity of freshly prepared lymph node, thymus and bone marrow cells to mediate cytotoxicity when plated directly on labeled test monolayers is presented in Fig. 1. The results demonstrate that insignificant lysis is obtained with nontreated lymph node cells, whereas con A-treated lymph node cells show considerable lytic capacity. On the other hand, thymus or bone marrow cells, either treated or nontreated with con A, do not manifest lytic capacity. In experiments similar to the one described in Fig. 1, no significant lysis was detected when bone marrow or thymus cells were treated with 1, 5, 10 or 25 µg/ml of con A.

The lytic capacity of con A-treated rat lymph node, bone marrow and thymus cells following sensitization on monolayers of mouse fibroblasts is shown in Fig. 2. Lymph node and bone marrow cells were incubated on C3H fibroblast monolayers for 5 days while thymus cells were incubated for 6 days. All 3 groups of cells were transferred to C3H monolayers, and lysis was measured in the presence or absence

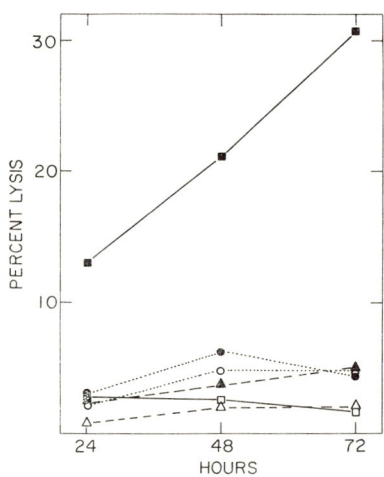

FIG. 1. The effect of con A on the rate of lysis of lymph node, bone marrow and thymus cells. 4 × 10⁶ Lewis lymph node cells □——□, bone marrow cells ○---○, or thymus cells △---△ were cultured directly on C3H test monolayers. Con A was added to several of the plates (■, ▲, ●). Percent lysis was measured after 24, 48 and 72 hr of incubation.

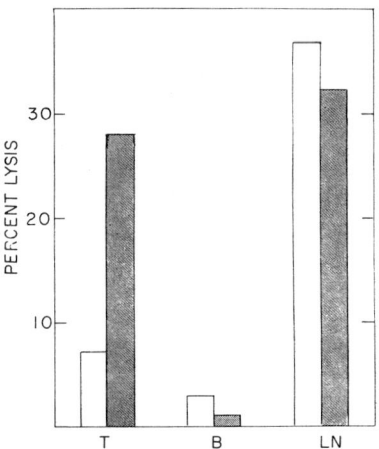

FIG. 2. The effect of con A on the rate of lysis of antigenically sensitized cells. 30×10^6 Lewis lymph node cells (LN), bone marrow cells (B) or thymus cells (T) were cultured on C3H fibroblast monolayers. On the 5th day the lymph node cells and the bone marrow cells were collected and 3.5×10^6 cells were cultured on C3H test monolayers. The thymus cells were collected and cultured on the 6th day. Percent lysis was measured 24 hr later. White bars—no con A added to the test monolayers; dark bars—50 μg/ml con A added to the test monolayers.

of con A. While lymph node cells in the absence of con A caused the release of over 30% of the ^{51}Cr, thymus cells caused the release of only 7%. However, in the presence of con A the release of ^{51}Cr by thymus cells reached 28%. The rate of lysis mediated by bone marrow cells was under 3%, which is below statistical significance. Thus, after a period of interacting with fibroblast monolayers and then with con A, lymph node and thymus cells can mediate cytotoxicity while bone marrow cells cannot. As shown in an earlier work (22), lysis mediated by antigenically sensitized lymph node cells is almost unaffected by con A added during lysis.

The picture obtained in Fig. 2 differs from the one in Fig. 1; thymic cells sensitized on mouse fibroblasts respond to con A by lysing the target cells (Fig. 2), whereas thymus cells which were not sensitized, do not lyse these target cells when treated with con A (Fig. 1). This difference should be related to the changes occurring in the lymphoid cell population during sensitization. The number of lymph node and thymus cells decreased considerably during this period. The changes in population size, as a function of incubation time under the conditions employed here, have been described previously (13, 22, 23). It was found that when thymus and lymph-node cell populations are plated on a fibroblast monolayer they first decrease (the loss of thymus cells is greater than that of lymph node cells) and then increase (lymph node cells from Day 4 on and thymus cells from Day 5 on) as a result of proliferation of the surviving sensitized cells. The cytolytic capacity of the transformed, sensitized thymus cells which were selected during 6 days of culture, is different from the original cell population.

It has been suggested that the thymus cells determine the immunospecificity of cellular immune reactions (15). Accordingly, experiments were conducted to test whether the con A-induced lysis of sensitized thymus cells is antigenically specific. Thymus cells were incubated for 6 days on one type of monolayer and their capacity to mediate cytotoxicity to monolayers of different antigenic composition was assayed. Lack of immunospecificity was observed in all the combinations tested (Table 1).

The lack of lytic capacity of bone marrow cells described in Fig. 1 could be attributed to the possibility that only a very small fraction of this population is capable of effecting lysis. Therefore, the experiments described in Figs. 1 and 2 were repeated with higher concentrations of cells (up to 6×10^6 nucleated cels per test culture). However, the rate of lysis was essentially the same for all the different cell numbers tested. Hence, it appears that lymphoid cells within the bone marrow population cannot mediate cytotoxicity. It could be argued that the presence of other cell types inhibit the lytic action of the bone marrow lymphocytes. To test this, lymph node and bone marrow cells were mixed in equal proportions and then seeded onto fibroblast monolayers. After 5 days the cytolytic capacity of the mixture was compared with the capacity of the lymph node and bone marrow cells, again in the presence or absence of con A. The results (Table 2) rule out the possibility that the cytolytic capacity of lymphocytes is severely impaired by bone marrow cells. Taken together, the experiments performed in this study indicate that the cells residing in the bone marrow are incapable of effecting lysis.

DISCUSSION

Con A causes transformation of lymph node cells as well as of thymus cells within 48 hr. Nevertheless, only con A-treated lymph node cells demonstrated significant lysis, once more indicating that transformation itself does not necessarily lead to acquisition of lytic capacity (24). Effector cells in the thymus cell population were observed only after the original population had undergone a process of sensitization and selection of fibroblast monolayers. The population of thymus cells

TABLE 1

Nonspecific Lysis of Target Cells by Con A-Treated Thymus Cells

Type of monolayer		Percent lysis	
Sensitizing [b]	Test [c]	Untreated	Con A-treated (50 µg/ml)
C3H	C3H	11.2	24.2
	Wistar	7.0	25.8
	Lewis	9.7	34.2
Wistar	C3H	13.5	26.8
	Wistar	13.0	23.0

[a] Measured 48 hr after transfer to test monolayers.
[b] Lewis thymus cells were cultured on either C3H or Wistar sensitizing monolayers for 6 days.
[c] On the 6th day the cells were collected and 3×10^6 cells were transferred to either C3H, Lewis or Wistar test monolayers.

TABLE 2

TARGET CELL LYSIS MEDIATED BY A MIXTURE OF LYMPH NODE AND BONE MARROW CELLS

Origin of cells[a]	Percent lysis[b]	
	Untreated	Con A-treated (50 μg/ml)
Bone marrow	1.6	1.6
Bone marrow + lymph node	24.6	21.2
Lymph node	38.6	37.2

[a] 15×10^6 bone marrow cells and 15×10^6 lymph node cells were cultured on sensitizing monolayers in the presence or absence of 50 μg/ml of con A. On the 5th day the cells were collected and 3×10^6 cells were transferred to each test monolayer.

[b] Measured 24 hr after transfer to test monolayer.

manifesting lysis on Day 6 was in fact derived from a very small number of cells. It appears that the intact population of thymus cells contains a relatively small number of potential effector cells. The percent of these cells increases *in vitro* as a result of a higher selective value of the potential effector cells. Thymus effector cells do, however, differ from lymph node effector cells in their inability to cause lysis in the absence of con A. Mouse fibroblast antigens can trigger lysis in lymph node cells but they are incapable of doing so to thymus cells even when the latter are selected on an antigenic monolayer. This implies that antigenically sensitized thymus cells, although inherently capable of fibroblast lysis, by themselves lack the capacity to respond to the antigenic signal.

REFERENCES

1. Taylor, R. B., *Transplant. Rev.* **1**, 114, 1969.
2. Miller, J. F. A. P., and Mitchell, G. F., *Transplant. Rev.* **1**, 3, 1969.
3. Davies, A. J. S., *Transplant. Rev.* **1**, 43, 1969.
4. Claman, N. H., and Chaperon, E. A., *Transplant. Rev.* **1**, 92, 1969.
5. Talmage, D. W., Radovich, J., and Hemmingsen, H., *Advan. Immunol.* **12**, 271, 1970.
6. Argyris, B. F., *Transplantation* **8**, 538, 1969.
7. Cantor, H., and Asofsky, R. J., *J. Exp. Med.* **131**, 235, 1970.
8. Globerson, A., and Auerbach, R. E., *J. Exp. Med.* **126**, 223, 1967.
9. Barchillon, J., and Gershon, R. K., *Nature* **227**, 71, 1970.
10. Abdou, N. J., and Richter, M., *Advan. Immunol.* **12**, 202, 1970.
11. Cerottini, J. C., Nordin, A. A., and Brunner, K. T., *Nature* **227**, 72, 1970.
12. Lonai, P., Clark, W. R., and Feldman, M., *Nature* **229**, 566, 1971.
13. Ginsburg, H., Immunology **14**, 621, 1968.
14. Berke, G., Ax, W., Ginsburg, H., and Feldman, M., *Immunology* **16**, 643, 1969.
15. Lonai, P., and Feldman, M. *Transplantation* **10**, 372, 1970.
16. Lonai, P., and Feldman, M., *Transplantation* **11**, 446, 1971.
17. Summer, J. B., Gralen, N., and Eriksson-quensel, I. B., *J. Biol. Chem.* **125**, 45, 1938.
18. Goldstein, I. J., Hollerman, C. E., and Merrick, J. M., *Biochim. Biophys. Acta* **97**, 68, 1965.
19. So, L. L., Goldstein, I. J., *Biochim. Biophys. Acta* **165**, 398, 1968.
20. So, L. L., and Goldstein, I. J., *Immunology* **99**, 158, 1967.
21. Yariv, J., Kalb, A. J., and Levitzki, A., *Biochim. Biophys. Acta* **165**, 303, 1968.
22. Stavy, L., Treves, A. J., and Feldman, M., *Nature* **232**, 56, 1971.
23. Berke, G., Yagil, G., Ginsburg, H., and Feldman, M., *Immunology* **17**, 723, 1969.
24. Perlmann, P., Nilsson, H., and Leon, M. A., *Science* **168**, 1112, 1970.

Cell-Mediated Immune Response *In Vitro*:
II. The Role of Thymus and Thymus-Derived Lymphocytes [1]

HERMANN WAGNER, ALAN W. HARRIS AND MARC FELDMANN

INTRODUCTION

The sequence of events in the cell-mediated immune response to tissue antigens is less well understood than in the humoral response, chiefly due to the lack of sensitive assay methods and experimental models. In the humoral system there is clear evidence that the effector cells (antibody-producing cells) are immediate descendants of bone marrow-derived (B) lymphocytes (1). On the other hand, evidence is accumulating from *in vivo* studies that in cellular immune responses to allografts, the specific effector cells are thymus derived (T) lymphocytes (2–4).

[1] This work was supported by grants from National Health and Medical Research Council, Canberra, Australia, the Australian Research Grants Commission, and the National Institute of Allergy and Infectious Diseases (AI-0-3958) to Professor G. J. V. Nossal. This is publication No. 1591 from the Walter and Eliza Hall Institute of Medical Research.

Recently, methods for obtaining cell-mediated immune responses *in vitro* have become available (5–7). For an *in vitro* response to xenogeneic cells it has been reported that thymocytes alone do not differentiate into effector cells (8) in contrast to thymocytes cultured together with spleen cells or bone marrow-derived cells (9). These results obtained in a xenograft system are clearly at variance with those obtained from *in vivo* allograft situations (2–4).

We have approached the question of the independent differentiation of thymocytes into cytotoxic effector cells by using an *in vitro* allograft system for the generation of a cell-mediated immune response (7). The technique is modeled on a one-way mixed lymphocyte reaction, performed in modified Marbrook–Diener culture flasks. This communication describes experiments which demonstrate that in mouse spleen cells, the precursors of cytotoxic lymphocytes, and the effector cells themselves, are thymus-derived (T) cells. Furthermore, it was found that thymocytes alone when immunized *in vitro* give rise to killer cells, no cooperation with bone marrow-derived cells being necessary. Of the various lymphoid cell populations tested, cortisone-resistant thymocytes and purified splenic T cells were the most active source of precursor cells.

MATERIALS AND METHODS

Animals. CBA/H-Wehi, BALB/c, (CBA × BALB/c) F1, C57 BL, and A/J mice of both sexes, 50–100 days of age were used. CBA thymocyte suspensions were prepared from female CBA mice, age 35–55 days.

Cell suspensions. Mice were killed by cervical dislocation. The spleen, thymus, or axillary and inguinal lymph nodes were excised under aseptic conditions, minced and strained through an 80-gauge stainless-steel sieve into cold culture medium. Care was taken to avoid the removal of mediastinal lymph nodes together with the thymus. To remove cell clumps, the cell suspensions were placed in a conical tube over 1 ml of fetal calf serum (FCS) obtained from Commonwealth Serum Laboratories, Parkville, Australia, for 5 min at 4° (10). The supernatant fraction, a single-cell suspension was then taken and its viability determined by the eosin dye-exclusion method (11).

Culture medium. Eagle's minimal essential medium with nonessential amino acids (Grand Island Biological Co., Grand Island, NY, Catalog No. F-15) was used. This was supplemented with 100 units/ml of penicillin G, 100 μg/ml of streptomycin, and 5% FCS, and buffered with sodium bicarbonate.

Tissue culture. The *in vitro* allograft system used is basically a one-way mixed lymphocyte reaction in which CBA mouse lymphocytes are cultured together with mitomycin C-treated allogeneic BALB/c lymphocytes. The conditions were previously described in detail (7). The culture technique used is based on that described by Marbrook (12), Diener and Armstrong (13), as recently modified by Wagner and Feldmann (7).

Usually 60 × 10^6 viable CBA lymphocytes (either spleen cells or thymus cells) were mixed with 15 × 10^6 viable mitomycin C-treated BALB/c spleen cells (30 min at 37° at a final concentration of 40 μg/ml) in 3 ml of medium and placed in a glass tube sealed off by a dialysis membrane and suspended from the stopper of an Erlenmeyer flask containing tissue culture medium. Cultures were incubated in a humidified incubator at 37° gassed with 10% CO_2 in air for various periods of time. In this system maximal cell proliferation as measured by ^{3}H-thymidine incorporation occurred between Day 3 and Day 4 of culture (7). However, maximal cytotoxicity against BALB/c allogantigens ($H2^d$) of lymphocytes immunized *in vitro* occurred at Day 6. Since it was demonstrated that mitomycin C-treated BALB/c spleen cells do not survive for 6 days in culture (7), all viable cells remaining after 6 days are assumed to be of CBA origin.

Cytotoxicity Assay

Source of target cells. As BALB/c and DBA/2 mice are of the same H-2 specificity ($H-2^d$) most of the cytotoxicity tests were performed using the DBA/2 mastocytoma P815X2 line (14) as target cells. These cells were cultured in Dulbecco's fortified Eagle's medium (FEM, Grand Island Biological Co.) with 10% fetal calf serum and were harvested during the exponential growth phase. In some experiments inguinal and axillary lymph node cells of BALB/c, C57 BL, and A/J mice were used as target cells.

Labeling of target cells. Target cells ($3-5 \times 10^6$) in 1 ml of FEM, supplemented with 15% heat-inactivated FCS were incubated with 100 μCi of ^{51}Cr-chromate (CEA, Gif-Sur-Yvette, France) for 30 min at 37° in a plastic petri dish (35×10 mm, Falcon Plastics Inc., Los Angeles). The dish was placed in an airtight box, gassed with 10% CO_2 in air and placed on a rocking platform. Afterward the cells were washed twice and adjusted to 5×10^5 viable cells/ml.

Assay. The radiochromium release assay was performed as described previously (7). Briefly, cells were harvested from the tissue cultures, washed twice, and their viability determined by eosin dye exclusion. Mixtures of cultured lymphocytes and labeled target cells were incubated on a rocking platform in an atmosphere of 10% CO_2 in air at 37°. The cells were then transferred into a plastic tube with 1 drop of 25% sheep erythrocytes and centrifuged for 5 min at 600g. The pellet and supernatant fluid were counted separately in automatic well-type gamma radiation counter. Each determination was set up in triplicate. The results were expressed as percentage of the maximal ^{51}Cr-release, which was determined by freezing and thawing 5×10^4 ^{51}Cr-labeled target cells.

Irradiation. Six- to nine-week-old (CBA × BALB/c) F1 mice of either sex were exposed to total body irradiation in a Phillips RT 250 machine. The dose used was 750-800 rad to midpoint with maximum scatter at 15 mA and half-value layer of 0.8 mm Cu.

Immunization of thymocytes in vivo by a graft versus host reaction. F1 (CBA × BALB/c) mice were lethally irradiated (750-800 rad) and within 3 hr injected i.v. with 10^8 CBA thymocytes. At various times, the animals were killed, the spleens removed, and single cell suspensions prepared.

Preparation of cortisone-resistant CBA thymocytes. Female CBA mice 35- to 55-days old were injected ip. with 1.5 mg cortisone acetate suspended in phosphate-buffered saline. Twenty-four hours later, the thymuses were removed under sterile conditions and a single cell suspension prepared. Corticosteroid injection resulted in a 75-85% depletion of thymus lymphocytes.

Preparation of thymus-derived (T) cells from the spleen. An enriched splenic T cell population was prepared according to the column-adherence technique of Basten et al. (15). This technique is based upon the fact that bone marrow (B)-derived lymphocytes have a receptor for antigen antibody complexes on their surface. Thus, under appropriate conditions, antibody-coated B cells in a spleen cell population will adhere to antigen-coated glass beads in a column, whereas T cells will not. The recovery of T cells in the filtrate fraction was usually 20–30% of total cells, which corresponds to 50–80% of T cells.

Complement-dependent cytotoxic tests for θ-positive lymphocytes. Viable lymphocytes ($50-100 \times 10^6$) were suspended in 1 ml of AKR anti-θ C_3H serum (diluted 1:2 with Dulbecco's phosphate-buffered saline) and incubated for 30 min at 37°. The cells were washed once through FCS and resuspended in 1.5 ml of agarose-absorbed (16) guinea pig serum (final dilution 1:4). After incubation for an additional 30 min at 37°, the cells were twice washed and were either cultured or assayed for cell-mediated cytotoxicity.

RESULTS

Nature of the Cytotoxic Effector Cells

Discrimination between T and B cells using the θ antigen marker. We have previously reported (7) that when CBA mouse spleen cells ($H-2^k$) are cultured *in vitro* together with mitomycin C-treated BALB/c spleen cells ($H-2^d$), cell-mediated cytotoxic activity is demonstrable against ^{51}Cr-labeled target cells of $H-2^d$ specificity (7). The maximal immune response occurred at Day 6 of culture when started with 60×10^6 lymphocytes plus $15-20 \times 10^6$ mitomycin C-treated allogeneic cells. Since the spleen contains a mixture of different lymphoid cell populations, it was necessary to establish whether the cytotoxic lymphocytes were thymus-derived (T) cells, or bone marrow-derived (B) cells. A pool of CBA spleen cells was divided into three parts. One part was treated with AKR anti θ C_3H serum and complement, a second part treated with normal AKR serum plus complement, and the third part remained untreated. All three samples were then cultured with mitomycin C-treated BALB/c spleen cells for 6 days. Cells were harvested, washed twice, and their cytotoxic activity determined at various ratios of lymphocytes to target cells for 150 min. Treatment with normal AKR serum did not diminish the cytotoxic activity of the cultured cells (Table 1), whereas anti θ serum abolished the cytotoxic activity of CBA spleen. Thus θ-bearing cells were necessary for the generation of "killer" activity *in vitro*.

To determine the nature of the effector cells in CBA spleen, spleen cells were cultured for 6 days with mitomycin C-treated BALB/c spleen cells. The cells were harvested, washed, counted, and divided into three parts. One part was treated with AKR anti-θ C_3H serum plus complement, one part with normal AKR serum plus complement, while the rest remained untreated. As shown in Table 2, anti-θ treatment abolished the cytotoxic activity, whereas normal AKR serum did not. This demonstrates that cytotoxic effector cells possess the surface antigen marker θ, and are thus thymus-derived lymphocytes.

The generation of cytotoxic activity from thymus cells. Experiments were performed to determine whether thymus cells, in the absence of other lymphoid cells, could differentiate into cytotoxic lymphocytes. Sixty million viable normal CBA

TABLE 1

Effect of AKR Anti-θ C3H Serum on the Capacity of CBA Spleen Cells to Generate Cytotoxic Lymphocytes[a]

Ratio lymphocytes to target cells	Not treated	AKR anti-θ serum plus complement	AKR serum plus complement
	% Lysis (± SEM)	% Lysis (± SEM)	% Lysis (± SEM)
100:1	100 ± 3	1 ± 4	100 ± 2
25:1	100 ± 5	0	99 ± 3
5:1	60 ± 3	0.5 ± 3	54 ± 4

[a] A pool of CBA spleen cells was divided into three parts, one remained untreated, one was treated with AKR anti-θ C3H serum plus complement (Methods), and one with AKR serum plus complement. In three different sets of cultures, the cells were immunized *in vitro* against H-2^d antigens. At Day 6, cells were harvested and assayed for cytotoxicity at various ratios for 150 min. Nonspecific lysis was subtracted.

mouse thymocytes were cultured with 15×10^6 mitomycin C-treated BALB/c spleen cells for 6 days. Cells were harvested, washed twice, and counted. Viability ranged between 10 and 20% of the initial cell concentration. Since mitomycin C-treated BALB/c spleen cells do not survive for 6 days in culture (7), these viable cells were of CBA thymus origin. Cytotoxic activity was clearly demonstrable when the cultured cells were assayed against ^{51}Cr-labeled mastocytoma target cells (H-2^d) (Table 3). Even at a lymphocyte-to-target cell ratio as low as 12 to 1, almost 100% lysis occurred within the assay time of 150 min.

The capacity of cortisone-resistant thymocytes to generate cytotoxic activity in vitro. Cortical thymocytes are destroyed *in vivo* by corticosteroids more readily than are medullary thymocytes (17, 18). Thus, the administration of corticosteroids causes within 12–48 hr a relative enrichment of medullary thymocytes (19). To investigate whether the precursors of cytotoxic lymphocytes predominantly exist in the medulla of the thymus, cells from the thymuses of cortisone-treated CBA mice prepared as described in Materials and Methods were tested for responsiveness to H-2^d antigens *in vitro* under the same conditions as the previous experiments with spleen cells. After 6 days the viability ranged between 15 and

TABLE 2

Effect of AKR Anti-θ Serum upon *in Vitro* Immunized Cytotoxic Lymphocytes[a]

Ratio lymphocytes to target cells	Not treated	AKR anti-θ C3H serum plus complement	AKR serum plus complement
	% Lysis	% Lysis	% Lysis
100:1	100 ± 0.9	4.2 ± 1.5	100 ± 1
25:1	92 ± 2	0	87 ± 0.5
5:1	53 ± 3	0	50 ± 2

[a] CBA spleen cells, immunized *in vitro* against H-2^d antigens, were harvested at Day 6 of culture and divided into three parts. One part remained untreated, one part was treated with anti-θ serum, and one part with normal AKR serum (Methods). The residual cells were assayed for cytotoxicity at the dilution, which resulted in the untreated cells in a ratio of lymphocytes to target cells of 100, 25, and 5 to 1. Nonspecific lysis (background) was subtracted.

TABLE 3

Cytotoxic Activity Derived from *in Vitro*-Immunized Thymocytes[a]

Ratio lymphocytes to target cells	% Specific lysis	
	Normal thymocytes	Cortisone-resistant lymphocytes
100:1	100	100
25:1	58	100
5:1	22	90
1:1	0	49
0.5:1	0	20

[a] Dispersed CBA thymocytes and cortisone-resistant thymocytes were immunized against H-2^d allo antigens *in vitro*. Cells harvested at Day 6 were assayed for cytotoxicity at various ratios of lymphocytes to target cells over 150 min. Nonspecific lysis was subtracted.

25%. These surviving medullary thymocytes proved to be far more active in the cytotoxic test than normal thymus cells immunized by the same method. Even at a ratio of one cultured viable cell per two target cells, 20% specific lysis occurred within 150 min. At a lymphocyte-to-target cell ratio of 5:1, 90% lysis occurred (Table 3). Proof that the cytotoxic activity generated was due to activated T cells rather than due to humoral factors was obtained by abolition of the cytotoxicity by treatment with anti-θ serum and complement.

Specificity of the cytotoxic effect of in vitro-immunized thymocytes. To establish that the lytic activity of medullary thymocytes immunized *in vitro* was immunologically specific, assays were performed against ^{51}Cr-labeled lymph node cells of different H-2 types. Cultured CBA medullary thymus cells immunized against BALB/c (H-2^d) allo antigens, harvested at day 6, did not lyse syngeneic (CBA) target cells (H-2^k), but lysed BALB/c (H-2^d) target cells (Table 4). In addition, A/J target cells (H-2^a), which share with BALB/c eight out of nine H-2 specificities not present on CBA cells were also lysed. C57 BL (H-2^b) target cells were not lysed to a significant extent. These share five out of eight H-2 specificities with H-2^d.

TABLE 4

Cytotoxic Specificity of the Cells Derived from *in Vitro*-Immunized Cortisone-Resistant Thymocytes[a]

^{51}Cr-labeled lymph node target cells	% Specific lysis	
Mouse strain	Expt 1	Expt 2
CBA (H2^k)	0	0
Balb/c (H2^d)	21	22
C57 BL (H-2^b)	1	0
A/J (H-2^a)	20	18

[a] Cortisone-resistant CBA thymocytes were immunized *in vitro* against H-2^d allo antigens. Cells harvested at Day 6 were assayed for cytotoxicity against various ^{51}Cr-labeled lymph node target cells at a ratio of lymphocytes to target cells of 100 to 1. Incubation time was 4 hr.

Kinetics of the in Vitro Generation of Cytotoxic Lymphocytes from Thymus Cells

Comparison between in vivo and in vitro immunization. A graft-versus-host model was chosen for the immunization of CBA thymocytes against H-2^d allo antigens *in vivo* (2). Cytotoxic activity generated over a 7-day period was compared with the activity obtained by immunization *in vitro*. Both sets of immunized lymphocytes were assayed at the same lymphocyte-to-target cell ratio of 100 to 1. The cytotoxic activity generated *in vitro* was twice that of *in vivo*-immunized cells (Fig. 1). Whereas peak *in vivo* cytotoxicity occurred at Day 5, the *in vitro* activity peaked at Day 6.

The enhanced capacity of medullary thymocytes to differentiate *in vitro* into cytotoxic effector cells is demonstrated in Fig. 2. As with CBA thymocytes (Fig. 1) and spleen cells (7), the peak cytotoxic activity occurred at Day 6. Within 150 min, 90% lysis occurred at a lymphocyte-to-target cell ratio as low as 3 to 1.

Comparison of the rate of lysis caused by in vitro-immunized normal thymocytes and medullary thymocytes. CBA thymocytes and cortisone-resistant thymocytes were immunized *in vitro* against BALB/c spleen cells. At Day 6 of culture, the cells were assayed in a cytotoxicity test at a lymphocyte-to-target cell ratio of 100 to 1. The lytic process was stopped at various time intervals of 5–150 min. The rate of lysis caused by both thymus cell populations followed a sigmoid curve (Fig. 3). Whereas cytotoxic lymphocytes derived from normal thymocytes lysed 50% of the target cells in 70 min, cortisone-resistant thymocytes were more efficient, lysing 50% of the target cells within 30 min.

Quantitation of the lytic capacity of various cytotoxic lymphocyte populations. It has been found that at a given incubation time a linear relationship exists between the percentage of lysis of target cells and the logarithm of the ratio of lymphocytes

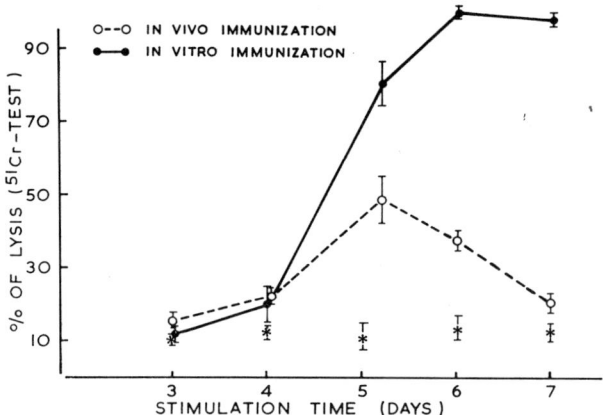

FIG. 1. Comparison of *in vivo* and *in vitro* immunization of CBA thymocytes against H-2^d allo antigen. Cytotoxic activity was assayed at a lymphocyte-to-target cell ratio of 100 to 1 for 150 min under identical conditions. Each point represents the mean of three determinations ± SEM. The single points represent lysis of target cells in the absence of added lymphocytes (background).

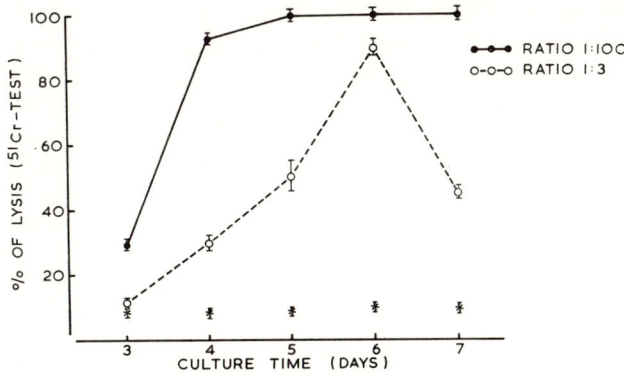

FIG. 2. *In vitro* immunization of cortisone-resistant thymocytes against H-2^d allo antigen. At the given time, cytotoxicity was assayed for 150 min at a target cell-to-lymphocyte ratio 1 to 100 and 1 to 3. Each point represents the mean of three determinations ± SEM. The single points represent background lysis.

to target cells (7, 20). Thus, it is possible to compare the lytic capacity of various populations of cytotoxic lymphocytes by comparing the ratio of lymphocytes to target cells required to obtain 50% lysis of target cells. Experiments were performed to compare the lytic activity of *in vitro* immunized CBA mouse thymus cells, medullary thymocytes, spleen cells, and purified T cells prepared from CBA spleens by the method of Basten *et al.* (15). The criterion for the functional purity of the splenic T-cell preparation was their capacity to act as helper cells, but not to give rise to antibody-plaque-forming cells after *in vitro* immunization with sheep red

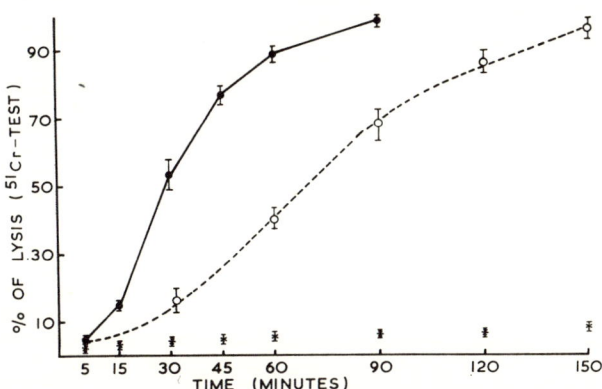

FIG. 3. Kinetic of the lytic reaction by *in vitro*-immunized CBA thymocytes (O–O–O) and cortisone-treated CBA thymocytes (●–●–●). Target cell-to-stimulated cell ratio was 1 to 100. Each point represents the mean of three determinations ± SEM. The single points represent background lysis.

cells (21). The four different lymphocyte preparations were cultured with mitomycin C-treated BALB/c cells, harvested at Day 6 and assayed for 150 min against ^{51}Cr-labeled target cells at various lymphocyte-to-target cell ratios (Fig. 4). All four cytotoxic lymphocyte populations demonstrated the linear relationship between cytotoxicity and the logarithm of the ratio of lymphocytes to target cells. It was striking that the values obtained for purified T cells from the spleen and medullary thymocytes were identical. Both cell populations had the same lytic activity, namely, 50% lysis at a ratio of 0.9–1.0. Spleen cells when cultured under identical conditions were 3-fold less effective (50% lysis at a ratio of 3:1) and thymocytes 10- to 12-fold less active (50% lysis at a ratio of 12:1), than medullary thymocytes or splenic T cells.

DISCUSSION

In a recent communication, a new technique for the induction of an allograft response *in vitro* was reported (7). Basically, it consists of a one-way mixed lymphocyte reaction using inbred mouse spleen lymphocytes. Between 5–7 days in culture, cells causing immunologically specific lysis of ^{51}Cr-labeled target cells were detected. Unlike previously described *in vitro* cell-mediated responses (5, 6, 22), the cytolytic capacity of the cultured cells was very high, in that 100% lysis of the target cells occurred even at a lymphocyte-to-target cell ratio of 25 to 1, in as brief a time as 200 min. This is a degree of cytolytic activity as high as any previously reported in animal experiments (3).

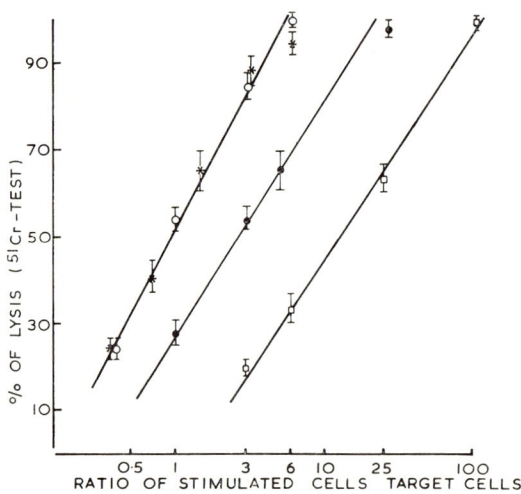

FIG. 4. Quantitative comparison of the lytic capacity of 6-day *in vitro*-immunized CBA thymocytes (□-□-□), spleen cells (●-●-●), cortisone-resistant thymocytes (○-○-○), and purified splenic T lymphocytes (*-*-*). The immunized cells were assayed for 150 min at various ratios of stimulated lymphocytes to target cells. Each point represents the means of three determinations ± SD.

This culture system was thus well suited for an investigation of some of the questions concerning the cellular basis of a cell-mediated response. The first problem approach was identification of the nature of the cell in a CBA spleen which are necessary for the development of the cell-mediated immune response.

Treatment of cytotoxic lymphocytes with AKR anti-θ C_3H serum and complement which Raff (23) and Schlesinger (24) have shown to kill thymus-derived cells, abolished the lytic capacity (Table 2), thus identifying the cytotoxic lymphocytes as thymus-derived cells. Moreover, anti-θ serum plus complement destroyed the capacity of spleen lymphocytes to be immunized, and to give rise to cytotoxic lymphocytes against a given allo-antigen (Table 1.) These experiments established that the precursors of killer cells in CBA spleen cells were thymus-derived cells. It could be demonstrated (Table 3) that thymus cells alone when immunized *in vitro* against alloantigens, differentiate into θ antigen-positive cytotoxic cells. These results confirm the identity of cytotoxic lymphocytes as thymus-derived cells and demonstrate that there is no need for interaction with bone marrow-derived cells.

The results obtained from the present *in vitro* system are consistent with those obtained by *in vitro* immunization. Cerottini *et al.* (3, 35), Blomgren *et al.* (2), and Sprent and Miller (4) have demonstrated in a graft-versus-host system that thymocytes alone may give rise to killer cells. The failure of Lonai and Feldman (8, 9) to generate a cytotoxic effect *in vitro* from rat thymocytes immunized against mouse fibroblasts may reflect either a difference in culture conditions, or in the nature of the response (xenograft versus allograft).

The time course of generation of cytotoxic activity *in vitro* was the same with CBA thymocytes (Fig. 1) as with CBA spleen cells (11). This suggests that the process of immunization is similar in both circumstances. In order to determine which group of cells in the thymus participate in the allograft response, use was made of the relative resistance of medullary thymocytes to the lympholytic action of cortisone (17). Cortisone-resistant thymocytes have been demonstrated to be more active, on a cell-for-cell basis in graft versus host reactions (19) and helper cell systems (26). Cortisone-resistant thymocytes cultured with BALB/c spleen cells gave rise to a much more active cell-mediated response. Fifty percent lysis of the target cells occurred in 30 min compared with 70 min by immunized normal thymocytes (Fig. 3). However, the time of generation of cytotoxic activity was the same in both cell populations with maximal activity at day 6. This supports the concept that the responding cells in normal thymus were in fact the cortisone-resistant cells probably medullary thymocytes.

The capacity of various lymphoid cell populations to give rise to cytotoxic effector cells *in vitro* was compared, using as a criterion the ratio of lymphocytes to target cells necessary to cause 50% lysis in 150 min. It was found that spleen cells were three times as active as thymocytes. However cortisone-resistant thymocytes and splenic T cells obtained by the method of Basten (15) were 12-fold more active than normal thymocytes. These two populations gave identical results, suggesting a functional relationship.

One of the features of this work was the high lytic capacity of some cultured cell populations. For example medullary thymocytes caused 50% lysis within 150 min at a lymphocyte-to-target cell ratio of 1 to 1 or less, an activity higher than any previously reported. Other *in vitro* systems for a cell-mediated response, such as those of Wunderlich and Canty (22) yielded only 8% lysis in 4 hr of the EL4 lymphoma by mouse spleen cells at a ratio of 100 lymphocytes per target cell. Ax *et al.* (6) reported 70% lysis of mouse fibroblasts by mouse spleen cells in 6 hr. Since these experiments involved target cells with differing susceptibility to cytotoxic lysis, it is more meaningful to compare results obtained with the same line of target cells, P815X2. Cerottini *et al.* (25) reported 50% lysis in 6 hr at a 50 to 1 ratio by *in vivo*-immunized thymocytes. It was thought possible that the same tumour cell line maintained in our laboratory was more susceptible to lysis. However, two experimental findings negate this possibility. The background lysis (no immune cells) was very low (Fig. 3), and the lysis caused by thymocytes immunized *in vivo* by the method of Cerottini *et al.* was similar to the published data (25). Figure 2 shows that the *in vitro*-immunized cells were much more lytic than the *in vivo*-immunized cells. The reason for the very high capacity is not yet known, but may be due to the tendency of activated lymphocytes to survive better than nonactivated cells *in vitro*. Thus the viable cells at the end of a 6-day culture period represent a highly selected sample of activated lymphocytes.

The functional capacity of cells immunized *in vitro* has recently been demonstrated in *in vivo* assay systems. It was found that cortisone-resistant thymocytes, immunized *in vitro,* were highly active in tumour allograft rejection in irradiated mice (27). These cells were also found to be capable of rejecting skin grafts in neonatally thymectomized mice, and in inducing a graft-versus-host reaction in F_1 hybrids (Rouse and Wagner, in preparation).

By demonstrating that cells immunized *in vitro* are active *in vivo,* and that cellular requirements of the allograft response *in vivo* and *in vitro* are the same, we can validly use this culture system to analyze in detail the sequence of events culminating in the production of cytotoxic lymphocytes, antigen recognition, cell proliferation, and differentiation into effector cells. These questions will be the topic of a subsequent communication.

ACKNOWLEDGMENTS

The authors gratefully acknowledge the advice and encouragement by Professor G. J. V. Nossal during the course of this work; Dr. A. Basten for providing splenic T cells purified by his antigen-binding column method, Dr. B. Byrd for stimulating discussions and Mrs. S. Owen and M. Odgers for their excellent technical assistance.

REFERENCES

1. Mitchell, G. F., and Miller, J. F. A. P., *J. Exp. Med.* **128**, 821, 1968.
2. Blomgren, H., Takasugi, M., and S. Friberg, Jr., *Cell. Immunol.* **1**, 619, 1970.
3. Cerottini, J. C., Nordin, A. A., and Brunner, K. T., *Nature London* **227**, 72, 1970.
4. Sprent, J., and Miller, J. F. A. P., *Cell. Immunol.* (in press).
5. Ginsberg, H., *Immunology* **14**, 621, 1968.
6. Ax, W., Koren, H. S., and Fischer, H., *Exp. Cell Res.* **64**, 439, 1971.
7. Wagner, H., and Feldmann, M., *Cell. Immunol.* (in press).
8. Lonai, P., and Feldmann, M., *Transplantation* **10**, 372, 1970.
9. Lonai, P., and Feldmann, M., *Transplantation* **11**, 446, 1971.
10. Shortman, K., Williams, N., and Adams, P., *J. Immunol. Methods* (in press).
11. Hanks, J. H., and Wallace, J. H., *Proc. Soc. Exp. Biol. Med.* **98**, 188, 1950.

12. Marbrook, J., *Lancet* **2**, 1279, 1967.
13. Diener, E., and Armstrong, W. D., *J. Exp. Med.* **129**, 591, 1969.
14. Dunn, T. B., and Potter, M., *J. Nat. Cancer Inst.* **18**, 587, 1957.
15. Basten, A., Sprent, J., and Miller, J. F. A. P., *Nature London* (in press).
16. Cohen, A., and Schlesinger, M., *Transplantation* **10**, 130, 1970.
17. Ishidate, M., and Metcalf, D., *Aust. J. Exp. Biol. Med. Sci.* **41**, 637, 1962.
18. Dougherty, T. F., Berliner, M. L., Schneebeli, G. L., and Berliner, D. L., *Ann. N.Y. Acad. Sci.* **113**, 825, 1964.
19. Blomgren, H., and Andersson, B., *Exp. Cell. Res.* **57**, 185, 1969.
20. Canty, T. G., and Wunderlich, J. R., *J. Nat. Cancer Inst.* **45**, 761, 1970.
21. Feldmann, M., and Basten, A., *Europ. J. Immunol.* (in press).
22. Wunderlich, J. R., and Canty, T. G., *Nature London* **228**, 63, 1970.
23. Raff, M. C., and Wortis, H., *Immunology* **18**, 931, 1970.
24. Schlesinger, M., *Nature London* **226**, 1255, 1970.
25. Cerottini, J. C., Nordin, A. A., and Brunner, K. T., *Nature London* **228**, 1308, 1970.
26. Cohen, J. J., and Claman, H. N., *J. Exp. Med.* **133**, 1026, 1971.
27. Rouse, B. T., Wagner, H. and Harris, A. W., *J. Immunol.* (in press)

Thymus-derived Cells as Killer Cells in Cell-mediated Immunity

By J. F. A. P. MILLER, K. T. BRUNNER, J. SPRENT, P. J. RUSSELL AND G. F. MITCHELL

CELLULAR IMMUNITY is mediated by specifically altered or "sensitized" lymphocytes and is thymus-dependent. Thus, neonatally thymectomized or thymectomized irradiated rodents have a diminished number of recirculating small lymphocytes and an impaired ability to undertake delayed hypersensitivity reactions or to reject allografts of normal or neoplastic tissue.[1] On the other hand, cells involved in the synthesis of classical immunoglobulin molecules and in the production of humoral antibody can be generated in the absence of thymus tissue. Yet, it has been clearly demonstrated that collaboration between thymus-derived lymphocytes and nonthymus-derived antibody-forming cell precursors is essential for a normal antibody response to a variety of antigens in mice.[2] The question as to whether collaboration between thymus-derived and nonthymus-derived cells is required for certain types of cellular immune responses is the subject of the present investigation.

Lymphocytes from specifically immunized mice can, in vitro, destroy target cells if these bear the histocompatibility antigens against which sensitivity was induced.[3,4] The cytotoxic effect can be quantitated by measuring the radioactivity released in the supernatant of ^{51}Cr-labeled target cells. The reaction is immunologically specific since lymphocytes from donors immunized to antigens not present on target cells do not exert a cytotoxic effect. For the reaction to occur there must be effective contact between lymphocytes and target cells, but complement or serum need not be used. Addition of alloantibody directed against the target cell, in the absence of added complement, inhibits lymphocyte-mediated target cell killing. This is presumably because there is competition between alloantibody and sensitized lymphocytes for antigenic sites on target cells.

Since graft rejection is thymus-dependent, it was of interest to determine whether killer lymphocytes generated in specifically sensitized mice were thymus-derived or not. The source of killer cells could be identified in thymus cell-reconstituted neonatally thymectomized mice if the donor of the thymus cells had histocompatibility antigens lacking in the host. Since anti-target cell antibody raised in the strain of mice sensitized to the target cells impairs killer cell activity, one should be able to determine, by the use of inhibition tests with appropriate antisera, whether the killer cells had the antigenic specificity of the donor of the thymus cells or of the recipient.

Sensitization of Normal Mice to DBA/2 Mastocytoma

Intact CBA and (A × CBA)F$_1$ hybrid mice were sensitized to DBA/2 mastocytoma and their spleen cells tested 11 days later for capacity to lyse ^{51}Cr-labeled mastocytoma cells in vitro, using methods previously described.[3] It can be seen from the percentage of ^{51}Cr released at 3 and 6 hours, that sensitization was effective in intact, nonthymectomized mice (Table 1). An A-anti-DBA/2 serum will cover H2 specificity 31 against which (A × CBA)F$_1$ cells are sensitized and should thus inhibit

---

From the Walter and Eliza Hall Institute of Medical Research, Royal Melbourne Hospital, Melbourne, Australia, and Institut Suisse Expérimentale du Cancer, Lausanne, Switzerland.

This is Publication 1456 from the Walter and Eliza Hall Institute of Medical Research.

Table 1. – DBA/2 Target Cell Destruction by Sensitized Spleen Cells from Intact and Neonatally Thymectomized Mice

Group	Serum added	% ^{51}Cr release at	
		3 hours	6 hours
Intact (A x CBA)F$_1$	-	24	44
	A anti-DBA/2	2	7
	C3H anti-DBA/2	0	3
Intact CBA	-	56	73
	A anti-DBA/2	45	63
	C3H anti-DBA/2	28	40
Neonatally thymectomized CBA	-	0.5	0.7

lysis of DBA/2 target cells by (A × CBA)F$_1$ sensitized cells but not by CBA sensitized cells (since sensitization of CBA against DBA/2 produces cells recognizing H2 specificities 4, 6, 10, 13, 14, 27, 28, 29 and 31, so that the A anti-DBA/2 serum cannot inhibit as it reacts with only one of the nine sites involved[4]). By contrast, a C3H-anti-DBA/2 serum should inhibit lysis by both CBA and (A × CBA)F$_1$ sensitized cells. As predicted, the C3H-anti-DBA/2 serum did inhibit lysis by both sensitized CBA and (A × CBA)F$_1$ cells and the A-anti-DBA/2 serum inhibited lysis by (A × CBA)F$_1$ sensitized cells, but caused only slight inhibition of lysis by CBA sensitized cells. The use of A-anti-DBA/2 serum should thus allow the identification of the killer cells: inhibition of lysis identifies the cell as (A × CBA)F$_1$ whereas either no or only slight inhibition establishes the cell as CBA.

Susceptibility of Thymectomized CBA Mice to DBA/2 Mastocytoma

It is evident from Table 1 that spleen cells from neonatally thymectomized mice challenged with DBA/2 mastocytoma, did not cause any significant lysis of the target cells in vitro. In one experiment, 65 per cent of mastocytoma inoculated neonatally thymectomized CBA mice were dead by 11 days due to the dissemination of the tumor. All the survivors, used as donors of spleen cells 11 days after tumor injection, had ascites.

Reconstitution of Thymectomized Mice by Thymus-derived Lymphocytes

As shown in Table 2, a single injection of

Table 2. – DBA/2 Target Cell Destruction by Sensitized Spleen Cells from Neonatally Thymectomized CBA Mice Reconstituted with (A x CBA)F$_1$ Lymphocytes

	Reconstitution regime	Serum added	% ^{51}Cr release at	
			3 hours	6 hours
thoracic duct lymphocytes	one injection of 20 x 10^6 cells 1 week before challenge	normal A	11.4	22.2
		normal C3H	7.9	17.8
		A anti-DBA/2	0.5	3.5
		C3H anti-DBA/2	2.4	6.5
	one injection of 40 x 10^6 cells 1 week before challenge	-	28	46
		A anti-DBA/2	8	17
		C3H anti-DBA/2	5	11
thymus lymphocytes	one injection of 10 x 10^6 cells 1 week before challenge	-	1.6	1.0
	several injections totalling 250 x 10^6 cells 1 - 3 weeks before challenge	-	35	54
		A anti-DBA/2	8	19
		C3H anti-DBA/2	8	18

Table 3. - DBA/2 Target Cell Destruction by Sensitized Spleen Cells from Lethally Irradiated (CBA x BALB/c)F_1 Recipients of CBA Thymus Cells

Group	% ^{51}Cr release at:		
	3 hours	6 hours	9 hours
CBA thymus ⟶ irradiated CBA	0.1	0.0	0.9
CBA thymus ⟶ irradiated (CBA x C57BL)F_1	-	0.8	-
CBA thymus ⟶ irradiated (CBA x BALB/c)F_1	9.0	18.4	21.9

either 20 or 40 million normal (A × CBA)F_1 thoracic duct lymphocytes (TDL) allowed effective sensitization, even though the cells were given one week before challenge. By contrast, 100 million (A × CBA)F_1 thymus cells given one week before challenge failed to reconstitute. On the other hand, several injections of up to 250 million thymus cells, given from 1 to 3 weeks prior to challenge, did allow sensitization. A-Anti-DBA/2 serum clearly inhibited lysis of target cells by spleen cells from reconstituted mice. The extent of inhibition was the same with A-anti-DBA/2 as with C3H anti-DBA/2 sera. This indicates that the killer cells were (A × CBA)F_1 and thus derived, not from the neonatally thymectomized hosts, but from the inoculated TDL or thymus lymphocytes.

Education of CBA Thymus Cells by Histocompatibility Antigens

Thymus lymphocytes react with histocompatibility antigens by transforming to large pyroninophilic cells which proliferate to a progeny that is much more active in undertaking graft-versus-host reactions than the original, unstimulated, thymus cells.[5] It was of interest to determine whether thymus lymphocytes could, following activation with specific histocompatibility antigens, become killer cells. CBA thymus cells were thus injected into lethally irradiated CBA, (CBA × C57BL)F_1 or (CBA × BALB/c)F_1 (BALB/c and DBA/2 share the same H2 antigens). Five days later a cell suspension made from the spleens of these recipients was incubated in vitro with ^{51}Cr-labeled DBA/2 mastocytoma cells. The data in Table 3 indicate a definite specific enhancement of killer cell activity with spleen cells of irradiated (CBA × BALB/c)F_1 recipients of CBA thymus cells, and not with spleen cells obtained from other mice.

Discussion and Conclusions

These results clearly identify thymus-derived cells as killer cells in cell-mediated immunity. Thymectomy depletes the recirculating lymphocyte pool and this can be reversed by injecting thymus lymphocytes. Such cells can be identified in the pool in experiments in which genetically marked cells are used, and it is those cells which initiate graft-versus-host reactions.[5] Hence, both the cells which provoke allograft reactions and which, in vitro, act as killer cells are originally derived from the thymus. No evidence has been obtained for interactions between thymus-derived and non-thymus-derived cells in the in vitro lymphocyte-target cell reaction. Whether collaboration occurs between different classes of thymus-derived cells, as in graft-versus-host reactions,[6] has not been determined.

REFERENCES

1. Miller, J. F. A. P., and Osoba, D.: Physiol. Rev. 47:437, 1967.
2. Miller, J. F. A. P., and Mitchell, G. F.: Transplantation Rev. 1:3, 1969.
3. Brunner, K. T., Mauel, J., Cerottini, J.-C., and Chapuis, B.: Immunology 14:181, 1968.
4. Mauel, J., Rudolf, H., Chapius, B., and Brunner, K. T.: Immunology 18:517, 1970.
5. Sprent, J., and Miller, J. F. A. P.: Unpublished.
6. Cantor, H., and Asofsky, R.: J. Exp. Med. 131:235, 1970.

Potentiation of Cultured Mouse Thymocyte Responses by Factors Released by Peripheral Leucocytes[1]

I. GERY, R. K. GERSHON AND B. H. WAKSMAN

Lymphoid cell interactions in the immune response, both *in vivo* and *in vitro*, have been the subject of much interest recently (1, 2). In this regard, substances have been found in supernatants of cell cultures which can affect the response of other lymphoid cells (3, 4). The following report describes a new effect wherein mouse thymocytes are highly stimulated by a combination of nonspecific stimulants and substances released by human leucocytes.

Five $\times$ 10^6 thymus or spleen cells from male CBA/H or CBA/J mice, aged 6 to 12 weeks, were cultured in duplicate in plastic tubes (Falcon #2001) in 1.0 ml MEM-S (Microbiological Associates, Bethesda, Md., with added antibiotics and *l*-glutamine), supplemented with 8% normal human serum. These cultures were stimulated by the following, added singly or in combination: a) 1.0 µl phytohemagglutinin-P (PHA, Difco Laboratories, Detroit, Mich.); b) different concentrations of human white blood cells (obtained by gravitational sedimentation of the erythrocytes); c) supernatants (SUP) from cultures of human leucocytes. The latter were prepared by incubating 1.5 $\times$ 10^6 human leucocytes in 2.0 ml of the above medium with or without stimulants for 24 hr, then removing the cells centrifugally and storing at -20°C. These human cultures were stimulated by 1.0 µl PHA or 100 µg endotoxin (LPS, Difco, lipopolysaccharide B, *Escherichia coli* 0111:B4). The supernatants at various dilutions were added in a volume of 0.5 ml to the mouse cells in the same volume. Treatment with mitomycin C (MIT, Nutritional Biochemicals Corp., Cleveland, Ohio) was carried out by incubating mouse thymocytes (40 $\times$ 10^6/ml) or human leucocytes (15 $\times$ 10^6/ml) with the drug (final concentration 100 µg/ml) for 30 min at 37°C. The cells were then spun down and washed twice with the medium. All cultures were incubated for 72 hr at 37°C in 5% CO$_2$ in air. A pulse of tritiated thymidine (^{3}HT, Schwarz BioResearch, Orangeburg, N.Y. 0.5 or 1.0 µCi) was given during the last 24 hr of incubation. Incorporation of ^{3}HT was determined by washing the cells twice with saline, followed by precipitation with trichloroacetic acid. The precipitates were dissolved in 0.4 ml formic acid and 3.0 ml ethanol and counted with 10 ml scintillation fluid (PPO, 0.5% and POPOP, 0.025% in toluene) in a Nuclear Chicago (Des Plaines, Ill.) Mark I scintillation counter. Counts in duplicate cultures regularly differed from the mean value by less than 15%, except with counts below 1000. The data recorded below are from representative experiments; the results were found to be reproducible in repeated tests

RESULTS AND DISCUSSION

Mouse thymus cells incorporated minute amounts of ^{3}HT when cultured without any stimulant; there was only a small increment in uptake after PHA was added (Table I). The uptake of ^{3}HT was markedly increased by the addition of 150,000 human leucocytes, whereas the addition of 30,000 or less had little effect. The addition of PHA to the leucocyte-thymocyte mixtures, however, strikingly enhanced the ^{3}HT incorporation at all leucocyte doses studied; a significant increase in the response was provoked by as few as 6000 human leucocytes. The values of ^{3}HT uptake in the PHA-stimulated mixed cultures were far greater than the sum of values obtained in the mixed cultures and the individual PHA-stimulated cultures.

The high incorporation of ^{3}HT in PHA-stimulated mixed cultures was mainly by the mouse thymocytes. Treatment of the human leucocytes with MIT abolished most of their proliferative activity but not their synergistic effect.

[1] Supported by United State Public Health Service Research Grants AI-06112, AI-06455 and CA-08593.

TABLE I

Synergy between human leucocytes and PHA in stimulation of mouse lymphocytes

Stimulant		Mouse Cells in Culture			
Human leucocytes	PHA	None[a]	Thymus	MIT-thymus[b]	Spleen
None	−	−	62[c]	8	4,277
None	+	−	258	11	31,843
Normal, 6,000	−	18	56	ND[b]	ND
Normal, 6,000	+	230	1,430	ND	ND
Normal, 30,000	−	6	384	17	5,198
Normal, 30,000	+	2,307	27,770	2,026	30,395
Normal, 150,000	−	22	19,612	278	7,198
Normal, 150,000	+	18,126	50,957	12,601	57,531
MIT-treated, 30,000	−	10	73	ND	ND
MIT-treated, 30,000	+	15	8,603	ND	ND
MIT-treated, 150,000	−	11	5,771	35	ND
MIT-treated, 150,000	+	373	42,028	522	ND

[a] Only human cells were tested in these cultures.
[b] MIT, mitomycin C; ND, not done.
[c] Incorporation of ³HT, presented as mean of CPM in duplicate cultures.

MIT treatment of the thymocytes, on the other hand, abolished the synergistic reaction with untreated human leucocytes and PHA.

The response of mouse spleen cells was greatly different from that of thymocytes. They responded much more to PHA when cultured alone and their response was not appreciably boosted by the addition of human cells to the culture. Indeed, the values of ³HT incorporation in the spleen cultures with human leucocytes and PHA were not appreciably higher than those in similarly stimulated thymus cultures.

The ability of human leucocytes to potentiate the reactivity of mouse thymocytes was further established by the use of supernatants of human leucocyte cultures stimulated with PHA or LPS. These gave increased ³HT uptake equal in magnitude to that triggered by the intact human cells (Table II). The synergy between the supernatants and PHA became more apparent with diluted supernatants, as reflected by an increase in statistical significance. Release of the potentiating substances by the human blood cells was clearly independent of the proliferative response of these cells. Cultures stimulated with LPS endotoxin produced great amounts of active substances despite very low values of ³HT incorporation.

Moreover, potentiating activity was found even in supernatants of unstimulated leucocyte cultures from some individuals (Exp. II; Table II). The latter finding suggests that the effects of the supernatants from stimulated cultures do not depend on carryover of stimulant, an assumption which is also supported by the following: 1) A significant potentiation of the PHA response was obtained with a 1:8 dilution of supernatant, which represents a 1:32 dilution of the PHA put into the thymocyte cultures; 2) LPS is a minimal stimulant of mouse thymocytes, yet the supernatant of LPS-stimulated leucocytes both were stimulatory on their own and also potentiated the PHA response. While it remains possible that PHA and LPS are altered by their interaction with human leucocytes and become more mitogenic, this argument cannot apply to the effects of supernatants from unstimulated leucocyte cultures.

The nature of the material in the supernatants that potentiates mouse thymocyte responses is at present under investigation. Preliminary results suggest that it is made by adherent cells of human blood and also of syngeneic spleen and thus may be related to potentiating factors which have recently been described in *in vitro* responses of

TABLE II

Effects of supernatants (SUP) from human leucocytes on mouse thymus cells

Exp.	Human Leucocyte Cultures[a] (Source of SUP)			Dilution of SUP	Mouse Thymus Cultures (Target for SUP)		p <	
	Cells	Stimulant	³HT uptake		Stimulant	HT uptake (CPM)	a[b]	b[c]
			cpm					
I	—	—	—	—	—	29		
					PHA	202	0.05	
					LPS	98	N.S.[d]	
					PHA + LPS	586	0.02	
	+	—	63	Undiluted	—	28		
					PHA	488	0.01	0.05
	+	PHA	64,492	Undiluted	—	18,546		
					PHA	37,205	0.05	0.001
				1:8	—	144		
					PHA	5,976	0.01	0.01
	+	LPS	747	Undiluted	—	13,426		
					PHA	53,898	0.01	0.01
				1:8	—	8,589		
					PHA	39,819	0.001	0.001
II	—	—	—	—	—	18		
					PHA	132	0.05	
	+	—	121	Undiluted	—	16		
					PHA	4,693	0.01	0.01
	+	PHA	62,309	Undiluted	—	16,482		
					PHA	42,239	0.01	0.01

[a] The cultures used for production of SUP were harvested after 24 hr of incubation; those tested for ³HT uptake—after 72 hr.

[b] p calculated for comparison between cultures with and without additional stimulant.

[c] p calculated for comparison with thymocytes cultured with PHA alone.

[d] N.S., not significant (p > 0.05).

peripheral cells to antigens (5–8). Whatever its nature, it has led to the demonstration that normal mouse thymocytes, which have previously been considered to be poor responders to PHA, have the potential to respond as well as spleen cells, provided they are assisted by products of other cells.

REFERENCES

1. Möller, G., editor, *Antigen Sensitive Cells*, Transplant. Rev., *1:* 1–149, 1969.
2. Playfair, J. H. L., Clin. Exp. Immun., *8:* 839, 1971.
3. Lawrence, H. S. and Landy, M., editors, *Mediators of Cellular Immunity*, Academic Press, New York, 1969.
4. Lawrence, H. S. and Valentine, F. T., Amer. J. Path., *60:* 437, 1970.
5. Janis, M. and Bach, F. H., Nature, *225:* 238, 1970.
6. Bach, F. H., Alter, B. J., Solliday, S., Zoschke, D. C. and Janis, M., Cell Immun., *1:* 219, 1970.
7. Dutton, R. W., McCarthy, M. M., Mishell, R. I. and Raidt, D. J., Cell. Immun., *1:* 196, 1970.
8. Hoffmann, M. and Dutton, R. W., Science, *172:* 1047, 1971.

Ontogeny of Cellular Immunity: Development in Rat Thymocytes of Mixed Lymphocyte Reactivity to Allogeneic and Xenogeneic Cells [1]

STELLA C. KNIGHT AND G. JEANETTE THORBECKE

INTRODUCTION

It has been suggested that there might be a basic similarity in the origin of the diversity in the amino acid sequence of the variable regions of the immunoglobulin molecules and of the diversity in cell surface antigens of the histocompatibility system (1). Jerne (personal communication) has proposed a more detailed relationship between these two, in a hypothesis stating that the germ line carries a set of v-genes coding for the variable portion of those antibody molecules which are directed against the histocompatibility antigens of the species. Support for a close connection between the histocompatibility antigens and antibody production has come from a number of recent publications showing linkage between the H-2 types and immune responsiveness to certain antigens in mice (2, 3) and guinea pigs (4).

Jerne further suggests that cells with the ability to recognize H antigens of their own species are present almost throughout ontogeny, and that only those cells

[1] Supported by Grant AI-3076 from the United States Public Health Service.

among this population which do not meet with their corresponding antigen within the individual survive, unhindered, the ontogenic process. His theory readily accounts for the relative preponderance in peripheral blood of cells responsive to allogeneic H-2 antigens (1-2%) which was suggested by results from studies on graft-versus-host (GVH) reactivity (5) and on mixed lymphocyte reactions (MLR) (6). Other explanations for a high incidence of such cells can be found in the stimulation by cross-reacting antigens from the intestinal flora (7, 8). It would be of great interest to determine whether a detectable level of reactivity to allogeneic antigens is present among lymphoid cells of neonatal animals. Moreover, a comparison with reactivity to xenogeneic antigens might give some insight into the range of specificities represented early in ontogeny.

It has previously been shown that neonatal mouse thymocytes are equally as effective as adult thymocytes in initiating GVH reactions (9). In addition, adult rat thymocytes give excellent mixed MLR *in vitro* (10). In the present experiments a comparative study was made of the MLR obtained with thymus cells from neonatal and from adult rats. Various forms of cellular immunity including graft rejection (11, 12), delayed-type sensitivity (13), MLR (14), and GVH (11) reactivity are known to be properties of thymus-derived cells. The thymus would, therefore, appear to be the site at which cells recognizing H-2 antigens proliferate during ontogeny before peripheralization of the mature lymphoid cells. For this reason thymus was chosen as likely to have the highest content of H-2 responsive cells in the neonate.

MATERIALS AND METHODS

Animals. Swiss Webster (S.W.) mice and Sprague Dawley (S.D.) rats (Blue Spruce, Altamont, N.Y.), A/J and LAF_1/J mice (the F_1 hybrid between A/J and $C_{57}L/J$) (Jackson Laboratories, Bar Harbor, Maine), ACI and Fischer (F) rats (Microbiological Associates, Wash.), and ACI × Fischer F_1 hybrids (bred in these laboratories) were used. ACI and Fischer rats differ at the major Ag-B histocompatibility locus (J. Palm and G. Black, personal communication). In a few experiments young adult New Zealand rabbits and White Leghorn chickens were used as donors of thymocytes.

Thymus cell suspensions. Rat or mouse thymuses were removed sterilely and teased in Hanks' balanced salt solution. Cells were filtered through gauze and the number of viable cells were counted using trypan blue dye exclusion (final concentration of dye 0.4%).

Graft-versus-host activity. Viable thymus cells (5×10^7) from adult or neonatal rats or from adult mice were injected intravenously into neonatal rats or mice (less than 24 hr of age). The reaction was assessed using Simonsen's spleen assay (15). On the 9th or 10th day after injection, spleen indices were calculated by dividing the spleen weight/body weight ratio for each experimental animal by the mean value of such ratios for littermate noninjected or saline-injected controls.

Mixed lymphocyte reactions. Cell cultures were set up in triplicate in plastic tubes (10 × 75 mm, Falcon plastics). Cells (5×10^6) were cultured in 1 ml of RPMI-1640 or Dulbecco's medium (Grand Island Biologicals, Grand Island, N.Y.) supplemented with 10-15% fresh pooled serum from Sprague Dawley rats (16).

Cultures contained 1 ml of cell suspension from one source or 0.5 ml of each of two different cell suspensions. In many experiments one-way MLR were obtained by preincubation of $0.5–1 \times 10^7$ of the stimulating cells with mitomycin C (Nutritional Biochemical Corp., Cleveland, Ohio) at a concentration of 25 µg/ml for 15 min at 37° (16). Cultures were incubated in a 5% CO_2 in air atmosphere for 5 days and the proliferative activity assessed by the uptake of tritiated thymidine (1 µCi of ^{3}H-thymidine, 0.36 Ci/mM, Schwarz Bioresearch, Orangeburg, N.Y.) during the last 24 hr of the culture period. Radioactivity of the perchloric acid-precipitable material was measured in counts per minute (cpm) using a Tri-Carb liquid scintillation counter (Packard Instrument Co., Downers Grove, Ill.). Increments in counts per minute due to mixing two cell suspensions were calculated by subtracting half the sum of the counts per minute incorporated by each cell suspension separately from the actual counts per minute incorporated by the mixture.

Stimulants. Staphylococcal filtrate (0.1 ml) (kindly provided by Dr. N. R. Ling, Department of Experimental Pathology, Medical School, Birmingham, England) prepared as described previously (17) was added to some cultures. Dr. M. A. Leon (St. Luke's Hospital, Cleveland, Ohio) provided the concanavalin A (18). It was made up to 0.2 mg/ml in saline, and 0.1 ml of this solution was added to 1-ml cultures.

RESULTS

Conditions for optimal one- and two-way MLR with rat thymocytes. It was initially determined that $5–10 \times 10^6$ adult rat thymocytes per culture tube gave excellent responses to staphylococcal filtrate (as do rabbit thymocytes) (19) and to concanavalin A when cultured in 1 ml of Dulbecco's medium or RPMI-1640 containing 10–15% pooled fresh rat serum. Peak responses of thymus cells to concanavalin appeared before the second day of culture and amounted to increments of 89,000 cpm of ^{3}H-thymidine incorporated as compared to thymocytes without additive. This observation adds thymocytes to the list of lymphoid cells known to give a proliferative response to this agent (18).

When cells from the two different rat strains were mixed in culture, thymocytes gave excellent MLR (Fig. 1). The peak of the response appeared during the 4–5-day period of culture; at this time increments as high as 50,000 cpm were seen. The response of adult rat spleen cells in MLR over the 4–5-day culture time was only slightly higher than that of thymus cells of the same animal set up at the same initial cell concentration (Fig. 2). This suggests that rat thymus cells under the culture conditions employed here may show a comparatively better survival than rabbit thymocytes *in vitro* (19).

When a variety of media, all with 10% fresh rat serum, were compared for their ability to support proliferation of rat thymocytes *in vitro* the media were of decreasing effectiveness in the following order: Medium RPMI-1640, Dulbecco's medium (Table 1), minimum essential medium (Eagle), and medium 199. Medium 199 allowed increments of approximately 3,000 cpm with the same thymocyte mixtures that produced increments of 15,000 cpm in Dulbecco's medium.

Incubation of both thymocyte populations with 25 µg/ml of mitomycin C for 10 or 20 min at 37° resulted in a marked reduction in their proliferation. The remain-

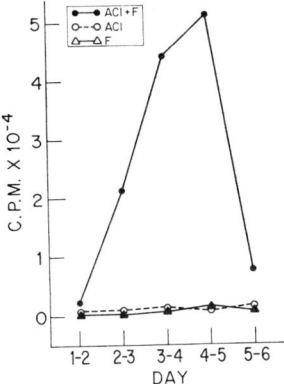

FIG. 1. Uptake of ^{3}H-thymidine by 10^7 adult rat thymocytes expressed as total counts per minute (cpm) per culture incorporation over the culture period indicated (Day 1–2 = period between 24th and 48th hr of culture, etc.).

ing response was usually under 3% of the total reaction although in an occasional experiment a response of up to 10% was seen (Table 1). The ability to stimulate MLR in untreated cells, however, remained intact, thus resulting in one-way MLR (Table 1). It was noted in some experiments that mitomycin-treated thymocytes tend to lose their effectiveness as stimulants when incubated for 2–3 hr at 37° in medium before mixing. Using RPMI-1640 medium in which a very high two-way stimulation was observed, a large fraction of the two-way reaction tended to be lost after mitomycin treatment, but in Dulbecco's medium the sum of the two components of the reaction frequently totalled or even exceeded the two-way reaction (Table 1). Similarly, as shown in Table 2 the sum of the components in the reaction of parental to F_1-hybrid thymocytes equalled or exceeded the two-way reactivity of the mixture of the two parent strains' thymocytes. It is possible that,

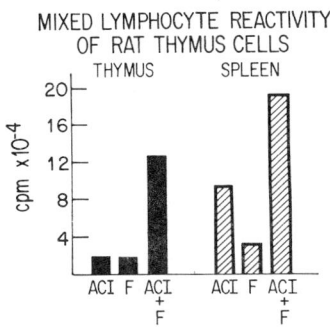

FIG. 2. Uptake of ^{3}H-thymidine by 10^7 adult rat thymus or spleen cells from ACI and F strains, and by mixed cells from the two rat strains. Expressed as counts per minute (cpm) incorporated per total culture during the last day of a 5-day incubation period.

TABLE 1

REACTIVITY OF THYMOCYTES FROM ACI AND FISCHER RATS IN
THE ONE-WAY MIXED LYMPHOCYTE REACTION

Reacting cells	Mitomycin-treated thymocytes	Increments (cpm) [a] in:	
		RPMI-1640	Dulbeccos
ACI × F	—	168,514	34,810
F	ACI	45,767	26,660
ACI	F	28,003	23,090
—	ACI × F	5,677	865

[a] ^{3}H-thymidine incorporation measured over the 96–120-hr period of incubation. Increment in cpm = cpm in mixed cells − sum of cpm in each cell type incubated separately.

particularly in Dulbecco's medium, a "ceiling effect" is obtained for the ^{3}H-thymidine incorporation under the culture conditions used.

Effect of age of reacting rat thymocytes on their one-way responsiveness towards allogeneic and xenogeneic cells. Using thymocytes from adult Fischer or ACI rats as reacting cells, the increments in counts per minute on addition of mitomycin-treated or F_1-hybrid allogeneic cells were always above 3,000 cpm although they varied considerably to a maximum of 45,000 cpm. The degree of stimulation varied between 6.8 and 117 times background, i.e., a rather wide range. It was nevertheless clear that thymocytes from neonatal animals responded well but to a lesser extent in this interaction; the increments varying from 1,500 to 5,500 cpm and the degrees of stimulation from 2.4 to 12.7 (Table 3). It should be noted that thymocytes taken from rats younger than 2 hr of age still gave a response. When thymocytes from neonatal and adult Fischer rats were compared for their reactivity within individual experiments, the difference was much more evident in the one-way than in the two-way reaction (Table 2). This lack of difference in the two-way reaction was possibly due to some limitation imposed by the culture conditions.

A comparison was next made of the ability of Fischer rat thymocytes to be stimulated by allogeneic rat or by xenogeneic mouse cells (Table 4). It was found that adult Fischer rat thymocytes reacted to a similar degree to both, and with peak proliferation occurring around the same time of culture. However, although neonatal cells again responded to the allogeneic stimuli, they failed to proliferate

TABLE 2

MIXED LYMPHOCYTE REACTIVITY OF THYMOCYTES FROM NEONATAL AND ADULT RATS
OF PARENTAL STRAIN WITH F_1-HYBRID THYMOCYTES

Reacting cells	Type of reaction	Increment (cpm) [a]
F (<12 hr) × Hybrid	One-way	5,269
F (<12 hr) × ACI	Two-way	38,686
ACI × Hybrid	One-way	33,082
F × ACI	Two-way	31,877
F × Hybrid	One-way	16,435

[a] ^{3}H-thymidine incorporation measured over the 96–120-hr of incubation. Increment in cpm = cpm in mixed cells − sum of cpm in each cell type incubated separately.

TABLE 3

REACTIVITY OF THYMOCYTES FROM ACI AND FISCHER RATS OF VARIOUS AGES IN THE ONE-WAY MIXED LYMPHOCYTE REACTION

Reacting cells		Stimulating cells	Increment (cpm) [a]	Degree of stimulation [b]
Strain	Age			
F	<2 Hr	ACI (m) [c]	1,566	3.8
	<10 Hr	ACI (m)	2,506	2.4
	<12 Hr	ACI (m)	5,367	12.7
	<12 Hr	F_1 hybrid	5,269	3.3
F	Adult	ACI (m)	25,660	44.8
		ACI (m)	11,900	11.4
		ACI (m)	45,767	8.0
		F_1 hybrid	16,435	8.1
ACI	Adult	F (m)	28,003	19.7
		F (m)	23,090	60.2
		F (m)	7,085	6.8
		F (m)	15,739	14.4
		F (m)	3,232	27.3
		F (m)	16,403	117.2

[a] Calculated as in Table 1.
[b] Degree of stimulation = ^{3}H-thymidine incorporation by mixed cells/sum of ^{3}H-thymidine incorporation by each cell population alone.
[c] m indicates mitomycin-treated cell population.

in response to mitomycin-treated mouse cells. This differential responsiveness was still observed with thymocytes from 2-day-old rats but cells from 7-day-old animals responded approximately equally well to both xenogeneic and allogeneic stimulants.

In a few experiments other xenogeneic stimulating cells were also used. It was found that both mitomycin-treated thymocytes from chicken and rabbits caused severe inhibition or only very slight stimulation of adult rat thymocytes. This was

TABLE 4

ONE-WAY RESPONSE OF THYMOCYTES FROM FISCHER RATS OF VARIOUS AGES TO ALLOGENEIC AND XENOGENEIC THYMOCYTES

Age of reacting cells	Allogeneic stimulant	Increment (cpm) [a]	DS [b]	Xenogeneic stimulant	Increment (cpm) [a]	DS [b]
< 6 Hr	F_1 hybrid	11,176	2.8	S.W. (m) [c]	−2,209	0.6
<12 Hr	F_1 hybrid	952	1.4	S.W. (m)	−410	0.7
2 Days	ACI (m)	1,554	7.8	S.W. (m)	−32	0.9
1 Week	ACI (m)	3,451	4.6	S.W. (m)	6,567	7.9
1 Week	F_1 hybrid	19,918	12.6	S.W. (m)	15,916	13.9
Adult	F_1 hybrid	4,459	3.9	S.W. (m)	2,432	7.1
Adult	F_1 hybrid	16,755	6.3	S.W. (m)	16,663	11.0

[a] ^{3}H-thymidine incorporation measured over the 96–120-hr period of incubation. Increment in cpm = cpm in mixed cells − sum of cpm in each cell type incubated separately.
[b] Degree of stimulation = ^{3}H-thymidine incorporation by mixed cells/sum of ^{3}H-thymidine incorporation by each cell population alone.
[c] m indicates mitomycin-treated cell population.

found using measurements of ^{3}H-thymidine incorporation over the 96–120-hr period of incubation. A possible earlier peak of stimulation by such xenogeneic cells would have been missed under these conditions.

Reactivity of mouse thymocytes in the one-way response towards allogeneic and xenogeneic cells. Preliminary experiments suggested that mouse thymocytes survived very well in RPMI-1640 medium containing 10% fresh rat serum. This medium was, therefore, used in a few experiments in which the reactivities of strain A mouse thymocytes against F_1-hybrid (LAF1) cells and against mitomycin-treated Fischer rat thymus cells were compared. Adult and 2-day-old mouse thymocytes reacted equally well to both these stimuli (Table 5).

Graft-versus-host (GVH) reactivity of rat and mouse thymocytes in neonatal animals of both species. Both neonatal and adult mouse thymocytes are known to induce GVH reactions in neonatal mice (9), whereas adult rat thymocytes are ineffective in neonatal rats (20). An attempt was made to induce such reactions by using thymocytes from rats into mice and vice versa.

Neonatal Fischer rats were injected intravenously with 5×10^7 thymocytes from adult ACI rats or LAFI mice. Control neonates were injected with Fischer rat thymocytes. Spleen indices, determined 9 days later, showed no significant differences between these three groups (Table 6).

When neonatal S.W. mice received a similar number of thymocytes from either adult rat of outbred S.W. mice a significant incidence of splenomegaly was observed. In control mice, receiving no cells at birth, a spleen index greater than 1.2 was seen only in 2 out of 59 mice, whereas approximately 50% of the mice receiving adult rat cells had spleen indices greater than 1.2. Thymocytes obtained from Sprague Dawley rats under 24 hr of age induced a similar degree of splenomegaly in neonatal mice as did thymocytes from adult rats (Table 7).

DISCUSSION

The present results establish that the ability of rat thymus cells to give a proliferative response upon mixing with allogeneic thymus cells differing in the major histocompatibility antigens is present in the neonate, although somewhat lower than in the adult. Development of mixed lymphocyte reactivity of rat thymocytes to

TABLE 5

One-Way Response of Thymocytes from A Strain Mice of Various Ages to Allogeneic and Xenogeneic Thymocytes

Age of reacting cells	Allogeneic stimulant	Increment (cpm)[a]	DS[b]	Xenogeneic stimulant	Increment (cpm)[a]	DS[b]
2 Days	F_1 hybrid	18,015	8.5	Fischer (m)[c]	15,819	16.1
Adult	F_1 hybrid	6,693	4.5	Fischer (m)	13,264	25.5
Adult	F_1 hybrid	8,497	3.2	Fischer (m)	8,851	3.3

[a] ^{3}H-thymidine incorporation measured over the 96–120-hr period of incubation. Increment in cpm = cpm in mixed cells − sum of cpm in each cell type incubated separately.

[b] Degree of stimulation = ^{3}H-thymidine incorporation by mixed cells/sum of ^{3}H-thymidine incorporation by each cell population alone.

[c] m indicates mitomycin-treated cell population.

TABLE 6

GVH Reactivity of 5×10^7 Thymus Cells in Neonatal Fischer Rats

Thymus donor	Spleen index	
	Mean and SE	>1.2 [a]
None	1.00 ± 0.04	1/12
Adult F. rat	1.00 ± 0.03	0/10
Adult ACI rat	1.03 ± 0.02	0/11
Adult LAF1 mouse	0.94 ± 0.08	1/8

[a] Number of spleens out of total in that group with spleen indices greater than 1.2.

allogeneic cells precedes reactivity to mouse cells. These findings are consistent with Jerne's hypothesis which postulates an early presence of cells reactive to H-2 antigens within the species (personal communication). It might be suggested that the thymus is the site at which cells entering from the circulation are stimulated to divide, nonspecifically, and where only those cells reactive to self antigens are destroyed.

The present results do not establish the earliest time during ontogeny at which cells reactive to allogeneic antigens can be detected in the rat thymus, nor do they allow a conclusion as to the stage of development, prior to day 2 of age, at which reactivities to allogeneic or xenogeneic cells begin in the mouse thymus. Cells reactive to H-2 antigens of other species might be present early because of cross-reactivity between H-2 antigens of different species, or may develop early after birth because of stimulation by floral or other environmental antigens cross-reacting with H-2 antigens. Even though such cells would be produced in peripheral lymphoid tissue some could certainly enter the circulation and reach the thymus. A similar process might also explain the increase in thymocyte reactivity to allogeneic cells in the rat during the first week of life seen in the present studies. Findings of Claman et al. (21) on synergism between thymus and bone marrow in the antibody response suggest that reactivity of thymocytes to sheep erythrocytes in mice also develops during the first week of life.

While there was a difference between neonatal and adult rat thymocytes in their ability to give MLR with mitomycin-treated mouse thymocytes, both appeared equally effective in producing splenomegaly in neonatal mice. These results cannot

TABLE 7

GVH Reactivity of 5×10^7 Thymus Cells in Neonatal S.W. Mice

Thymus donor	Spleen index	
	Mean and SE	>1.2 [a]
None	1.00 ± 0.02	2/59
Neonatal S.D.	1.37 ± 0.72	10/13
Adult S.D.	1.30 ± 0.11	14/31
Adult S.W.	1.86 ± 0.21	6/7

[a] Number of spleens out of the total initial group with spleen indices greater than 1.2.

be readily interpreted since the contributions of donor and host to the proliferative process in the spleen were not evaluated. Another puzzling result was the observation that both rat and mouse thymus cells could induce splenomegaly in neonatal mice but not in neonatal rats, even though both populations were equally responsive to allogeneic and xenogeneic cells in MLR. It seems likely that, when inoculated with a similar cell dose, the neonatal rat with its larger body weight would be less sensitive to induction of splenomegaly than the neonatal mouse. However, there may be other factors involved, since adult rat spleen cells can readily induce splenomegaly in neonatal rats (20). It is possible that neonatal rats (but not mice) lack a cooperating cell such as the macrophage which may be needed in the induction of GVH reactions and is absent from thymus cell suspensions. It should be noted that MLR requirements for macrophages *in vitro* have not been noted except by investigators who have spread the cells over the bottom of culture dishes (22) rather than concentrating them in culture tubes such as was done in the present experiments.

There are several genetically determined cell surface-mediated properties of thymus cells which appear linked to the H-2 locus.

(1) Susceptibility to infection with Gross virus (23) as evidenced by susceptibility to Gross virus-induced, thymus-dependent (24) leukemia.

(2) Presence of TL thymus-specific antigen which is located on the cell surface in close proximity to the H-2 antigens (25).

(3) Mixed lymphocyte reactivity, also a property of the thymus-dependent population, can usually not be demonstrated unless there are major histocompatibility differences (28).

(4) The ability to give a complete immune response, including delayed-type sensitivity to 2,4-dinitrophenyl–poly-L-lysine (DNP–PLL) in the guinea pig (4). The immunogenicity of PLL is required to mediate the carrier function (26) when an analysis of the so-called "helper-mechanism" in the immune response is made according to Mitchison *et al.* (27). These helper cells or carrier-sensitized cells appear to belong to the thymus-derived population of lymphoid cells (27). Although it has not been established as yet that this function of thymus-derived cells is mediated through interaction of the cell surface with the antigens, it appears likely enough to warrant inclusion of this property in this list.

It seems, therefore, that H-2 variability may be intimately related to that part of the immune response which is thymus-dependent and involves thymus or thymus-derived cells. However, a clear relationship with the other cell type involved in the immune response, the actual antibody-producing cell, has not yet been demonstrated. If it could be shown that cells of thymic origin have immunoglobulin (Ig) molecules or parts thereof on their surface, a direct link with antibody structure would be provided. Although suggestive evidence that some thymus-dependent functions are inhibited by anti-Ig antisera has been presented (29, 30), such findings still need to be confirmed and extended before it can be regarded as proven that the specificity of thymus-derived cells in interaction with antigens is primarily the result of antibody on their cell surface. At this time the evidence for the presence of Ig determinants on the cell surface of the precursors of antibody-forming cells is much stronger (31–35).

ACKNOWLEDGMENTS

The competent technical assistance of Miss Judy Chapman is gratefully acknowledged.

REFERENCES

1. Burnet, F. M., *Nature London* **226**, 123, 1970.
2. McDevitt, H. O. and Tyan, M. L., *J. Exp. Med.* **128**, 1, 1968.
3. Vaz, N. M., and Levine, B. B., *Science* **168**, 852, 1970.
4. Ellman, L., Green, J., Martin, W. J., and Benacerraf, B., *Proc. Nat. Acad. Sci U.S.A.* **66**, 322, 1970.
5. Nisbet, N. W., Simonsen, M., and Zaleski, M., *J. Exp. Med.* **129**, 459, 1969.
6. Wilson, D. B., and Nowell, P. C., *J. Exp. Med.* **131**, 391, 1970.
7. Rapaport, F. T., Markowitz, A. S., and McCluskey, R. T., *J. Exp. Med.* **129**, 623, 1969.
8. Rapaport, F. T., *In* "Cross-Reacting Antigens and Neoantigens" (J. Trentin, Ed.). Williams and Wilkins, Baltimore, Md., 1967.
9. Cohen, M. W., Thorbecke, G. J., Hockwald, G. M., and Jacobson, E. B., *Proc. Soc. Exp. Biol.* **114**, 242, 1963.
10. Schwarz, M. R., *Immunology* **10**, 281, 1966.
11. Cooper, M. D., Peterson, R. D. A., South, M. A., and Good, R. A., *J. Exp. Med.* **123**, 75, 1966.
12. Warner, N. L., Szenberg, A., and Burnet, F. M., *Aust. J. Exp. Biol.* **40**, 373, 1962.
13. Arnason, B. G., Jankovic, B. D., Waksman, B. H., and Wennersten, C., *J. Exp. Med.* **116**, 177, 1962.
14. Kisken, W. A., and Swenson, N. A., *Nature London* **224**, 76, 1969.
15. Simonsen, M., *Prog. Allergy* **6**, 349, 1962.
16. Wilson, D. B., *J. Exp. Med.* **126**, 625, 1967.
17. Ling, N. R., Spier, E., James, K., and Williamson, N., *Brit. J. Haematol.* **11**, 421, 1965.
18. Powell, A. E., and Leon, M. A., *Exp. Cell Res.,* in press.
19. Knight, S. C., and Ling, N. R., *Clin. Exp. Immunol.* **4**, 667, 1969.
20. Billingham, R. E., Defendi, V., Silvers, W. K., and Steinmuller, D., *J. Nat. Cancer Inst.* **28**, 365, 1962.
21. Claman, H. N., Chaperon, E. A., and Triplett, R. F., *J. Immunol.* **97**, 828, 1966.
22. Twomey, J. J., Shankey, O., Jr., Brown, J. A., Laughter, A. H., and Jordon, P. H., Jr., *J. Immunol.* **104**, 845, 1970.
23. Lilly, F., Boyse, E. Z., and Old, L. J., *Lancet* **2**, 1207, 1964.
24. McEndy, D. P., Boon, M. C., and Furth, J., *Cancer Res.* **4**, 377, 1944.
25. Boyse, E. A., and Old, L. J., *Ann. Rev. Genet.* **3**, 187, 1970.
26. Paul, W. E., Katz, D. H., Goidl, E. A., and Benacerraf, B., *J. Exp. Med.* **132**, 283, 1970.
27. Mitchison, N. A., Rajewsky, K., and Taylor, R. B., *In* "Developmental Aspects of Antibody Formation and Structure" (J. Sterzl and H. Riha, Eds.). Czechoslovakian Academy of Science, Academic Press, New York, in press.
28. Amos, D. B., and Bach, F. H., *J. Exp. Med.* **128**, 623, 1969.
29. Mason, S., and Warner, N. L., *J. Immunol.* **104**, 762, 1970.
30. Greaves, M. F., Torrigiani, G., and Roitt, I. M., *Nature London* **222**, 885. 1969.
31. Mage, R. G., and Dray, S., *J. Immunol.* **95**, 525, 1965.
32. Daguillard, F., and Richter, M., *J. Exp. Med.* **131**, 119, 1970.
33. Raff, M. C., Sternberg, M., and Taylor, R. B., *Nature London* **225**, 553, 1970.
34. Thorbecke, G. J., Takahashi, T., and McArthur, W. P., *In* "Lymphatic Tissue and Germinal Centers in Immune Reactions" (K. Lindahl-Kiessling and M. G. Hanna, Eds.). Plenum Press, New York, in press.
35. Alm, G. V., and Peterson, R. D. A., *J. Exp. Med.* **129**, 1247, 1969.

Thymus Dependence of the Immune Response: Response to the Haptenic Determinant NIP in Mice

Jennifer Aird

INTRODUCTION

In mice, the expression of humoral immunity to most antigens so far tested, has been shown to depend upon a population of lymphocytes which have been influenced by the thymus and are therefore known as thymus derived (Leuchars, 1970). Experiments have shown that although both thymus derived and bone marrow derived cells are required for antibody production to sheep red blood cells (SRBC), only marrow derived cells produce detectable antibody (Davies, Leuchars, Wallis, Marchant and Elliott, 1967). The precise function of thymus derived cells in this system remains to be established. However, in relation to the response to hapten-carrier complexes it has been suggested that thymus derived cells are responsible for carrier recognition (Taylor, 1969). Since the response to some of the macromolecular protein antigens used as carriers has already been shown to depend upon the presence of the thymus (Taylor, 1963), it was of interest to discover whether the response to the hapten NIP conjugated to one such carrier was also thymus dependent. The thymus dependence of the anti-hapten response was also tested in relation to variations in hapten density on the carrier molecule.

MATERIALS AND METHODS

Antigen

The hapten used was 3-iodo-4-hydroxy-5-nitrophenylacetic acid (NIP). Two preparations of NIP coupled to bovine serum albumin (BSA) were used for immunization: $NIP_{1.5}BSA$ containing one and a half moles of NIP per molecule of BSA, and $NIP_{34}BSA$ containing 34 moles of NIP per molecule of BSA. NIP coupled to T_2 bacteriophage was used for the antibody assay by the phage inactivation technique (Mäkelä, 1966) and

NIP coupled to ε-amino-n-caproic acid (NIP-cap, 10^{-6}M) for hapten inhibition. The preparation of NIP and NIP conjugates has previously been described (Brownstone, Mitchison and Pitt-Rivers, 1966).

Animals

Male mice of an inbred CBA strain were used. Mice were either thymectomized at 6–8 weeks of age (Miller, 1960) or left untreated as normal controls. Thymectomized mice were irradiated 1 week after thymectomy with a mean dose of 880 rad at a dose rate of 148 rad/min, from a Siemens Gammatron-1 cobalt unit. Within 2 hours after irradiation all mice received an intravenous injection of 5×10^6 syngeneic CBA bone-marrow cells. Some of the mice were grafted 1 day later with a single lobe of CBA neonatal thymus which was implanted under the left kidney capsule. These mice will be referred to as reconstituted mice. The remaining thymectomized irradiated mice which did not receive a thymus graft will be referred to as deprived mice. The method of preparation of the chimaeras has been described in detail elsewhere (Davies, Leuchars, Wallis and Koller, 1966).

Immunization

All mice were immunized 4 weeks after irradiation. Of the three experimental groups of normal, deprived and reconstituted mice, half of each group received an intraperitoneal injection of 100 μg alum precipitated $NIP_{1.5}BSA$ with 10^9 *Haemophilus pertussis* organisms as adjuvant, and the remaining half received 100 μg alum precipitated $NIP_{34}BSA$ with the same adjuvant, by the same route. Mice were bled at various intervals after immunization and the sera stored at $-20°$ for later study.

Antigen dose in deprived mice

Based on the findings of the first experiment groups of deprived mice (prepared as described above) were injected with either 500 μg, 1500 μg or 5000 μg of alum precipitated $NIP_{1.5}BSA$ with pertussis as adjuvant, or the same doses of $NIP_{34}BSA$, plus adjuvant.

Antibody assay

The phage inactivation technique using $NIP-T_2$ phage has previously been described (Mäkelä, 1966). The relative proportions of IgG and IgM were determined by the combined 2 ME-reduction-hapten-inhibition method (Kontiainen and Mäkelä, 1967) based on the finding that IgG anti-hapten antibodies are more easily inactivated by free hapten than IgM anti-hapten antibodies, and that IgM antibody activity is abolished by 2-mercaptoethanol (0·2 M). Antibody titres, expressed as the reciprocal of the serum dilution inactivating 50 per cent of the $NIP-T_2$ phage PFU, were calculated and statistically analysed by the Computing Centre of Helsinki University. In the Tables figures are expressed as $\log_{10}$ values of geometric means ± the standard deviations. All figures have been corrected to two decimal places.

RESULTS

NORMAL MICE

The response of normal mice to NIP following immunization with 100 μg $NIP_{1.5}BSA$ or $NIP_{34}BSA$, differed in both the quality and quantity of the antibody produced accord-

TABLE 1

MEAN ANTI-NIP TITRES OF NORMAL, DEPRIVED AND RECONSTITUTED MICE INJECTED WITH 100 μg ALUM PRECIPITATED $NIP_{1.5}BSA$ PLUS 10^9 *Haemophilus pertussis* ORGANISMS

Day	Experimental group	No. mice	Antibody titre ($\log_{10}$) IgM	Antibody titre ($\log_{10}$) IgG	Per cent IgM
14	Normal	10	4.15 ± 0.31	4.52 ± 0.58	27
	Deprived	9	3.24 ± 0.48	2.63 ± 0.64	80
	Reconstituted	9	3.97 ± 0.48	3.96 ± 0.78	40
21	Normal	10	4.42 ± 0.37	4.78 ± 0.66	37
	Deprived	6	3.09 ± 0.30	2.28 ± 0.86	65
	Reconstituted	6	3.82 ± 0.59	4.44 ± 0.89	13
28	Normal	9	3.94 ± 0.27	$\underline{5.00 \pm 0.59}$	11
	Deprived	4	2.99 ± 0.20	$\underline{2.32 \pm 0.11}$	49
	Reconstituted	5	3.53 ± 0.16	$\underline{4.78 \pm 0.42}$	5
35	Normal	7	3.80 ± 0.33	4.78 ± 0.65	8
	Deprived	4	3.03 ± 0.35	2.49 ± 0.29	31
	Reconstituted	4	3.27 ± 0.10	4.85 ± 0.06	3
	Uninjected controls	9	2.83 ± 0.37	1.30 ± 0.51	

Figures underlined $P < 0.001$.

TABLE 2

MEAN ANTI-NIP TITRES OF NORMAL, DEPRIVED AND RECONSTITUTED MICE INJECTED WITH 100 μg ALUM PRECIPITATED $NIP_{34}BSA$ PLUS 10^9 *Haemophilus pertussis* ORGANISMS

Day	Experimental group	No. mice	Antibody titre ($\log_{10}$) IgM	Antibody titre ($\log_{10}$) IgG	Per cent IgM
14	Normal	10	5.17 ± 0.37	5.05 ± 0.25	50
	Deprived	9	3.32 ± 0.30	1.92 ± 0.22	95
	Reconstituted	10	4.63 ± 0.34	4.60 ± 0.30	46
21	Normal	9	5.09 ± 0.20	5.27 ± 0.55	35
	Deprived	6	$\underline{3.30 \pm 0.18}$	$\underline{2.35 \pm 0.42}$	87
	Reconstituted	8	$\underline{4.42 \pm 0.31}$	$\underline{4.98 \pm 0.34}$	21
28	Normal	7	4.82 ± 0.26	5.32 ± 0.47	28
	Deprived	5	3.29 ± 0.25	1.67 ± 0.24	97
	Reconstituted	7	4.89 ± 0.40	5.51 ± 0.32	20
35	Normal	7	4.27 ± 0.30	5.05 ± 0.24	13
	Deprived	5	2.77 ± 0.13	1.46 ± 0.26	97
	Reconstituted	7	4.35 ± 0.31	4.43 ± 0.12	43
	Uninjected controls	9	2.83 ± 0.37	1.30 ± 0.51	

Pairs of figures underlined $P = < 0.001$.

ing to whether the mice were immunized with mainly monovalent ($NIP_{1.5}$) or polyvalent (NIP_{34}) conjugate. The results are shown in Tables 1 and 2. Sera of the mice immunized with $NIP_{1.5}BSA$ had a lower mean total antibody titre (Table 3) throughout the experiment, the peak response occurred at 28 days compared to a 21-day peak response to $NIP_{34}BSA$, which was about twice as high as the peak response to $NIP_{1.5}BSA$.

Since 100 μg of $NIP_{34}BSA$ is more immunogenic than the same dose of $NIP_{1.5}BSA$, the finding that the peak IgM response to $NIP_{34}BSA$ is about five times higher than the peak response to $NIP_{1.5}BSA$ may not be very significant. Consequently the expression of IgM as a percentage of the total antibody produced at each time gives a more accurate picture of the relative proportions of IgM and IgG in the sera at these times.

DEPRIVED MICE

The response to 100 μg $NIP_{1.5}BSA$ and $NIP_{34}BSA$ was severely depressed in mice in the absence of the thymus. Mean titres of deprived mice were significantly lower ($P<0.001$) than those of normal or reconstituted animals at all times, and generally lower than one

TABLE 3
MEAN TOTAL ANTI-NIP TITRES OF NORMAL, DEPRIVED AND RECONSTITUTED MICE INJECTED WITH 100 μg ALUM PRECIPITATED $NIP_{1.5}BSA(A)$ OR $NIP_{34}BSA(B)$ PLUS 10^9 *Haemophilus pertussis* ORGANISMS

Day	Experimental group	Total antibody titre ($\log_{10}$)
14	Normal A	4·72 ± 0·47
	Normal B	5·46 ± 0·23
	Deprived A	3·16 ± 0·51
	Deprived B	3·34 ± 0·29
	Reconstituted A	4·37 ± 0·43
	Reconstituted B	4·96 ± 0·24
21	Normal A	4·97 ± 0·51
	Normal B	5·54 ± 0·35
	Deprived A	3·16 ± 0·51
	Deprived B	3·37 ± 0·12
	Reconstituted A	4·68 ± 0·57
	Reconstituted B	5·10 ± 0·30
28	Normal A	5·05 ± 0·54
	Normal B	5·46 ± 0·38
	Deprived A	3·16 ± 0·56
	Deprived B	3·30 ± 0·25
	Reconstituted A	4·81 ± 0·40
	Reconstituted B	5·61 ± 0·33
35	Normal A	4·85 ± 0·57
	Normal B	5·14 ± 0·18
	Deprived A	3·17 ± 0·82
	Deprived B	2·79 ± 0·13
	Reconstituted A	4·86 ± 0·06
	Reconstituted B	4·71 ± 0·17

$\log_{10}$ above the background response of uninjected controls. Figs 1 and 2 show the differences in IgG and IgM antibody titres of normal and deprived mice immunized with $NIP_{1.5}BSA$ and $NIP_{34}BSA$.

The total antibody titres in both groups of deprived mice were rather similar (Table 3), so that the polyvalent conjugate containing a higher density of NIP per molecule of BSA was no more effective in immunizing these mice than the mainly monovalent conjugate, at least not at a dose of only 100 μg of protein.

ANTIGEN DOSE IN DEPRIVED MICE

By increasing the dose of $NIP_{1.5}BSA$ and $NIP_{34}BSA$ in deprived mice, the response to the mainly monovalent conjugate up to a dose of 5000 μg, was no greater than the response to 100 μg of the same conjugate. The response to the polyvalent conjugate, however, showed an increase of about one $\log_{10}$ in total antibody titre when the dose was increased to only 500 μg; there was a slight further increase at 1500 μg but 5000 μg gave more or less the same response as 500 μg.

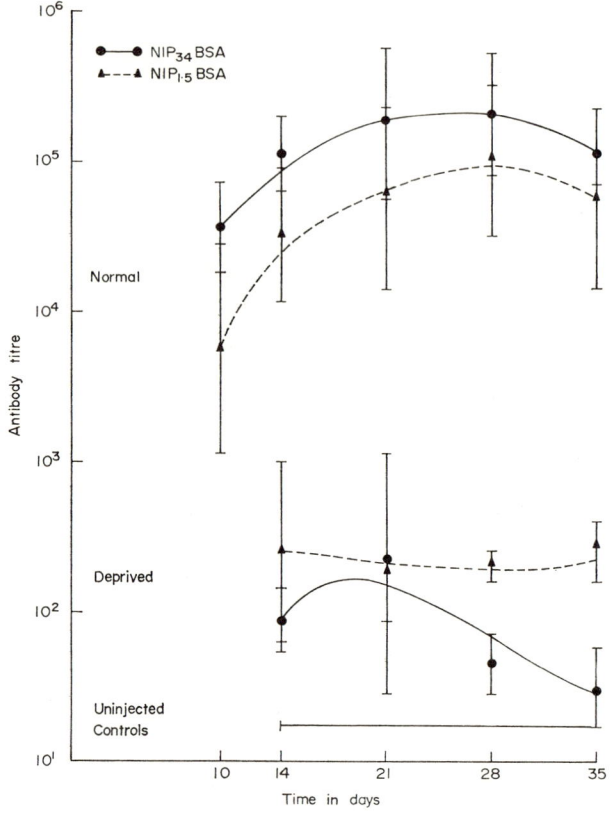

Fig. 1. Mean anti-NIP IgG titres of normal and deprived mice injected with 100 μg alum precipitated $NIP_{1.5}BSA$ or $NIP_{34}BSA$ and 10^9 *Haemophilus pertussis* organisms.

As the results in Table 4 indicate, at 21 days there was a significant difference between the responses to $NIP_{1.5}BSA$ and $NIP_{34}BSA$, at all doses above 100 μg.

RECONSTITUTED MICE

The response of reconstituted mice to both conjugates of NIP-BSA was mostly lower than the response of normal mice, particularly at early times after immunization, but still significantly higher than the response observed in the deprived animals. The peak total

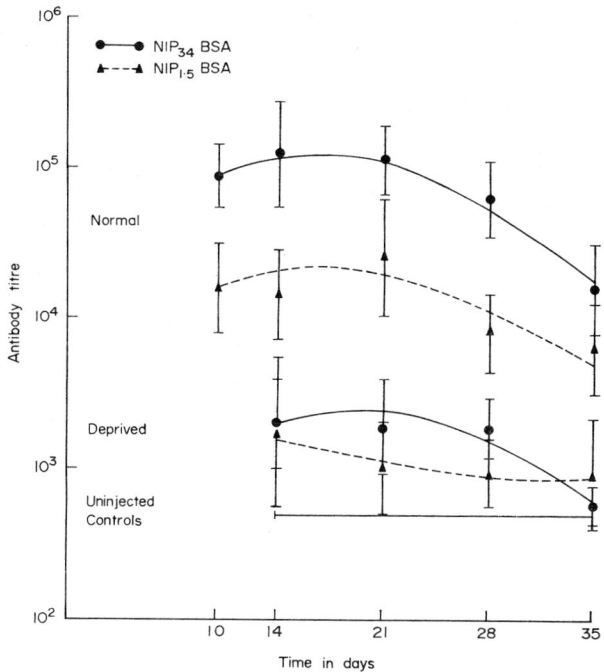

Fig. 2. Mean anti-NIP IgM titres of normal and deprived mice injected with 100 μg alum precipitated $NIP_{1.5}BSA$ or $NIP_{34}BSA$ and 10^9 *Haemophilus pertussis* organisms.

TABLE 4

MEAN ANTI-NIP TITRES OF DEPRIVED MICE 21 DAYS AFTER INJECTION OF VARIOUS DOSES OF ALUM PRECIPITATED $NIP_{1.5}BSA$ OR $NIP_{34}BSA$ AND 10^9 *Haemophilus pertussis* ORGANISMS

	100 μg	500 μg	1500 μg	5000 μg
$NIP_{1.5}BSA$				
IgM titre	3·21 ± 0·30	3·14 ± 0·09	3·42 ± 0·53	3·63 ± 0·25
IgG titre	2·70 ± 0·86	1·60 ± 0·15	2·44 ± 0·88	1·64 ± 0·46
Total Ab. titre	3·40 ± 0·51	3·15 ± 0·09	3·54 ± 0·50	3·64 ± 0·25
$NIP_{34}BSA$				
IgM titre	3·30 ± 0·18	4·10 ± 0·19	4·61 ± 0·71	4·05 ± 0·19
IgG titre	2·35 ± 0·42	2·21 ± 1·26	3·26 ± 0·86	2·24 ± 0·68
Total Ab. titre	3·37 ± 0·11	4·18 ± 0·29	4·64 ± 0·70	4·06 ± 0·20

The difference between all doses of $NIP_{1.5}BSA$ and $NIP_{34}BSA$ above 100 μg (total antibody titre) was significant.

antibody response to both conjugates occurred at 28 days (Table 3) and was little more than half the response of the normal mice in relation to $NIP_{1.5}BSA$, but almost half as high again compared to normal in the mice immunized with $NIP_{34}BSA$. By day 35, however, the response of the mice which had received $NIP_{1.5}BSA$ was almost equal to the value for normal mice, while the response of the mice which had received $NIP_{34}BSA$ was now only half of the normal value. In these mice there was an even smaller percentage of IgM in the group immunized with $NIP_{1.5}BSA$ than was observed in normal mice, particularly at the late bleedings. On day 35 only 3 per cent of the total antibody produced was attributable to IgM in mice immunized with $NIP_{1.5}BSA$, whereas in the mice immunized with $NIP_{34}BSA$ almost half the total antibody (43 per cent) was IgM.

DISCUSSION

Thymus dependency shows variability both in relation to the responding organism and the nature of the antigenic stimulus. In birds, for example, cells which derive from the thymus are important in cell-mediated immunity whereas responses which involve humoral antibody production are dependent on a population of cells which derives from the bursa of Fabricius (Warner and Szenberg, 1964). In mammals, however, this division of labour amongst cells of the lymphoid series is less well defined, and as the present study illustrates certain humoral antibody responses are very clearly thymus dependent.

Taylor and Wortis (1968) have shown that different immunoglobulin classes produced in a response to SRBC in mice vary in their relative thymus dependency; IgM and IgG_{2a} production were found to be less thymus dependent than the production of IgG_1, when thymectomized, irradiated mice were given increasing doses of SRBC. The results which have been presented here tend to support some of these findings in that higher doses of polyvalent $NIP_{34}BSA$ led to an increase in the response of deprived mice, but only in terms of IgM antibodies.

It has been shown that variations in hapten density on the carrier molecule affect the quality of the antibody produced in relation to the hapten. Polyvalent conjugates, such as $NIP_{34}BSA$, give rise to a higher proportion of IgM than monovalent or mainly monovalent conjugates (Mäkelä, 1970). It may be for this reason, therefore, that the response of deprived mice to $NIP_{34}BSA$ appears to be less thymus dependent than the response to $NIP_{1.5}BSA$. However, it can also be argued that because different numbers of NIP molecules are being introduced with the same amount of protein carrier, then still higher doses of $NIP_{1.5}BSA$ may be required to elicit a response comparable to the response to 500 μg $NIP_{34}BSA$. At present, immunogenically equivalent doses (i.e. doses of the two conjugates which will give the same total antibody titre) have not been fully determined. It still seems valid, however, to predict that the response to the polyvalent conjugate will be less thymus dependent because of the relative thymus independence of IgM antibody production. Since it has been proposed that receptor antibodies on the surface of lymphocytes are similar to the resulting humoral antibodies (Mäkelä, 1970), it is interesting to speculate that the relative thymus independence of IgM production may in some way be related to the antigen focusing mechanism which has been proposed as a function of thymus derived cells (Miller and Mitchell, 1969; Taylor, 1969). In the absence of this device, in deprived mice, it may be possible for 'IgM-like' receptors on precursors of antibody producing cells to concentrate their own antigen by virtue of their large number of combining sites when compared with IgG receptors.

In relation to normal and reconstituted mice the most interesting finding was that these results confirmed those described earlier by Mäkelä, Cross and Ruoslahti (1969), in that there was always a higher percentage of IgM in the mice immunized with the polyvalent conjugate. In reconstituted mice the responses were more variable and tended to be slightly lower and later than those of normal mice. This apparent weakness may have been due to the combined effects of irradiation and surgery and to the fact that only a single lobe of thymus tissue was grafted into these mice. No satisfactory explanation can be offered for the greater relative difference in the proportions of IgM in the response to both conjugates compared with normal mice. It is possible that inadequate numbers, either, of available stem cells from the bone marrow, and/or of thymus derived cells released from the graft, may in some way have affected the quality of the antibody produced.

There is evidence to show that co-operation takes place between thymus derived and bone marrow derived cells in the humoral antibody response to SRBC (Claman, Chaperon and Triplett, 1966). Recent transfer experiments described by Mitchison (1969) have also provided strong evidence for co-operation between cells of different specificities in the response of mice to hapten-protein conjugates. More recently Raff (1970), using anti-θ serum in a similar transfer system, has shown that the cells responsible for carrier recognition are also thymus derived.

Experiments which have indicated the importance of the carrier in hapten specific immunity suggest that the failure of deprived mice to respond to the hapten, as illustrated here, is due to an initial failure to respond to the carrier.

ACKNOWLEDGMENTS

I wish to thank Professor Olli Mäkelä for his help and advice and Dr Tony Davies for the original suggestions. This work has been supported by the U.S.P.H.S. (grant GM-12046) and the Finnish Medical Research Council.

REFERENCES

BROWNSTONE, A., MITCHISON, N. A. and PITT-RIVERS, R. (1966). 'Chemical and serological studies with an iodine-containing synthetic immunological determinant 4-hydroxy-3-iodo-5-nitrophenyl-acetic acid (NIP) and related compounds.' *Immunology*, **10**, 465.

CLAMAN, H. N., CHAPERON, E. A. and TRIPLETT, R. F. (1966). 'Thymus-marrow cell combinations—synergism in antibody production.' *Proc. Soc. exp. Biol. (N.Y.)*, **122**, 1167.

DAVIES, A. J. S., LEUCHARS, E., WALLIS, V. and KOLLER, P. C. (1966). 'The mitotic response of thymus derived cells to antigenic stimulus.' *Transplantation*, **4**, 438.

DAVIES, A. J. S., LEUCHARS, E., WALLIS, V., MARCHANT, R. and ELLIOTT, E. V. (1967). 'The failure of thymus derived cells to produce antibody.' *Transplantation*, **5**, 222.

KONTIAINEN, S. and MÄKELÄ, O. (1967). 'Determination of 19S and 7S components in an antihapten antibody.' *Ann. Med. exp. Fenn.*, **45**, 472.

LEUCHARS, E. (1970). 'Spectrum of thymus dependency.' Symposium on the role of lymphocytes and macrophages in the immunological response. XIII *International Congress of Haematology* (Ed. by D. C. Dumonde). Springer Verlag, Berlin.

MÄKELÄ, O. (1966). 'Assay of anti-hapten antibody with the aid of hapten coupled bacteriophage.' *Immunology*, **10**, 81.

MÄKELÄ, O. (1970). 'Analogies between lymphocyte receptors and the resulting humoral antibody.' *Transplantation Rev.*, **4**, 3.

MÄKELÄ, O., CROSS, A. and RUOSLAHTI, E. (1969). 'Similarities between the cellular receptor antibody and the secreted antibody.' *Cellular Recognition* (Ed. by R. T. Smith and R. A. Good).

MILLER, J. F. A. P. (1960). 'Studies on mouse leukaemia: The role of the thymus in leukaemogenesis by cell-free leukaemic filtrates.' *Brit. J. Cancer*, **14**, 93.

MILLER, J. F. A. P. and MITCHELL, G. F. (1969). 'Thymus and antigen-reactive cells.' *Transplantation Rev.*, **1**, 3.

MITCHISON, N. A. (1969). *Immunological Tolerance* (Ed. by M. Landy and W. Braun), p. 149. Academic Press, London and New York.

RAFF, M. C. (1970). 'The role of thymus derived lymphocytes in the secondary humoral immune response in mice.' *Nature (Lond.)*, **226**, 1257.

TAYLOR, R. B. (1963). 'Immunological competence of thymus cells after transfer to thymectomized recipients.' *Nature (Lond.)*, **199**, 873.

TAYLOR, R. B. (1969). 'Cellular cooperation in the antibody response of mice to two serum albumins: Specific function of thymus cells.' *Transplantation Rev.*, **1**, 114.

TAYLOR, R. B. and WORTIS, H. H. (1968). 'Thymus dependence of antibody response: Variations in the dose of antigen and class of antibody.' *Nature (Lond.)*, **220**, 927.

WARNER, N. L. and SZENBERG, A. (1964). *The thymus in Immunobiology* (Ed. by R. A. Good and A. E. Gabrielson), p. 395. Harper and Row, New York.

The Thymus and Pathogenic States

Effects of Infant Thymectomy and Antilymphocyte Serum on Xenotransplantation of a Human Leukemia in the Hamster [1]

Linda Poole Merk and Richard A. Adams

INTRODUCTION

Xenograft rejection is traditionally considered to be mediated by humoral antibody, and its immunological nature has been reaffirmed recently by the demonstrations that heterotransplantation of human melanoma (13) or choriocarcinoma (3) in the hamster cheek pouch and a rat carcinosarcoma in the mouse (7) are facilitated by ALS[2] administration. A more recent study involving suppression of rat-to-mouse skin xenograft rejection by ALS has been interpreted by Lance (8) to imply a certain degree of

---

[1] These studies were supported in part by Research Grant C-6516 from the National Cancer Institute and FR-05526 from the Division of Research Facilities and Resources, NIH.

[2] The abbreviation used is: ALS, antilymphocyte serum.

mediation of such rejection by cells. As further evidence, thymic-dependent, cytotoxic cellular immunity to a mouse mastocytoma has been directly demonstrated in rats by Jose and Good (6).

In our laboratories, experience with more than 30 neoplasms of human lymphoid origin in serial transplantation in hamsters indicates that such tumors are transplantable only in hamsters younger than 3 to 4 days and that ALS treatment is required for the progressive growth of most of these tumors. Hamsters that reject such tumors contain serum antibodies specific for human cells that are detectable by immunofluorescence techniques (4), and antiserum raised in adult hamsters against the human leukemic cells can confer on newborn hamsters the ability to reject a human leukemic xenograft (unpublished data). Further, heterologous rabbit antiserum or spleen cells from specifically sensitized or normal hamster donors also protect newborn hamsters in the same manner (1).

The purpose of the present study was to determine the extent to which thymic-dependent mechanisms are involved in the acceptance or rejection of such human tumor xenografts. Neonatal hamsters were thymectomized, subjected to various regimens of ALS treatment, and challenged with an ALS-dependent tumor at various times up to 30 days of age, well beyond the age at which normal hamsters have developed immunocompetence. Thymectomy was found to potentiate the facilitative effects of ALS on growth of the test human tumor.

MATERIALS AND METHODS

Thymectomy. Pregnant hamsters (strain LVG:LAK, a noninbred but closed colony) were obtained from Lakeview Hamster Colony, Newfield, N.J. Infant hamsters were thymectomized at 1 to 3 days of age by standard aspiration techniques under light Nembutal anesthesia (approximately 0.1 ml Diabutal (Diamond Laboratories, Des Moines, Iowa), diluted 1:60 in sterile water). Operative mortality was negligible. Sham-thymectomized hamsters and normal controls were included in each litter.

Antilymphocyte Serum. Antihamster thymus serum was prepared in these laboratories by giving New Zealand white rabbits injections of hamster thymic cells as described previously (2). All hamsters received the same dose of ALS (0.05 ml i.p.), regardless of age or weight.

Treatment with ALS Alone. ALS was administered to 3 groups of animals. One group (111 hamsters) received ALS only at time of tumor inoculation (Regimen A); a 2nd group (55 hamsters) received ALS only at birth (Regimen B); and a

3rd group (120 hamsters) received 2 doses of ALS, once at birth and again at time of tumor inoculation (Regimen C) (see Table 1).

Treatment with Thymectomy and ALS. Three groups of thymectomized and control animals were used. One group (79 hamsters) was thymectomized only; no ALS was administered. Group 2 (93 hamsters) received ALS once, at time of tumor inoculation; and the 3rd group (161 hamsters) received 2 doses of ALS, 1 on day of thymectomy and 1 on day of tumor inoculation (see Table 2).

Tumor. H-HM-1, the ALS-dependent tumor selected for study, was originally established by direct i.p. implantation into ALS-treated neonatal hamsters of bone marrow cells from a male pediatric patient with acute lymphoblastic leukemia, as described in further detail elsewhere (Ref. 9; R. A. Adams, L. Pothier, E. E. Hellerstein, and G. Bórleau, to be published). The tumor has been maintained by serial i.p. transplantation in neonatal hamsters treated with one 0.05-ml administration of ALS and is currently in its 55th passage. It progresses to acute leukemia in about 30% of implanted hamster neonates, with total white blood cell counts ranging from 20,000 to 400,000/cu mm or more. In the remainder, the solid tumor that grows in the peritoneal cavity invades most of the major organs, including liver, spleen, kidneys, and gonads, and metastasizes to deep and superficial lymph nodes, thymus, lung, and brain. Death generally occurs between 10 and 20 days postgrafting. Throughout serial transplantation, the tumor cells have retained human species-specific antigens at the cell surface, as demonstrated by immunofluorescence methods, and have retained a diploid male human karyotype.

For maintenance of the carrier line of tumor or for challenge of the experimental hamsters, tumor was dissected from the abdomen, minced in 2% penicillin : streptomycin in 0.9% NaCl solution, and injected i.p. in a concentration of approximately 20% (about 1.0×10^8 trypan blue unstained cells) in 0.2 ml inoculum. All hamsters received the same inoculum of tumor, regardless of age or weight. Successful implantation of tumor was defined as progressive growth of tumor to death of the host; in a few instances, tumor grew temporarily and then regressed, and these instances were classed as "no growth." The effectiveness of immunosuppression was evaluated in terms of the incidence of tumor and the prolongation of the time interval after birth at which tumor could be successfully transplanted.

RESULTS

Effects of ALS Treatment Alone on Tumor Implantation.

We examined 286 unthymectomized hamsters for the effects of varying the time of ALS and tumor administration. Three regimens were examined: ALS at time of tumor inoculation, ALS at birth, or ALS at birth and again at time of tumor inoculation (Table 1). When ALS was administered once at the time of tumor inoculation (Regimen A), tumor (which is normally transplantable in 100% of 0- to 24-hr-old neonates) was not transplantable in hamsters beyond 3 days of age. Of the hamsters given implants at 2 to 3 days, 32.6% died from their tumors. When ALS was administered immediately at birth (Regimen B), successful tumor implantation could be delayed to 4 to 5 days of age, while administration of ALS at birth and again at the time of tumor implantation resulted in progressive tumor growth, in some cases as late as 6 to 7 days of age. Hence, ALS has a definable effect in facilitating implantation of this tumor in the neonatal hamster.

Effects of Thymectomy and ALS Combined on Tumor Implantation. Table 2 illustrates tumor growth in thymectomized hamsters as compared with sham-thymectomized and normal control hamsters. These control data have been combined because no differences were found. The dependence of this tumor on ALS is clearly seen in the failure of the tumor to grow in either the thymectomized or control hamsters not given ALS (Table 2, Column 1). Clearly, thymectomy alone was totally ineffective in the 0- to 10-day age range, and thus

Table 1

Facilitative effects of rabbit anti-hamster thymocyte serum on xenotransplantability of human acute lymphoblastic leukemia H-HM-I in neonatal hamsters

Age at tumor implantation (days)	Tumor incidence[a]		
	Rabbit anti-hamster thymocyte serum at time of tumor inoculation (Regimen A)	Rabbit anti-hamster thymocyte serum at Day 0 (Regimen B)	Rabbit anti-hamster thymocyte serum at Day 0 and day of tumor inoculation (Regimen C)
0–1	28/28 (100%)		
2–3	15/46 (32.6%)	9/9 (100%)	22/28 (78.6%)
4–5	0/27	8/31 (25.8%)	18/42 (42.9%)
6–7	0/2	0/15	7/36 (19.4%)
>7	0/8		0/14

[a] Number of hamsters dying with tumor/total inoculated.

Table 2

Facilitative effects of neonatal thymectomy at 1 to 3 days and rabbit anti-hamster thymocyte serum combined on heterotransplantability of human acute lymphoblastic leukemia H-HM-1 in hamsters

Age at tumor implantation (days)	Tumor incidence[a]					
	No rabbit anti-hamster thymocyte serum		Rabbit anti-hamster thymocyte serum once at tumor transplantation		Rabbit anti-hamster thymocyte serum at thymectomy and tumor transplantation	
	Thymec-tomized	Control[b]	Thymec-tomized	Control	Thymec-tomized	Control
0–5	0/34	0/24	9/11 (81.8%)	1/5 (20.0%)	19/20 (95.0%)	1/10 (10.0%)
6–10	0/8	0/13	16/19 (84.4%)	0/15	19/35 (54.3%)	0/9
11–15			4/25 (16.0%)	0/12	4/23 (17.4%)	0/12
16–20			0/5	0/1	0/34	0/18
21–30						

[a] Number of hamsters dying with tumor/total inoculated.
[b] Sham-thymectomized + nonthymectomized.

did not substitute for the administration of ALS (see Table 1). By contrast, when thymectomy was coupled with any of the ALS regimens used in the study, significant prolongations in the period of susceptibility to tumor implantation could be demonstrated (Table 2, Columns 2 and 3). Infant thymectomy coupled with the most effective ALS regimen, *i.e.*, one administration at birth and another at tumor implantation, resulted in the most significant prolongation, tumor being transplantable in a low but significant percentage of thymectomized hamsters as late as 16 to 20 days of age.

White Blood Cell Counts and Histology. White blood cell counts and histological examinations were performed on selected animals. As with unthymectomized hamsters, metastatic foci occurred (Fig. 1), total white blood cell counts were significantly elevated in more than 50% of those examined, and conversion to leukemia was frequent (Fig. 2). In all tumors examined (usually 1 per litter), the tumor cells retained human species-specific antigens at the cell surface, as determined by immunofluorescence. Thus, these biological properties were not altered by the growth of this human tumor in older, thymectomized and/or ALS-treated hamsters.

DISCUSSION

The results of the present study indicate that multiple doses of ALS prolonged the period of perinatal susceptibility to implantation of a human tumor and that neonatal thymectomy significantly potentiated this suppressive effect of ALS on the host resistance to tumor implantation, but that thymectomy without ALS treatment was inadequate immunosuppression. Thus, analogous to the case of the humoral immune response to sheep erythrocytes in mice, for example (11), thymic-dependent mechanisms may figure significantly in the acceptance or rejection of these leukemic xenografts in the hamster.

It is not easy to understand how a thymic-influenced mechanism could be so difficult to demonstrate by thymectomy without adjunctive ALS treatment. One among the several possibilities is that the newborn hamster may contain sufficient numbers of thymic-dependent immunocompetent cells that, while thymectomy removes the source of the thymic-dependent reaction, ALS may be required to block or remove those thymic-dependent peripheral lymphoid cells still present after thymectomy. Other published evidence supports this argument; thymectomy alone in adult mice is ineffective in reducing immunological competence; however, coupled with ALS treatment, it produces a long-standing lymphopenia both in peripheral blood and in the lymphoid organs, as well as a significant impairment of the skin allograft rejection reaction (12). Such a mechanism might also underlie results recently reported with another allogeneic system (5), in which thymectomy was found to potentiate the effects of ALS in increasing the number of metastases associated with implantation of Sarcoma 180 in mice.

However effective thymectomy in combination with ALS treatment may be in prolonging the period of susceptibility to human leukemic grafts in the postnatal hamster, tumor failed to grow in animals older than 20 days. It is possible that weight-adjusted doses of ALS coupled with thymectomy might result in successful grafting in older hamsters. Another tumor, H-EB-3, derived from Burkitt lymphoma (2) can grow in comparably ALS-treated thymectomized hamsters when implanted as late as 30 days after birth (unpublished data). Such evidence might suggest that variable antigenicity of human tumor cells may also be an important factor. Experiments are in progress to elucidate the nature of thymic dependence in this xenogeneic system, further to define whether the thymus provides antigen-recognizing "helper" cells or effector "killer" cells (10) or whether both humoral and cellular mechanisms may function simultaneously. This technique is being utilized as well in attempts to facilitate the primary isolation of human tumors in hamsters.

REFERENCES

1. Adams, R. A., Flowers, A., Sundeen, R., and Merk, L. P. Chemotherapy and Immunotherapy of Three Human Lymphomas Serially Transplantable in the Neonatal Syrian Hamster. Cancer, *29:* 524–533, 1972.
2. Adams, R. A., Foley, G. E., Farber, S., Flowers, A., Lazarus, H., and Hellerstein, E. Serial Transplantation of Burkitt's Tumor (EB3) Cells in Newborn Syrian Hamsters and its Facilitation by Antilymphocyte Serum. Cancer Res., *30:* 338–345, 1970.
3. Davis, R. C., and Lewis, J. L., Jr. The Effect of Adult Thymectomy on the Immunosuppression Obtained by Treatment with Antilymphocyte Serum. Transplantation, *6:* 879–884, 1968.
4. Driscoll, M., and Adams, R. A. Antibody Response of Neonatal Hamsters towards Transplantable Human Leukemia Cells. Federation Proc., *27:* 667, 1968.
5. Isbister, W. H., Deodhar, S. D., and Crile, G., Jr. Effect of Adult Thymectomy and Antilymphocyte Globulin Treatment on Metastases in an Allogeneic Mouse Tumor System. Transplantation, *12:* 322–323, 1971.
6. Jose, D. G., and Good, R. A. Absence of Enhancing Antibody in Cell Mediated Immunity to Tumour Heterografts in Protein Deficient Rats. Nature, *231:* 323–325, 1971.
7. Kubista, T. P., Shorter, R. G., and Hallenbeck, G. A. Acceptance of

Walker 256 Carcinosarcoma by C57BL/6 Mice Treated with Rabbit Anti-Mouse Thymus Serum. Cancer Res., 27: 2072–2076, 1967.
8. Lance, E. M. Response of Mice to Xenografts of Skin. Transplant. Proc., 2: 497–501, 1970.
9. Merk, L. P., and Adams, R. A. Heterotransplantation of a Human Leukemia, H-HM-1: Effects of Thymectomy and Antilymphocyte Serum. Proc. Am. Assoc. Cancer Res., 12: 83, 1971.
10. Miller, J. F. A. P., Brunner, K. T., Sprent, J., Russell, P. J., and Mitchell, G. F. Thymus-derived Cells as Killer Cells in Cell-mediated Immunity. Transplant. Proc., 3: 915–917, 1971.
11. Miller, J. F. A. P., and Mitchell, G. F. Thymus and Antigen-reactive Cells. Transplant. Rev., 1: 3–42, 1969.
12. Monaco, A. P., Wood, M. L., and Russell, P. S. Adult Thymectomy: Effect on Recovery from Immunologic Depression in Mice. Science, 149: 432–435, 1965.
13. Sommers, S. C., Reeves, G., and Reeves, E. Immunologic and Chemotherapeutic Effects on Human Melanoma Heterotransplants. Proc. Soc. Exptl. Biol. Med., 123: 740–742, 1966.

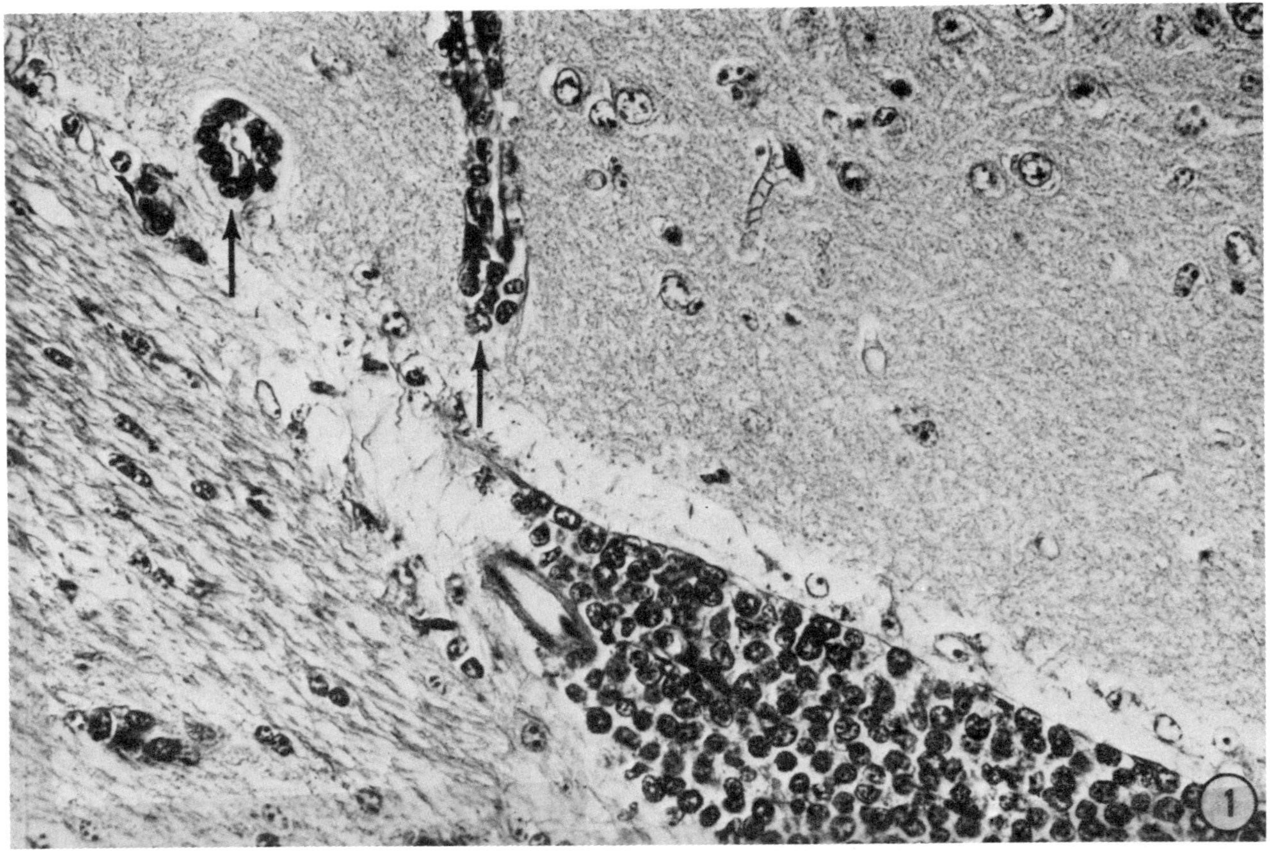

Fig. 1. Brain of neonatally thymectomized hamster 40 days after i.p. implantation of H-HM-1 tumor cells at 9 days of age. Note infiltration and perivascular cuffing (*arrows*) by tumor cells. H & E, × 500.

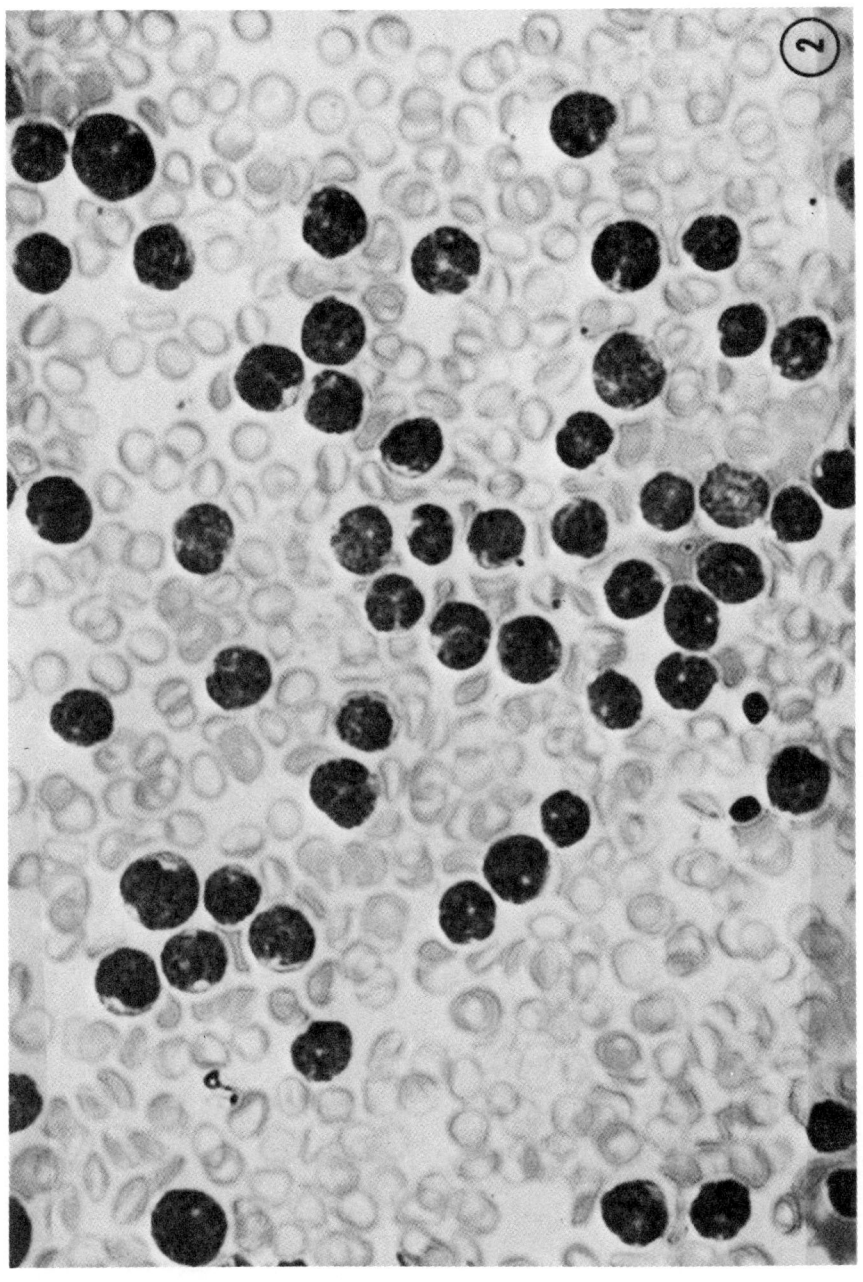

Fig. 2. Peripheral blood of neonatally thymectomized hamster 15 days after i.p. implantation of H-HM-1 tumor cells at 9 days of age. Total white blood cell count of this animal was 257,000/cu mm. Wright and Giemsa, × 800.

Thymoma Associated With Pancytopenia

Stanley Burrows, MD, and Robert Carroll, MD

MOST cases of severe pancytopenia that are not caused by leukemia or exposure to toxic chemicals have an unknown cause. There has been an increasing number of reports of hematologic abnormalities associated with thymoma, suggesting that some of these conditions of "idiopathic" aplastic anemia, neutropenia, and pancytopenia, together with immunoglobulin deficiencies, may be related to tumors of the thymus. We recently observed an elderly man with severe pancytopenia and mild immunoglobulin deficiency, in whom an invasive thymoma was discovered at postmortem examination.

Report of a Case

A 90-year-old man was first admitted to the Cooper Hospital on Dec 19, 1970, with the chief complaint of increasingly severe weakness for the previous ten days. An increasing number of petechiae and ecchymoses had appeared over the extremities during the four days prior to admission.

From the departments of pathology (Dr. Burrows) and hematology (Dr. Carroll), the Cooper Hospital, Camden, N.J.

He had been in good health until ten months before admission, when he developed mouth ulcers which improved upon treatment with nystatin. A nosebleed, requiring packing for control, led to his admission to another hospital one week later. A fall of hemoglobin concentration from 16 gm/100 ml to 10.8 gm/100 ml was attributed to blood loss, and he was discharged on a regimen of iron medication administered orally. Hemoglobin concentration rose to 12 gm/100 ml in one month, and iron medication was stopped five months later.

Physical examination showed that the patient had marked pallor, with numerous petechiae and ecchymoses of the buccal mucosa, nasopharynx, face, and lower extremities. Vital signs were normal. The spleen and liver were not palpable.

Laboratory studies included the following values: hemoglobin, 7 gm/100 ml; hematocrit reading, 21%; white blood cell count (WBC), 2,100/cu mm, with 41% neutrophils, 57% lymphocytes, and 2% monocytes; platelets, 2,000/cu mm. Urinalysis showed numerous red blood cells, (RBC). Additional values were as follows: serum calcium was 8.6 mg/100 ml; phosphorus, 3.9 mg/100 ml; blood urea nitrogen, 42 mg/100 ml; uric acid, 4.7 mg/100 ml; cholesterol, 146 mg/100 ml; protein, 6.0 gm/100 ml; creatinine, 1.1 mg/100 ml; alkaline phosphatase, 75 milliunits (normal, 30 to 85 milli-

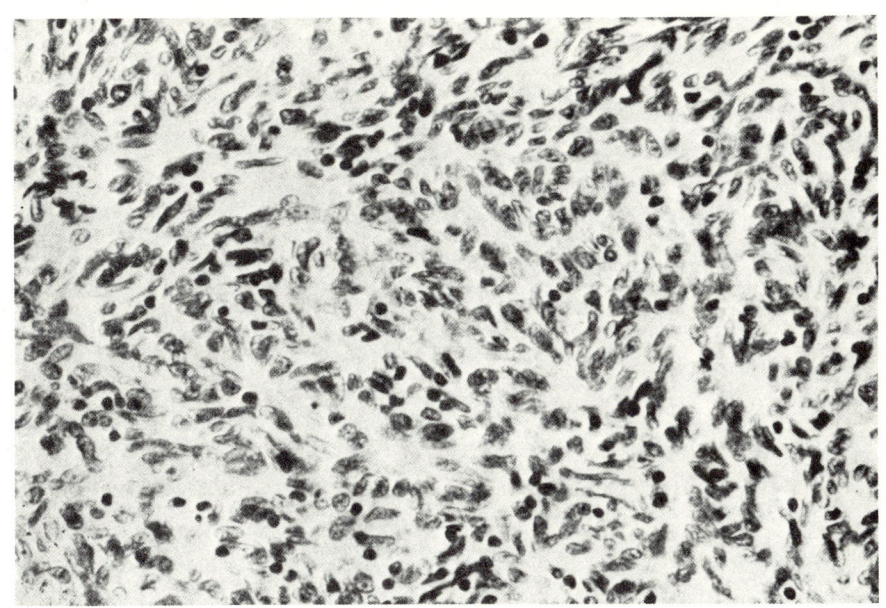

Fig 1.—Thymic tumor showing spindle cell pattern with scattered lymphocytes (hematoxylin-eosin, reduced from ×400).

units); lactic dehydrogenase, 132 milliunits (normal, 90 to 200 milliunits); serum glutamic oxaloacetic transaminase (SGOT), 37 units (normal, 10 to 40 units). Protein electrophoresis showed a slightly decreased γ-globulin fraction of 0.6 gm/100 ml. Bone marrow aspiration was interpreted as hypoplasia.

The clinical impression was pancytopenia due to hypoplasia of the bone marrow from an unknown cause. Therapy included corticosteroids, two units of packed RBC, and 10 units of platelet concentrates. Hematologic studies on the following day showed a rise in the following values: hemoglobin concentration to 10.4 gm/100 ml, hematocrit reading to 29%, WBC to 2,600/cu mm, and platelets to 75,000/cu mm. Hematuria stopped, and the patient was discharged on Dec 23, with similar hematologic values, except that the platelet count had fallen to 50,000/cu mm.

The patient was admitted for the second time on Jan 1, 1971, following recurrence of hematuria and epistaxis the previous night, followed by extreme weakness and leg pain. Petechiae and ecchymoses were again seen over the buccal mucosa and the skin.

Laboratory studies included the following values: hemoglobin, 10.6 gm/100 ml; hematocrit reading, 30.2%; WBC, 1,100/cu mm, with 15% neutrophils, 78% lymphocytes, and 8% monocytes; platelets, 1,000/cu mm. Serum chemistry studies were similar to the first admission, except for an increase of SGOT to 120 units.

Therapy included corticosteroids and 2 units of fresh blood. The patient's temperature rose to 103 F (39.4 C) on the third hospital day and he died.

Findings From Autopsy

The major gross finding was a somewhat irregular, flattened, firm gray-white tumor mass in the superior anterior mediastinum in the region of the thymus, measuring 4 cm in diameter and up to 1.5 cm in thickness. The tumor mass adhered to the adjacent innominate vein, and the vein was filled with moderately firm gray-white tissue measuring up to 1.5 cm in diameter. Other gross findings included moderate coronary artery athero-

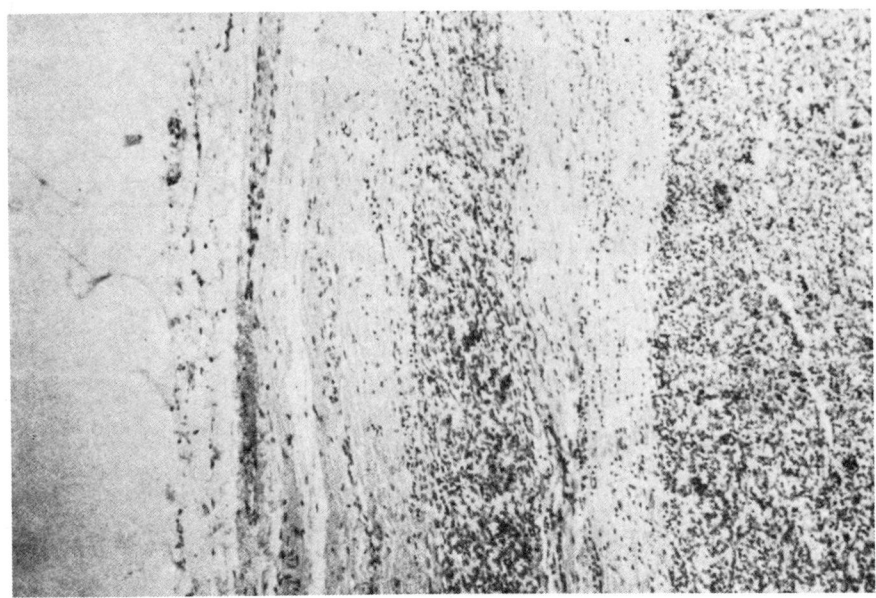

Fig 2.—Invasion of wall and occlusion of lumen of innominate vein by thymic tumor (hematoxylin-eosin, reduced from ×100).

sclerosis, moderate pulmonary fibrosis with emphysema, and moderately enlarged nodular prostate.

Histologic study of the mediastinal tumor showed a spindle cell pattern with scattered lymphocytes (Fig 1). Interlacing bands of fibrous tissue separated the tumor into nodules of various sizes. The wall of the adjacent innominate vein was invaded by a histologically similar tumor, and the tumor occluded the lumen of the vein (Fig 2). The vertebral bone marrow was markedly hypoplastic and largely fatty. Only scattered groups of lymphocytes and a few inactive, immature myeloid elements were seen in the bone marrow.

Comment

The association of thymoma with hematologic abnormalities may not be as rare as the limited number of reports indicate. Rubin et al[1] noted that recent reviews of clinical disorders associated with thymic tumors reported only 14 (3.5%) of 403 cases of thymomas associated with hematologic abnormalities, compared to 165 (40.9%) cases associated with myasthenia gravis. However, three (11.5%) of their own series of 26 patients with thymic tumors had hypoplastic anemia, whereas only two (7.7%) had myasthenia gravis, both after the removal of the thymomas.

Rogers et al[2] reviewed 61 cases of thymoma associated with hematologic abnormalities, as reported in the world literature. Anemia alone was the most common hematologic abnormality in 39 cases (64%); with associated neutropenia in 4 (7%) or thrombocytopenia in 7 (12%), occurring less frequently. Pancytopenia was the predominant hematologic abnormality in six (10%) of the cases, whereas anemia progressed to pancytopenia in an additional four (7%) of the cases. The bone marrow usually shows lymphocytosis, although a recent case[3] of thymoma, associated with agranulocytosis and a lesser degree of anemia and thrombocytopenia, exhibited a hyperplastic bone marrow with myeloid maturation arrest.

The age range of patients was from 20 to 78, making our patient the oldest. The syndrome occurred twice as frequently in women as in men. The most common symptom has been a developing anemia, although hemorrhage due to thrombocytopenia may be the first symptom. (Our patient had symptoms of hemorrhage related to severe thrombocytopenia. At the same time, he had pallor and weakness related to anemia. He died with the clinical evidence of sepsis, probably caused by the severe agranulocytosis.)

In all but three of the cases reviewed by Rogers et al[2] thymic tumors were noninvasive, and were usually asymptomatic, with incidental discovery in chest roentgenograms. Locally invasive thymomas may be associated with cough, pain, pleural effusion, or superior vena caval syndrome. Although the thymoma in our patient was locally invasive and obstructed the innominate vein, there were no localized symptoms caused by the thymoma.

Manifestations of auto-immune disease were noted in 26 (43%) of the cases. Myasthenia gravis occurred in eight cases, hypergammaglobulinemia in four, hypogammaglobulinemia in six, positive direct Coombs' test in six, antinuclear antibodies in four, positive LE preparation in two, false-positive results of serological studies in one, and malabsorption in one case. Our patient exhibited slight hypogammaglobulinemia. It is not surprising that patients with thymic tumors show an increased incidence of auto-immune disease, considering the vital role of the normal thymus in the development and maintenance of immunologic competence of the body.

The most common histologic type of thymoma associated with hematologic abnormalities has been the spindle cell type, similar to that seen in our patient. Improvement or cure of the hematologic abnormalities after thymectomy was most frequent in patients with only anemia, although corticosteroids were needed in several cases. Thymectomy was not helpful in patients with thrombocytopenia, pancytopenia, or complicating hemolytic anemia. Six cases of anemia occurred after thymectomy. Our patient's pancytopenia would probably not have been helped by thymectomy.

The cause of the hematologic abnormalities associated with thymoma is unknown. Clarkson and Prockop[4] could not demonstrate any change in the erythropoietic activity of a dog that received large amounts of saline extracts of a thymoma associated with aregenerative anemia, and concluded that the anemia was probably not caused by a tumor secretion. Further studies are needed to elucidate the thymic-hematopoietic relationships.

Thymic tumors may be small and easily overlooked on routine chest roentgenograms. The presence of thymomas should be considered in patients having "idiopathic" hypoplastic anemia, with or without neutropenia and thrombocytopenia. Special roentgenogram views are warranted to detect thymic tumors, particularly if auto-immune phenomena are also present. Once detected, the thymic tumors should be removed with the hope for cure, or improvement, of the hematologic abnormalities. The association of thymomas with hematologic abnormalities may prove to be more common than medical literature indicates, if the index of suspicion is high.

References

1. Rubin M, Straus B, Allen L: Clinical disorders associated with thymic tumors. *Arch Intern Med* **114:**389-398, 1964.

2. Rogers BHG, Manaligod JR, Blazer WV: Thymoma associated with pancytopenia and hypogammaglobulinemia: Report of a case and review of the literature. *Amer J Med* **44:**154-164, 1968.

3. Jacobson BM, Castleman, B: Case records of the Massachusetts General Hospital: Anemia, granulocytopenia and terminal sepsis in a 70-year-old woman. *New Eng J Med* **284:**39-47, 1971.

4. Clarkson B, Prockop DJ: Aregenerative anemia associated with benign thymoma. *New Eng J Med* **259:**253-258, 1958.

Malignant Thymoma in a Child

WILLIAM E. DEMUTH, JR., M.D., JAMES SMITH, M.D.

MALIGNANT thymic tumors in children are rare. Many reports of mediastinal tumors in children reported from institutions caring for large numbers of children describe no experience with malignant neoplasm of the thymus. In his classic book, Gross[4] reported only two instances, both admitted in extremis.

The controversy concerning the origin of malignant thymomas continues. Although the parent cell has never been conclusively proven, the consensus now seems to be that the tumor arises in the lymphoid elements of the thymus. Irrespective of its genesis, the rapid progression of airway and vena caval obstruction may give rise to great difficulty in management. Experience with such a case prompts this report.

Case Report

R. M. (A99266), a 9-year-old boy, was admitted to the Carlisle Hospital on August 29, 1969 because of noisy respiration. A week before, he played with other children and was normally active. He was seen by his family physician 5 days prior to admission and was treated for a supposed minor respiratory infection. During the subsequent 3 days, breathing became noisy, and on the night before admission breathing became labored and he did not sleep well. On the morning of admission, puffiness of the face and periorbital edema were noted. His appetite was good and he ate his usual breakfast 3 hours before admission. Prior to the present illness, the child was believed to be completely healthy without any history of illness except for the usual childhood diseases.

Physical Examination: Blood pressure 120/90 mm. Hg, temp. 98, pulse 110/min, respirations 20/min. He was a well-developed boy in moderate respiratory distress with moderate stridor. He preferred to sit up, his eyes and face were swollen, and conjunctivae were injected. Cervical veins were prominent and a hard mass extended to the midline low in the right anterior triangle of the neck. Firm bilateral anterior and posterior cervical nodes were palpable. Subcostal inspiratory retraction was present, but breath sounds were not diminished. Examination was otherwise unremarkable.

Chest x-ray (Fig. 1): A large mass was present in the anterior mediastinum. Both trachea and esophagus were displaced posteriorly.

Laboratory Data: Hemoglobin 13.0 Gm.; hematocrit 39%; WBC 5050, differential — polys 69, lymphocytes 26, monocytes 4, basophil 1; urine analysis — negative. Electrolytes — potassium 4.3 mEq., sodium 147 mEq., chloride 84 mEq., CO_2 37 m mol.

During the subsequent 2 hours respiratory distress increased and it was decided to proceed with tracheostomy in the hope that the airway might be improved. It was realized the obstruction may extend beyond the trachea and bronchoscopy was indicated.

Operation: Premedication consisted of 0.2 mg. scopolamine. Because of extreme agitation, endotracheal intubation was accomplished under nitrous oxide-oxygen-thiopental anesthesia. Tracheal intubation was easily carried out, but adequate inflation was impossible and a bronchoscope was hurriedly passed which provided better ventilatory exchange. Despite this, cardiac arrest ensued, and open cardiac massage was effective in re-establishing heart action. Tracheostomy was then performed and a plastic cuffed tracheostomy tube was passed downward approximately 10 cm. with better aeration resulting from intermittent positive pressure insufflation. At the conclusion of tracheostomy, the cervical mass was biopsied through the tracheostomy wound and the chest was closed after drainage tubes had been inserted.

In the course of thoracotomy for resuscitation, the huge, fixed anterior mediastinal mass was visualized and it was believed that irradiation afforded

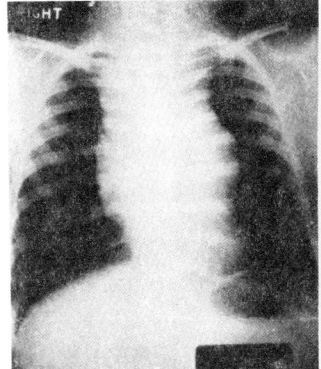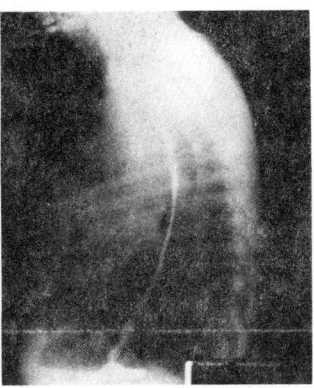

Fig. 1. PA (left) and lateral (right) roentgenograms of the chest.

the only hope for palliation. Consequently, he was immediately removed to the x-ray therapy department for treatment. Distention of the cervical veins and cyanosis of the lips and nail beds persisted despite the administration of oxygen. X-ray therapy was again given the following morning, but respiratory difficulty continued. The child responded only slightly and he died 40 hours after admission without overcoming respiratory or vena caval obstruction.

Microscopy of Biopsy Specimens: Cells were predominantly uniform, mononuclear, oval to round. Small clumps of cells containing larger reticular nuclei and abundant cytoplasm were present. Some contained PAS positive granules after diastase digestion. In the peripheral aspects of the tumor, a few structures which appeared to be remnants of Hassels corpuscles were present.

Autopsy: Except for findings within the thorax, both gross and microscopic findings were unremarkable. The face was swollen as described above.

Gross: A hard, nodular, gray tumor mass encircled the heart and great vessels. The aortic arch, superior vena cava and pulmonary artery were narrowed and irregularly indented by the encroaching tumor mass. The trachea and both main stem bronchi were incorporated in the tumor mass extending from the carotid bifurcation down to the pulmonary hila on both sides (Fig. 3). Marked narrowing of all involved airway structures was demonstrated and it was evident that the tracheostomy tube could not have reached beyond the obstruction which extended well beyond the carina on both sides. Margins of the tumor were indistinct. Although incompletely excised free of other structures, tumor weight was 310 Gm. The left lung and most of the right lower lobe were completely atelectatic.

Microscopic: Heart — no abnormalities. Lungs — alveoli were blood filled in many areas and extensive bilateral atelectasis was present. Hilar nodes were unremarkable. Tumor cells were seen in the outer muscular layer of the esophagus but no mucosal changes were present.

Sections of the neoplasm were substantially the same as those described for the material removed at biopsy. A diagnosis of malignant thymoma was made.

Discussion

Less than 100 malignant tumors of the thymus gland have been reported in children. Their tendency to encroach upon the superior mediastinal vessels and trachea usually produce a clinical picture of respiratory and superior vena caval obstruction. Bizarre cutaneous lesions,[9] petechia[10] and massive cervical lymphadenopathy[8] have been reported in association with thymic neoplasms in children.

In the past, benign thymic enlargement has been indicted as a cause of tracheal obstruction, which, if true, could pose a serious diagnostic problem in differentiating benign from malignant lesions. Hope et al.[7] reported in 1963 that no proven case of tracheal obstruction due to thymic hyperplasia had ever been recorded at the Philadelphia Children's Hospital. Other evidence[5,6] strongly supports this view. Caffery[2] emphasized the usefulness of a brief course of steroid therapy in rapidly reducing the size of the benign hyperplastic thymus which may prove helpful as a diagnostic test. Evidence of tracheal or bron-

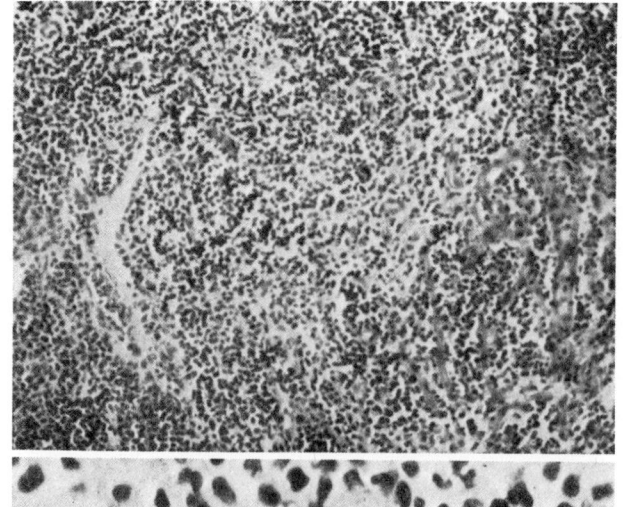

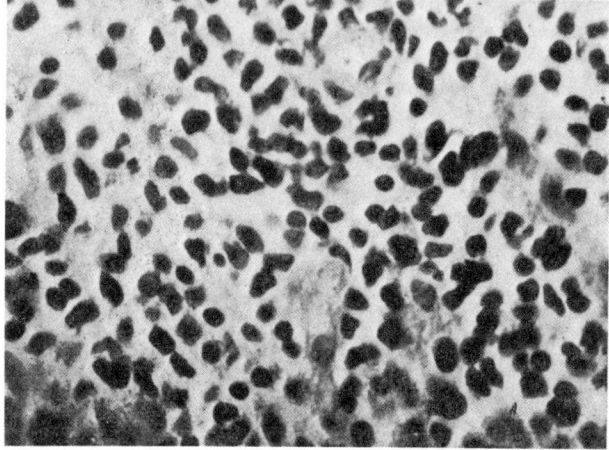

FIG. 2. Microscopic sections of biopsy specimens removed from the neck at time of tracheostomy (top × 100, bottom × 440).

chial obstruction should suggest the presence of a malignant neoplasm.

It is not possible to conclude that any form of therapy is very efficacious since many of the children reported died shortly after hospital admission. Bomze and Kirshbaum[1] reported rapid decrease in size of a malignant thymoma in a child following x-ray therapy, but Cutler[3] stated "usually those tumors which respond rapidly are so highly malignant that they are accompanied by a grave prognosis." Despite this, at present it appears that radiation therapy offers the best chance for palliation or cure.

At the stage when most of the diagnoses are made, resection would seem to be impossible even for palliation. If, as in our case, the tumor presents in the neck, biopsy can be performed and therapy instituted promptly.

Reports frequently have not included clinical details, but in those instances where the clinical course has been described, most appear to have run a very rapid course and, frequently the physician first examining the patient believes a minor respiratory infection to be present.

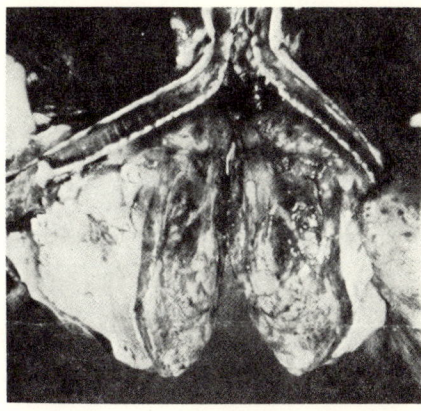

FIG. 3. Gross autopsy specimen demonstrating large mediastinal tumor. Bronchi and trachea have been opened. Note encroachment at carina.

References

1. Bomze, E. J., and J. D. Kirshbaum: Lymphosarcoma of the mediastinum (malignant thymoma). J. Lab. Clin. Med. **24**: 928, 1939.
2. Caffey, J.: Pediatric X-ray Diagnosis, ed. 4, Yearbook Medical Publishers, Inc., Chicago, 1961.
3. Cutler, M.: Lymphosarcoma, clinical, pathological and radiotherapeutic study with report of 30 cases. Arch. Surg. **30**: 445, 1935.
4. Gross, R. E.: The Surgery of Infancy and Childhood, W. B. Saunders Co., Philadelphia, Pa., 1954, pp. 773-774.
5. Haller, J. A., D. O. Mazur, and W. W. Morgan: Diagnosis and management of mediastinal masses in children. J. Thorac. Cardiovasc. Surg. **58**: 385, 1969.
6. Heimberger, I. L., and J. S. Battersby: Primary mediastinal tumors of childhood. J. Thorac. Cardiovasc. Surg. **50**: 92, 1965.
7. Hope, J. W., P. F. Borns, and C. E. Koop: Radiological diagnosis of mediastinal masses in infants and children. Radiol. Clin. N. Amer. **1**: 17, 1963.
8. Rogatz, J. L.: Pleomorpheus cell lymphosarcoma of the thymus. J. Pediat. **14**: 618, 1939.
9. Wasserman, P., and J. W. Epstein: Congenital carcinoma of the thymus with extensive generalized metastasis. J. Pediat. **14**: 798, 1939.
10. Wollstein, M., and S. McLean: Hodgkin's disease primary in the thymus gland. Amer. J. Dis. Child. **32**: 889, 1926.

Thymic Function, Immunologic Deficiency, and Autoimmunity

David Osoba, M.D., F.R.C.P.(C)

There has been a rapid expansion of knowledge relating to the functions of the thymus since the demonstration, 10 years ago, that the thymus plays an important role in immunity.[88, 100] From experiments in mice[18, 61, 109] and in cell culture systems,[70, 108, 112, 139] it is now evident that the formation of 19S hemolytic antibodies to sheep erythrocytes is dependent upon interactions between at least three separate classes of cells. These classes of cells, found in the spleen and lymph nodes, are "helper" T cells (derived from the thymus), B cells (probably derived from the bone marrow in mammals and from the bursa of Fabricius in birds), and A cells. Cell-mediated immune responses are dependent upon effector cells arising from thymus-derived T cells[16] that are probably different than the "helper" T cells involved in antibody formation.[84] The roles of these cells will be considered more fully in the sections dealing with humoral and cell-mediated immunity. From the study of immunologic deficiency diseases in man it has become evident that these diseases can be explained on the basis of knowledge derived from experimental animal models. This knowledge will lead to therapeutic strategies capable of curing, or at least controlling, most of these diseases in the near future. My purpose in this paper is to suggest a view of the pathogenesis of immunologic deficiency and autoimmune diseases, based upon current concepts of the development and differentiation of the immunologic system.

DEVELOPMENT OF THE IMMUNOLOGIC SYSTEM

In the human being, the epithelial rudiment of the thymus develops from clusters of cells in the foregut endoderm of the third and fourth

---

Portions of the work cited were supported by the Medical Research Council of Canada (MA-1609) and the Ontario Cancer Treatment and Research Foundation (Project No. 203).

pharyngeal pouches[67] at about the sixth week of gestation.[46] Initially, the primordia for the thymus, parathyroids, and great vessels are in close proximity, but by the eighth week the thymus begins to descend into the superior mediastinum. By the tenth week lymphocytes appear in the epithelial rudiment. Although the source of these first thymic lymphocytes in man is unknown, in chicken embryos they are derived from blood-borne cells[106] which probably originate in the blood islands.

Lymphocytic colonization of the thymus, with development of the characteristic medulla and cortex, proceeds rapidly during the next few weeks. Lymphocytes appear in the blood,[117] and thereafter lymphoid development of the spleen and lymph nodes occurs. Sequestration of stem cells by the thymus probably continues throughout fetal and neonatal life and, if experimental evidence in mice[38, 68] is also true for man, the thymus continues to receive stem cells from the bone marrow even during adult life.

In the mouse, cells colonizing the thymus are closely related to stem cells (colony-forming cells) responsible for the development of the myeloid component of the hematopoietic system.[145] Indeed, both may be the progeny of a single class of stem cells capable of giving rise to the entire myeloid and lymphoid systems. That a similar situation exists in man can be inferred from some diseases which affect these stem cells.

The thymus is the site of unusually active cellular proliferation,[96] probably under the control of genetic and thymic humoral factors,[101] since the rate of proliferation is independent of antigenic stimulation.[62] Apparently, most of the cells born in the thymus also die there, since only a small proportion leave the thymus.[95] The reasons for the high death rate are unknown, but this observation has contributed to a hypothesis that the thymus is a "mutant-breeding organ".[79]

Jerne postulates that the thymus, and perhaps the bone marrow (in mammals) and the bursa of Fabricius (in birds) are sites for the proliferation of clones of cells capable of reacting with environmental (exogenous) antigens, as well as with histocompatibility antigens of other members of the same species. These clones develop from precursor cells carrying genes coding for self-antigens, but as they proliferate in the thymus, some cells will sustain random somatic mutations rendering them no longer capable of self-reactivity. Such cells will now be capable of reacting with environmental antigens, and will be allowed to survive, but those that do not sustain mutations will be suppressed and die in the thymus. The surviving cells eventually migrate to and populate the peripheral lymphoid organs.

As yet, this hypothesis has not been adequately tested, but it provides an explanation for the development of tolerance to self-antigens at the same time as the development of diversity of immune reactivity to foreign histocompatibility antigens and to exogenous antigens. In addition, a failure of the mechanism for suppressing clones of cells with self-reactivity might explain the development of autoimmune diseases.

In mice, the lymphocytes in the thymus bear a specific alloantigen, called θ.[120] This marker also identifies thymus-derived lymphocytes (T cells) in the peripheral lymphoid organs. About 35 per cent of the cells in the spleen and Peyer's patches and 65 per cent of cells in the lymph nodes are θ-positive.[114, 119] As yet, a similar marker has not been demonstrated on human thymic lymphocytes.

The first indication that immunologic responsiveness in higher animals depends upon more than one class of cells arising in diverse anatomic structures came from experiments in chickens.[24, 49, 143] In addition to the thymus, chickens have a second structure, the bursa of Fabricius, necessary for full development of immune responsiveness. The bursa develops from the epithelial endoderm of the hindgut associated with the cloaca. The bursal lymphocytes are derived from blood-borne stem cells.[105] Cells leaving the bursa populate areas of the spleen and lymph nodes anatomically distinct from those populated by thymus-derived cells.[24, 77, 114] Although the equivalent of the bursa in rabbits may be the sacculus rotundus and Peyer's patches,[23] the bursal equivalent in most mammals, including man, is unknown. However, there is indirect evidence from experiments in mice[18, 109] and from experience with immunologic deficiency diseases in man[45] to suggest that the bone marrow itself has this function.

In mice, cells derived from the bone marrow (B cells) also bear a specific antigenic marker called MBLA (mouse-specific B lymphocyte antigen).[118] Thymus cells do not have this antigen, but approximately 40 per cent of the cells in the bone marrow are MBLA-positive. Peyer's patches, spleen, and lymph nodes also contain MBLA-positive cells (70, 55, and 30 per cent, respectively).

Although T and B cells develop in separate anatomical areas, it is likely that they are the progeny of a single class of stem cells capable of populating the entire lymphoid system.[33]

A third class of cells (A, or accessory cells) also participates in humoral antibody production.[50, 61, 107, 112, 125, 131] These cells are found in the spleen and lymph nodes and are probably derived from precursors present in bone marrow.[61, 113] Whether A-cell precursors are related to the precursors of T and B cells is unknown. The roles of B, T, and A cells in the two major types of immune response will now be considered more fully.

HUMORAL IMMUNE RESPONSES

Circulating antibodies are produced in response to immunization with soluble antigens, e.g. foreign erythrocytes. In mice, the response to foreign erythrocytes is dependent upon an interaction between B, "helper" T, and A cells (see references 110 and 124 for brief reviews). B cells bear specific surface receptors capable of binding antigens.[9, 60, 112] These receptors have some of the characteristics of light (κ and λ) and heavy chains (μ).[63, 64] Before antigenic stimulation, B cells do not produce significant quantities of antibody,[18, 102] but after stimulation they proliferate and mature into antibody-forming cells.[109] Thus, B cells are the immediate precursors of antibody-forming cells. Each clone of B cells is restricted with respect to the number of specific antigens to which it can respond.[1, 32, 102, 111, 112, 116] It is still uncertain whether or not a clone of B cells is class-restricted, even though its progeny produce antibody molecules of only a single class of immunoglobulin at any given time.[15, 66, 87]

"Helper" T cells also appear to bear specific receptors for antigens,[9, 65] but thus far these receptors have been shown only to have the characteristics of κ chains.[64] "Helper" T cells do not mature into antibody-forming cells.[109] Their exact function in the interaction with B cells in humoral responses is still unclear, but from secondary responses there is evidence that when antigens are composed of hapten-carrier moieties, "helper" T cells react with the carrier portion and B cells with the hapten portion of the immunogenic molecule.[11, 103]

In contrast to B and "helper" T cells, A cells need not proliferate during an immune response.[50, 61, 125] It has been suggested that they may play a role in "processing" certain antigens, rendering these antigens more immunogenic, but may not be necessary in the immune response to all antigens.[131] If A cells do play a role in processing antigen, then it is likely that they function during the first stage of an immune response. Presumably, "helper" T and B cells are triggered at later stages.

CELL-MEDIATED IMMUNE RESPONSES

Cell-mediated responses are characteristic of delayed hypersensitivity, homograft immunity, and graft-versus-host reactions. The effector ("killer") cells are found in the circulation, thoracic duct, spleen, and lymph nodes. The mechanism by which "killer" cells destroy allogeneic cells is unknown. Up to the present time, they have not been found to secrete any known class of immunoglobulin. The "killer" cells are derived from precursors originating in the thymus and proliferate in response to foreign histocompatibility antigens.[16] It is likely that the precursors of the "killer" cells are not identical to the "helper" T cells participating in humoral immune responses, since cells having these two functions appear to have different physical properties following separation on equilibrium density gradients.[84] It is still unclear whether or not the T-cell precursors of "killer" cells bear specific surface receptors for antigens or whether the "killer" function is specific. However, they do have surface receptors which combine with anti-light-chain antisera.[63] There is growing evidence that cell-cell interactions[73, 122, 129] or interactions with the products of other cells[6] may be required for the transition of T cells into "killer" cells.

A SUMMARY OF THE CELLULAR BASIS OF IMMUNOLOGICAL RESPONSIVENESS

The cells of the immunologic system can be considered to pass through three stages of differentiation during development (Fig. 1). Cellular proliferation is an important part of all of these stages. During the first stage, pluripotential stem cells give rise to cells capable of

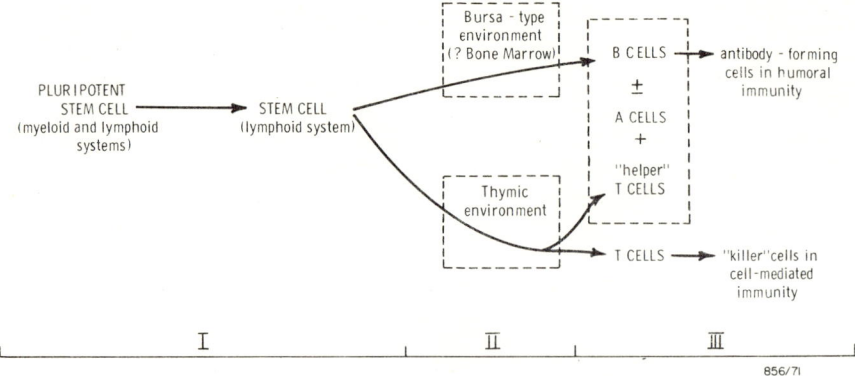

Figure 1. A schematic representation of a model depicting cellular differentiation in the development of the immunological system. The numerals I, II, and III refer to three distinct stages in the differentiation process.

populating the lymphoid system, and these migrate to the thymus and perhaps the marrow (the equivalent of the avian bursa). Under the influence of the thymic environment and the bursa-like environment in the marrow, cells in the thymus differentiate into T cells, and those in the marrow into B cells. Each clone of B cells is restricted in its capacity to react with a variety of antigens. Thus, these cells may be considered to be immunologically committed. Whether or not T cells are restricted in their capacity to react with a variety of antigens is still unclear. The third stage is the formation of effector cells.

In cell-mediated immune responses T cells having the capacity to react with histocompatibility antigens become "killer" cells. In humoral responses to environmental antigens, "helper" T cells interact with A cells and B cells, and the B cells mature into antibody-forming cells. T cells with "killer" potential and "helper" T cells are probably not identical. Whereas the proliferation in the first two stages is independent of antigen, that in the third stage is triggered by antigen, and therefore is antigen dependent.

TESTS OF IMMUNOLOGIC FUNCTION IN MAN

Immunologic responses in man, as in animals, are classified as being humoral and cell-mediated in type. However, both the identification of the number of classes of cells involved in each kind of response, and the characterization of these cells, beyond their general morphologic identification as lymphocytes, still require much further investigation. Studies of humoral immunity in man would be aided greatly by the development of cell culture systems for the generation of antibody-forming cells. At present, it is necessary to directly challenge a patient with antigens to determine if the capacity to form a primary humoral response is present. Although such tests are useful, they require a lengthy time interval between challenge and determination of serum antibody levels, and they do not give information about the number of cells producing a specific antibody at a given time, nor about the number of precursors and possible cell-cell interactions necessary for antibody production.

On the other hand, cell culture systems which test the capacity of lymphocytes to proliferate and to participate in cell-mediated immune responses are available. The addition of phytohemagglutinin (PHA) to peripheral blood cells stimulates lymphocytes to proliferate. It is likely that it is the T cells which undergo proliferation.[17, 27] The cells of patients[83] and mice[35] with congenital absence of the thymus usually do not respond to PHA. Although the PHA response is useful for determining whether or not thymus-derived cells capable of proliferation are present in the circulation, there is little evidence that this test gives any indication of the capacity of these cells to function immunologically. This latter information is given by the one-way mixed leukocyte reaction.[7] In this test, the peripheral blood lymphocytes of the individual to be tested are cultured in the presence of allogeneic cells which have been rendered incapable of proliferation by pretreatment with appropriate drugs or irradiation. It is likely that this test detects the presence of functional T cells capable of recognizing foreign histocompatibility antigens. The cells of patients and mice[35] with congenital absence of the thymus fail to respond. Tests of cellular migration out of capillary tubes in the presence or absence of antigen show promise of being useful,[26, 36] but at present it is still unclear just what functions these procedures are testing.

Finally, skin tests of delayed hypersensitivity to a variety of antigens are also useful, but again they suffer from the defects that they must be done directly on the patient, are time consuming, and do not give information about the cellular basis of these responses. At present, there do not seem to be any known tests of A-cell function in man. In spite of the lack of sufficient specific tests of the immunologic system in man, clinical experience from immunologic deficiency diseases correlated with knowledge obtained from animal experimental systems has allowed an inference of the cellular basis of many of these diseases.

IMMUNOLOGIC DEFICIENCY DISEASES

In the past it has been conventional to classify immunologic deficiency diseases into two broad groups—those which are probably genetically determined (primary) and those which are either associated with malignancy or are the result of immunosuppression (secondary). However, an alternative method of classifying these diseases (Table 1) is based upon a consideration of the cellular stage of development which appears to be affected in each condition. This latter method has the advantage of providing a functional basis for discussing these diseases, although it is still uncertain in some cases what the exact nature of the lesion is, or the exact stage which is affected. A recent article by Gatti and Good[44] provides an excellent review of the clinical features of these diseases.

Diseases Resulting from Defects in Stem Cells

In *reticular dysgenesis*[28, 48] both the myeloid and lymphoid systems fail to develop. Although this failure of development is probably the

Table 1. *Examples of Immunological Deficiency Diseases Reflecting Defects at Different Stages of Development of the Immunological System*

I. Defects in the Function of Stem Cells
   A. Stem cells of both the myeloid and lymphoid systems
      1. Reticular dysgenesis
   B. Stem cells of the lymphoid system
      1. Combined immunodeficiency syndromes (Swiss-type agammaglobulinemia, sex-linked lymphopenic agammaglobulinemia)

II. Defects in the Function of Thymic and Bursal-type (Bone Marrow) Environments
   A. Thymic environment
      1. III-IV pharyngeal pouch syndrome of diGeorge
      2. Ataxia telangiectasia
   B. Bursal-type environment
      1. Sex-linked agammaglobulinemia (Bruton-type)
      2. Late-onset agammaglobulinemia ("acquired")

III. Defects in the Function of B, T and A Cells
   A. Temporary
      1. After immunosuppressive therapy
      2. Associated with viral infections
   B. Persistent
      1. Associated with lymphoreticular malignancy (e.g., Hodgkin's disease, multiple myeloma, chronic lymphocytic leukemia)
      2. Deficiencies of single immunoglobulin classes
      3. Wiskott-Aldrich syndrome

result of an absence of pluripotent stem cells, it is conceivable that such stem cells are present but fail to differentiate because of a defect in their environment. (An example of the latter possibility, in the myeloid system, is the hereditary anemia of S1/S1^d mice. These mice have stem cells of the myeloid system, but they fail to function normally in the S1/S1^d environment. When transplanted into irradiated wild-type recipients, the S1/S1^d stem cells can fully repopulate the myeloid system.)[90] Only a few patients with reticular dysgenesis have been described, and all have died early in neonatal life, so that studies of their immune systems have not been possible. However, in addition to anemia and neutropenia, absence of the thymus and marked lymphopenia have also been present.

Combined immunodeficiency diseases include both *Swiss-type agammaglobulinemia*[20, 31, 71, 75, 77, 126] and *sex-linked lymphopenic agammaglobulinemia.*[47, 77, 127] These are probably variants of the same disease. Both are transmitted in a recessive fashion; the former is autosomal, affecting both males and females, and the latter is sex-linked, with expression in male infants. The adjective "combined" indicates that the end result of the lesion in these conditions is a loss of both T-cell and B-cell functions. Thus, affected children show a profound deficiency of both cell-mediated and humoral immune responses.

Although the lesion responsible for these defects could conceivably be affecting precursors of both T and B cells during their development in the thymic and bursal-type environments, it is more likely that the lesion is at an earlier stage of development, affecting stem cells responsible for development of the lymphoid system. Supporting this argument is the fact that some of these children have been treated successfully, with complete restoration of immunological functions, by grafts of histocompatible bone marrow.[45, 97] These results suggest that the thymic environment in these children is capable of giving rise to functioning T cells once it has been provided with the appropriate stem cells.

(An analogous situation in mice is found in the myeloid system of the W/W^v strain. These mice lack normal myeloid stem cells, and their bone marrow is unable to repopulate the myeloid system of irradiated wild-type recipients. However, the environment necessary for differentiation of myeloid stem cells is normal in W/W^v mice since the myeloid system in these mice can be restored by transplants of wild-type bone marrow.)[89]

Diseases Resulting from Defects in the Thymic and Bursal-type Environments

The *III-IV pharyngeal pouch syndrome of diGeorge*[30, 69, 81] is an example of a disease in which the thymic environment responsible for differentiation of stem cells into T cells is defective. In this condition, a lesion early in embryonic life affects the development of the epithelial anlage of the thymus, parathyroids, and great vessels. Consequently, these children exhibit a lack of functional T cells (with the concomitant inability to mount cell-mediated immune responses), hypoparathyroidism with tetany and, often, anomalies of the great vessels. Immunoglobulin levels are normal in these children, and they can form antibodies in response to some antigens.

An important result of the lack of T-cell functions in these children is that they are prone to graft-versus-host disease caused by viable allogeneic lymphocytes in fresh blood transfusions. Stem cells of the lymphoid system are presumably normal in these children, because these patients do exhibit normal B-cell functions, and because they can be treated successfully by a thymic graft and do not require a bone-marrow transplant.[5, 19] This situation in man is paralleled by the results of experiments in neonatally thymectomized mice.[101] These mice are unable to reject skin grafts, and their cells cannot give rise to graft-versus-host disease because their lymphoid organs lack T cells.

Ataxia telangiectasia[34, 37, 115] also appears to be a disease in which the thymic environment is faulty. However, the deficiency of T-cell function in these children does not become clinically evident until a few years after birth. Furthermore, although B-cell functions are apparently normal for a time, most of them eventually develop IgA and IgE[3] deficiency as well. Whether the immunoglobulin deficiencies are the result of a lack of "helper" T cells involved in antibody responses, or whether there is a separate lesion affecting B cells, is unknown. The latter situation is conceivable since the genetic defect in these children is pleomorphic, affecting blood vessels as well as the immune system.

It is noteworthy that these children are unusually prone to developing malignant tumors,[43] an association that, in conjunction with the results of experiments in neonatally thymectomized mice,[101] has been used as evidence to suggest that T cells may have a surveillance function in suppressing clones of malignant cells.[13]

The evidence that *sex-linked agammaglobulinemia*[12, 44, 56, 57, 59] represents the lack of a normal bursal-type environment is based primarily upon the results of bursectomy (surgical and hormonal) in chickens.[24, 49, 143] Chickens lacking a bursa are hypogammaglobulinemic and do not form antibodies, but cell-mediated immune responses dependent upon T cells remain intact. Boys affected with this disease are hypogammaglobulinemic, with subnormal or absent levels of all major classes of immunoglobulins, but they do have the capacity to produce delayed hypersensitivity reactions and can reject skin grafts. Furthermore, if untreated, they suffer almost entirely from bacterial rather than viral and fungal infections. Therapy with gamma globulin injections and antibiotics is simple and reasonably effective, and thus marrow transplants have not been attempted in these children.

Late-onset agammaglobulinemia[44, 58, 128, 144] has many of the hallmarks of the sex-linked variety of agammaglobulinemia, but the onset is usually in adult life. Since the relatives of many of these patients display various defects of the immune system, it is thought that the lesion is genetically-determined. T-cell functions are usually normal, and therapy with gamma globulin appears to be effective in decreasing the frequency and severity of further infections. If this condition is attributable to a failure of the bursal-type environment, then this failure occurs later in life, perhaps in some manner analogous to that of adult-onset diabetes mellitus.

Diseases Resulting from Defects in the Function of B, T, and A Cells

To classify a disease as representing either an absence or abnormal function of B, T or A cells, it is necessary to be certain that a normal lymphoid stem cell population is present and that the thymic and marrow environments function normally. Immunodeficiencies resulting from the use of *immunosuppressive therapy*[42, 121, 130, 132] and those associated with *viral infections*[133, 136, 142] fit into this category. During immunosuppressive therapy it is likely that the obligatory requirement of T and B cells to proliferate in response to antigens is suppressed. The antiproliferative effect of immunosuppressive agents is well known, and forms the basis for their use in allotransplantation. The chemotherapy of malignant diseases also produces the inadvertent side-effect of suppressing the normal immune response.

During certain viral infections, such as rubeola and rubella, the capacity to initiate immune responses requiring T cells is deficient, e.g. individuals with skin tests previously positive to PPD show negative skin tests. The addition of rubella virus to cells exposed in culture to PHA or allogeneic cells suppresses the response. Thus, it is likely that T cells are either temporarily absent or incapable of responding to antigens. This temporary deficiency is probably not the explanation for the high IgM levels found in neonates with congenital viral infections.[137]

In *lymphoreticular malignancies*[2, 21, 55, 74, 91, 99, 141] and *deficiencies of a single immunoglobulin class*,[4, 8, 134, 135] such as IgA, the exact stage of development affected is open to argument. In some lymphoreticular malignancies, e.g. Hodgkin's disease,[2, 55, 141] the defect seems to primarily affect T-cell functions, leaving B-cell functions intact. In others, e.g. multiple myeloma,[21, 91] the reverse situation is seen, while in chronic lymphocytic leukemia[21] both B-cell and T-cell functions are affected. However, the nature of these defects is not clear. T and B cells may develop normally, but replacement of the lymphoid tissues by malignant tissue might alter the environment in which these cells function. Another possibility is that T and B cells fail to develop normally because the malignancy affects the thymic or bursa-like environments. It is also possible that A-cell function may be abnormal.

Similarly, deficiencies of a single immunoglobulin class could arise as a result of defects at more than one stage of the development of the class of cells affected. It is still uncertain whether precursors of IgA-secreting cells are restricted to maturing only into IgA-secreting cells, or whether a switch-over from production of one immunoglobulin to another can occur within a single cell. If the former is true, then the most likely defect is a failure of differentiation in the IgA-cell line; if the latter, then a fault in the switch-over mechanism could account for isolated immunoglobulin class deficiencies.

Abnormal A-cell function may be the basis of the immunologic deficiency seen in the *Wiskott-Aldrich syndrome*.[22] Some of the patients studied have shown a deficiency in their capacity to process pneumococcal polysaccharide and Vi antigens and have low IgM, with high IgA, and normal or high IgG levels in the serum. In keeping with the postulate that A-cell function is abnormal, thus affecting the production of IgM antibodies, is the discovery that A cells are required for immune responses giving rise to at least some IgM antibodies in mice.[61, 112]

In these diseases, as in all the immunodeficiency diseases, investigations would be aided greatly by specific markers for B, T, and A cells and by precise quantitative assays capable of testing the function of each class of cells in cell culture.

AUTOIMMUNE REACTIVITY

The presence of autoimmune reactivity has been associated frequently with well documented cases of immunologic deficiency, e.g. isolated IgA deficiency[4, 39, 76] and late-onset agammaglobulinemia.[40, 41] There is reason to think that the development of autoreactive antibodies in these patients is an epiphenomenon caused by the action of environmental pathogens in an immunologically deficient milieu.

Mice that are thymectomized at birth and raised in a conventional environment frequently develop a "wasting disease," characterized by weight loss, diarrhea, and infections.[92] They are also predisposed to develop autoimmune manifestations such as dermatitis and Coombs-positive hemolytic anemia, as well as renal and hepatic lesions similar to those found in systemic lupus erythematosus.[29] However, neonatally thymectomized mice raised in a germ-free environment do not develop any of these manifestations until after they are placed in a conventional environment.[92] Thus, the exposure of such mice to environmental pathogens is almost certainly responsible for the development of "wasting disease."

It has been suggested that environmental pathogens also may be responsible for the development of autoimmune disease in immunologically deficient mice.[92] Furthermore, it is likely that viruses may be the etiologic agents responsible for the development of autoimmune hemolytic anemia, LE cells and immune-complex nephritis, as has been suggested in at least one experimental animal model, New Zealand mice.[93, 94, 138]

In humans, viral infections have often been associated with the subsequent development of autoimmune hemolytic disease.[25] It follows that the development of autoimmune reactivity in immunologically deficient patients could well be secondary to their inability to resist environmental pathogens.

It would seem reasonable to think that autoimmune reactivity in the diseases associated with "hyperplasia" of the thymus and with thymomas[52, 78] (Table 2) must have a different pathogenesis than does the development of autoimmune reactivity associated with known immunologic deficiency. At least two different mechanisms may be responsible in these diseases. In some, the autoimmune manifestations are probably secondary to immunologic deficiency, e.g. the hypogammaglobulinemia associated with thymoma.[52, 54, 86] These patients initially demonstrate deficient humoral antibody formation, but many subsequently also have deficient cell-mediated responses.[44, 140] The association of autoimmune reactivity with immunologic deficiency in the presence of a thymoma[104, 123] raises the question of whether or not some of the other autoimmune diseases associated with thymoma or "hyperplasia", such as rheumatoid arthritis, systemic lupus erythematosus, and autoimmune hemolytic anemia also may be epiphenomena superimposed on a background of immunologic deficiency. Rheumatoid arthritis has been associated with hypogammaglobulinemia in some patients. Autoimmune hemolytic anemia is known to occur in patients with chronic lymphocytic leukemia and Hodgkin's disease, both of which are frequently accom-

Table 2. *Diseases Associated with the Presence of Thymic Tumors and "Hyperplasia" of the Thymus*

Frequent Associations
  Hypogammaglobulinemia
  Myasthenia gravis
  Erythroid hypoplasia (pure red cell agenesis)

Rare Associations
  Systemic lupus erythematosus
  Rheumatoid arthritis
  Dermatomyositis, myositis and myocarditis
  Scleroderma
  Sjögren's syndrome
  Hyperglobulinemic purpura
  Cushing's syndrome
  Bullous dermatitis
  Autoimmune hemolytic anemia

panied by immunological deficiency. In New Zealand mice, aberrations in antibody formation and defects in cell-mediated immunity are present before the autoimmune manifestations appear.[14, 82, 138]

Whether or not heretofore unrecognized immunologic deficiency or other immunologic abnormalities play a role in the pathogenesis of rheumatoid arthritis, systemic lupus erythematosus, and autoimmune hemolytic anemia requires reappraisal. An indirect argument in support of this possibility is that relatives of patients with immunologic deficiency diseases have a very high frequency of autoimmune disease.[40] This suggests that a genetic lesion, perhaps one that predisposes to deficiencies of the immune system, may underlie all of these diseases.[39a]

Another mechanism operating in autoimmunity associated with morphological alterations in the thymus is exemplified by myasthenia gravis, and perhaps erythroid hypoplasia.[52] Evidence from experiments in guinea pigs suggests that a thymitis, induced by injections of autologous or heterologous striated muscle or thymus cells, results in the release of an agent capable of blocking neuromuscular transmission.[51, 53, 80] The experimental thymitis is probably caused by antibodies that react with myoid fibers normally present in the thymus. It has been suggested that a similar mechanism may operate in myasthenia gravis when a thymoma is present, since the thymic tissue surrounding a thymoma frequently shows the presence of lymphoid follicles and plasma cells.[52] Thus, in these conditions the thymus appears to be the target of antibodies with self-reactive properties.

Neither of the above mechanisms explains how clones of cells with self-reactive properties arise in the first place. The prevailing hypothesis is that during development and differentiation such clones have survived because of a failure in a suppressive mechanism whose function is to eliminate cells with potential for reactivity with self-antigens.[79]

Thus, the pathogenesis of autoimmune diseases, whether associated with abnormal thymic morphology or not, is still largely enigmatic, and further work is required to clarify the situation.

In the consideration of autoimmunity two further notes of caution are required. The first is the necessity to distinguish between autoantibodies capable of producing tissue injury and autoantibodies capable of combining with normal tissue but not producing any apparent injury. The former may truly result in autoimmune disease, while the latter may only reflect previous tissue damage.

The second is that it is not always clear whether or not so-called "hyperplasia" of the thymus is a pathologic state. Usually, the term "hyperplasia" is used to refer to a thymus containing lymph follicles with germinal centers. It has been stated that lymph follicles do not occur in the normal human thymus at any age.[85] However, several studies show that lymph follicles with germinal center formation are present in such diverse conditions as congenital heart disease, bronchogenic carcinoma, and healthy individuals killed in road accidents.[10, 72, 98] However, Henry[72] suggests that the extent of lymph follicle formation may be greater in those conditions we commonly think of as being autoimmune in nature than in the normal thymus.

REFERENCES

1. Ada, G. L., and Byrt, P.: Specific inactivation of antigen-reactive cells with ^{125}I-labelled antigen. Nature, 222:1291, 1969.
2. Aisenberg, A. C.: Quantitative estimation of normal and Hodgkin's disease lymphocytes with thymidine-2 ^{14}C. Nature, 205:1233, 1965.
3. Ammann, A. J., Cain, W. A., Ishizaka, K., Hong, R., and Good, R. A.: Immunoglobulin E deficiency in ataxia-telangiectasia. New Eng. J. Med., 281:469, 1969.
4. Ammann, A. J., and Hong, R.: Selective IgA deficiency: Presentation of 30 cases and a review of the literature. Medicine, 50:223, 1971.
5. August, C. S., Rosen, F. S., Filler, R. M., Janeway, C. A., Markowski, B., and Kay, H. E. M.: Implantation of a foetal thymus, restoring immunological competence in a patient with thymic aplasia (DiGeorge's syndrome). Lancet, 2:1210, 1968.
6. Bach, F. H., Alter, B. J., Solliday, S., Zoschke, D. C., and Janis, M.: Lymphocyte reactivity *in vitro*. II. Soluble reconstituting factor permitting response of purified lymphocytes. Cell. Immunol., 1:219, 1970.
7. Bach, F. H., and Voynow, N. K.: One-way stimulation in mixed leucocyte cultures. Science, 153:545, 1966.
8. Bachman, R.: Studies on serum γA-globulin level. III. Frequency of a-γA-globulinemia. Scand. J. Clin. Lab. Invest., 17:316, 1965.
9. Basten, A., Miller, J. F. A. P., Warner, N. L., and Pye, J.: Specific inactivation of thymus-derived (T) and non-thymus-derived (B) lymphocytes by ^{125}I-labelled antigen. Nature, 231:104, 1971.
10. Bhathal, P. S., and Campbell, P. E.: Eosinophil leucocytes in the child's thymus. Austral. Ann. Med., 14:210, 1965.
11. Boak, J. L., Mitchison, N. A., and Pattison, P. H.: The carrier effect in the secondary response to hapten-protein conjugates. III. The anatomical distribution of helper cells and antibody-forming-cell-precursors. European J. Immunol., 1:63, 1971.
12. Bruton, O. C.: Agammaglobulinemia. Pediatrics, 9:722, 1952.
13. Burnet, F. M.: Immunological Surveillance. Sydney, Pergamon Press (Australia) Ltd., 1970.
14. Cantor, H., Asofsky, R., and Talal, N.: Synergy among lymphoid cells mediating the graft-vs-host response. I. Synergy in graft-vs-host reactions produced by cells from NZB/B1 mice. J. Exper. Med., 131:223, 1970.
15. Cebra, J. J., Colberg, J. E., and Dray, S.: Rabbit lymphoid cells differentiated with respect to alpha, gamma, and mu heavy polypeptide chains and to allotypic markers Aa1 and Aa2. J. Exper. Med., 123:547, 1966.
16. Cerottini, J.-C., Nordin, A. A., and Brunner, K. T.: Specific *in vitro* cytotoxicity of thymus-derived lymphocytes sensitized to alloantigens. Nature, 228:1308, 1970.
17. Claman, H. N., and Brunstetter, F. H.: The response of cultured human thymus cells to phytohemagglutinin. J. Immunol., 100:1127, 1968.
18. Claman, H. N., Chaperon, E. A., and Triplett, R. F.: Thymus-marrow cell combinations. Synergism in antibody production. Proc. Soc. Exper. Biol. Med., 122:1167, 1966.
19. Cleveland, W. W., Fogel, B. J., Brown, W. T., and Kay, H. E. M.: Foetal thymic transplant in a case of DiGeorge's syndrome. Lancet, 2:1211, 1968.
20. Cole, R. B., D'Sousa, A., Good, R. A., Gatti, R. A., and Hoyer, J.: Lymphopenic agammaglobulinemia (Swiss type) in Chicago. Autosomal recessive form. Amer. J. Dis. Child., 17:22, 1961.
21. Cone, L., and Uhr, J. W.: Immunological deficiency disorders associated with chronic lymphocytic leukemia and multiple myeloma. J. Clin. Invest., 43:2241, 1964.
22. Cooper, M. D., Chase, H. P., Lowman, J., Krivit, W., and Good, R. A.: Wiskott-Aldrich syndrome – an immunologic deficiency disease involving the afferent limb of immunity. Amer. J. Med., 44:499, 1968.
23. Cooper, M. D., Perey, D. Y., McKneally, M. F., Gabrielsen, A. E., Sutherland, D. E. R., and Good, R. A.: A mammalian equivalent of the avian bursa of Fabricius. Lancet, 2:1388, 1966.
24. Cooper, M. D., Peterson, R. D. A., and Good, R. A.: Delineation of the thymic and bursal lymphoid systems in the chicken. Nature, 205:143, 1965.
25. Dacie, J. V.: III. Haemolytic anaemia following or associated with known virus infections. *In* The Haemolytic Anaemias. Part II. The Autoimmune Haemolytic Anaemias, 2nd ed., London, Churchill, 1965, p. 525.
26. David, J. R.: Macrophage migration. Fed. Proc., 27:6, 1968.
27. Davies, A. J. S., Festenstein, H., Leuchars, E., Wallis, V. J., and Doenhoff, M. J.: A thymic origin for some peripheral-blood lymphocytes. Lancet, 1:183, 1968.
28. DeVaal, O. M., and Seynhaeve, V.: Reticular dysgenesis. Lancet, 2:1123, 1959.
29. DeVries, M. J., van Putten, L. M., Balner, H., and van Bekkum, D. W.: Lésions suggérant une réactivité autoimmune chez des souris atteintes de la "runt disease" apres thymectomie néonatale. Rev. Franç. Etud. Clin. Biol., 9:381, 1964.

30. DiGeorge, A. M.: Congenital absence of the thymus and its immunologic consequences: Concurrence with congenital hypoparathyroidism. In Good, R. A., and Bergsma, D., eds.: Immunologic Deficiency Diseases in Man. Birth Defects Original Article Series, Vol. 4. New York, National Foundation Press, 1968, p. 116.
31. Donohue, W. L.: Alymphocytosis. Pediatrics, *11*:129, 1953.
32. Dutton, R. W., and Mishell, R. I.: Cell populations and cell proliferation in the in vitro response of normal mouse spleen to heterologous erythrocytes. J. Exper. Med., *126*:443, 1967.
33. Edwards, G. E., Miller, R. G., and Phillips, R. A.: Differentiation of rosette-forming cells from myeloid stem cells. J. Immunol., *105*:719, 1970.
34. Eisen, A. H., Karpati, G., Laszlo, T., Andermann, F., Robb, J. P., and Bacal, H. L.: Immunologic deficiency in ataxia-telangiectasia. New Eng. J. Med., 272:18, 1965.
35. El-Arini, M. O., and Osoba, D.: Unpublished observations.
36. Falk, R. E., Falk, J. A., and Zabriskie, J. B.: Reactivity of nonsensitized thymocytes to antigen: Release of specific lymphocyte-activating substances. Transpl. Proc., 3:841, 1971.
37. Fireman, P., Boesman, M., and Gillen, D.: Ataxis telangiectasia: A dysgammaglobulinemia with deficient gamma$_{1A}$ - (B_2A) - globulin. Lancet, *1*:1193, 1964.
38. Ford, C. E., Micklem, H. S., Evans, E. P., Gray, J. G., and Ogden, D. A.: The inflow of bone marrow cells to the thymus: Studies with part-body irradiated mice, injected with chromosome-marked bone marrow and subjected to antigenic stimulation. Ann. N.Y. Acad. Sci., *129*:283, 1966.
39. Fraser, K. J.: IgA immunoglobulins and autoimmunity. Lancet, 2:804, 1969.
39a. Fudenberg, H. H.: Genetically determined immune deficiency as the predisposing cause of "autoimmunity" and lymphoid neoplasia. Amer. J. Med., *51*:295, 1971.
40. Fudenberg, H. H., German, J. J., III, and Kunkel, H. G.: The occurrence of rheumatoid factor and other abnormalities in families of patients with agammaglobulinemia. Arth. Rheum., 5:565, 1962.
41. Fudenberg, H. H., and Hirschhorn, K.: Agammaglobulinemia: Some current concepts. MED. CLIN. N. AMER., *49*:1533, 1965.
42. Gabrielson, A. E., and Good, R. A.: Chemical suppression of adaptive immunity. Adv. Immunol., 6:92, 1967.
43. Gatti, R. A., and Good, R. A.: Occurrence of malignancy in immunodeficiency diseases: A literature review. Cancer, 28:89, 1971.
44. Gatti, R. A., and Good, R. A.: The immunological deficiency diseases. MED. CLIN. N. AMER., *54*:281, 1970.
45. Gatti, R. A., Meuwissen, H. J., Allen, H. D., Hong, R., and Good, R. A.: Immunologic reconstitution of sex-linked lymphopenic immunologic deficiency. Lancet, 2:1366, 1968.
46. Gilmour, J. R.: The embryology of the parathyroid glands, the thymus and certain associated rudiments. J. Path. Bact., *45*:507, 1937.
47. Gitlin, D., and Craig, J. M.: The thymus and other lymphoid tissues in congenital agammaglobulinemia. I. Thymic alymphoplasia and lymphocytic hypoplasia and their relation to infection. Pediatrics, 32:517, 1963.
48. Gitlin, D., Vawter, G., and Craig, J. M.: Thymic alymphoplasia and congenital aleukocytosis. Pediatrics, *33*:184, 1964.
49. Glick, B., Chang, T. S., and Jaap, R. C.: The bursa of Fabricius and antibody production. Poultry Sci., 35:224, 1956.
50. Goldie, J. H., and Osoba, D.: Requirement of a nonproliferating class of cells for generation of immune responses in cell culture. Proc. Soc. Exper. Biol. Med., *133*:1265, 1970.
51. Goldstein, G.: The thymus and neuromuscular function: A substance in thymus which causes myositis and myasthenic neuromuscular block in guinea pigs. Lancet, 2:119, 1968.
52. Goldstein, G., and MacKay, I. R.: The Human Thymus. London, Wm. Heineman Medical Books Ltd., 1969.
53. Goldstein, G., and Whittingham, S.: Experimental autoimmune thymitis: An animal model for myasthenia gravis. Lancet, 2:315, 1966.
54. Good, R. A.: Agammaglobulinemia: A provocative experiment of nature. Bull. Univ. Minn. Hosp., 26:1, 1954.
55. Good, R. A., and Finstad, J.: The association of lymphoid malignancy and immunologic functions. In Zarafonetis, C., ed.: Proceedings of the International Conference on Leukemia-Lymphoma. Philadelphia, Lea and Febiger, 1968, p. 175.
56. Good, R. A., and Finstad, J.: The Gordon Wilson Lecture: The development and involution of the lymphoid system and immunologic capacity. Trans. Amer. Clin. Climatol. Assoc., 79:69, 1968.
57. Good, R. A., Kelly, W. D., Rotstein, J., and Varco, R. L.: Immunological deficiency diseases. Progr. Allergy, 6:187, 1962.
58. Good, R. A., and Varco, R. L.: A clinical and experimental study of agammaglobulinemia. J. Lancet, 75:245, 1955.

59. Good, R. A., and Zak, S. J.: Disturbances in gammaglobulin synthesis as experiments of nature. Pediatrics, *18*:109, 1956.
60. Gorczynski, R. M., Miller, R. G., and Phillips, R. A.: Identification by density separation of antigen-specific surface receptors on progenitors of antibody-producing cells. Immunol., *20*:693, 1971.
61. Gorczynski, R. M., Miller, R. G., and Phillips, R. A.: In vivo requirement for a radiation-resistant cell in the immune response to sheep erythrocytes. J. Exper. Med., in press.
62. Gordon, H. A.: Morphological and physiological characterization of germ-free life. Ann. N.Y. Acad. Sci., *78*:208, 1959.
63. Greaves, M. F.: Biological effects of anti-immunoglobulins: Evidence for immunoglobulin receptors on T and B lymphocytes. Transplant. Rev., *5*:45, 1970.
64. Greaves, M. F.: Personal communication.
65. Greaves, M. F., and Möller, E.: Studies on antigen binding cells. I. The origin of reactive cells. Cell. Immunol., *1*:372, 1970.
66. Green, I., Vassali, P., Nussenzweig, V., and Benacerraf, B.: Specificity of the antibodies produced by single cells following immunization with antigens bearing two types of antigenic determinants. J. Exper. Med., *125*:511, 1967.
67. Hammar, J. A.: Zur Histogenese und Involution der Thymusdrüse. Anat. Anz., *27*:23, 41, 1905.
68. Harris, J. E., Ford, C. E., Barnes, D. W. H., and Evans, E. P.: Cellular traffic of the thymus: Experiments with chromosome markers. Evidence from parabiosis for an afferent stream of cells. Nature, *201*:886, 1964.
69. Harvey, J. C., Dungan, W. T., Elders, M. J., and Hughes, E. R.: Third and fourth pharyngeal pouch syndrome, associated vascular anomalies and hypocalcemic seizures. Clin. Pediat., *9*:496, 1970.
70. Haskill, J. S., Byrt, P., and Marbrook, J.: In vi.ro and in vivo studies of the immune response to sheep erythrocytes using partially purified cell preparations. J. Exper. Med., *131*:57, 1970.
71. Haworth, J. C., Hoogstraten, J., and Taylor, H.: Thymic alymphoplasia. Arch. Dis. Child., *42*:40, 1967.
72. Henry, K.: The thymus in rheumatic heart disease. Clin. Exper. Immunol., *3*:509, 1968.
73. Hersh, E. M., and Harris, J. E.: Macrophage-lymphocyte interaction in the antigen-induced blastogenic response of human peripheral blood leukocytes. J. Immunol., *100*:1184, 1968.
74. Hirschhorn, K., Schreibman, R. R., Bach, F. H., and Sitzbach, L. E.: In vitro studies of lymphocytes from patients with sarcoidosis and lymphoproliferative disease. Lancet, *2*:842, 1964.
75. Hitzig, W. H., Biro, Z., Bosch, H., and Huser, H. J.: Agammaglobulinämie und Alymphocytose mit Schwund des lymphatischen Gewebes. Helv. Paediat. Acta, *13*:551, 1958.
76. Hobbs, J. R., Hepner, G. W., Douglas, A. P., Crabbé, P. A., and Johansson, S. G. O.: Immunological mystery of coeliac disease. Lancet, 2:649, 1969.
77. Hoyer, J. R., Cooper, M. D., Gabrielsen, A. E., and Good, R. A.: Lymphopenic forms of congenital immunologic deficiency diseases. Medicine, *47*:201, 1968.
78. Irvine, W. J.: The thymus in autoimmune disease. Proc. Roy. Soc. Med., *63*:718, 1970.
79. Jerne, N. K.: The somatic generation of immune recognition. European J. Immunol., *1*:1, 1971.
80. Kalden, J. R., Williamson, W. G., Johnston, R. J., and Irvine, W. J.: Studies on experimental autoimmune thymitis in guinea-pigs. Clin. Exper. Immunol., *5*:319, 1969.
81. Kretschmer, R., Say, B., Brown, D., and Rosen, F. S.: Congenital aplasia of the thymus gland (DiGeorge syndrome). New Eng. J. Med., *279*:1295, 1968.
82. Leventhal, B. G., and Talal, N.: Response of NZB and NZB/NZW spleen cells to mitogenic agents. J. Immunol., *104*:918, 1970.
83. Lischner, H. W., Punnett, H. H., and DiGeorge, A. M.: Lymphocytes in congenital absence of the thymus. Nature, *214*:580, 1967.
84. MacDonald, H. R.: Personal communication.
85. MacKay, I. R.: Histopathology of the human thymus. In Wolstenholme, G. E. W., and Porter, R., eds.: The Thymus. London, Churchill, 1966, p. 449.
86. MacLean, L. D., Zak, S. J., Varco, R. L., and Good, R. A.: Thymic tumor and acquired immune agammaglobulinemia: Clinical and experimental study of immune response. Surgery, *40*:1010, 1956.
87. Mäkelä, O.: The specificity of antibodies produced by single cells. Cold Spring Harbor Symp. Quant. Biol., *32*:423, 1967.
88. Martinez, C., Kersey, J., Papermaster, B. W., and Good, R. A.: Skin homograft survival in thymectomized mice. Proc. Soc. Exper. Biol. Med., *109*:193, 1962.
89. McCulloch, E. A., Siminovitch, L., and Till, J. E.: Spleen-colony formation in anaemic mice of genotype W/W[v]. Science, *144*:844, 1964.
90. McCulloch, E. A., Siminovitch, L., Till, J. E., Russell, E. S., and Bernstein, S. E.: The cellular basis of the genetically-determined hemopoietic defect in anaemic mice of genotype S1/S1[d]. Blood, *26*:399, 1965.

91. McKelvey, E. M., and Fahey, J. L.: Immunoglobulin changes in disease; quantitation on the basis of heavy polypeptide chains IgG (gamma G), IgA (gamma A) and IgM (gamma M) and of light polypeptide chains type K (I) and type L (II). J. Clin. Invest., 44:1778, 1965.
92. McIntire, K. R., Sell, S., and Miller, J. F. A. P.: Pathogenesis of the post-neonatal thymectomy wasting syndrome. Nature, 204:151, 1964.
93. Mellors, R. C.: Autoimmune and immunoproliferative diseases of NZB/B1 mice and hybrids. Int. Rev. Exper. Pathol., 5:217, 1966.
94. Mellors, R. C.: Autoimmune disease and neoplasia of NZB mice: Experimental model and its implications. In Rose, N. R., and Milgrom, F., eds.: Immunology: Proceedings of the International Convocation on Immunology. New York, S. Karger, 1969, p. 222.
95. Metcalf, D.: Relation of the thymus to the formation of immunologically reactive cells. Cold Spring Harbor Symp. Quant. Biol., 32:583, 1967.
96. Metcalf, D.: The thymus and lymphopoiesis. In Good, R. A., and Gabrielson, A. E., eds.: The Thymus in Immunobiology, New York, Hoeber-Harper, 1964, p. 150.
97. Meuwissen, H. J., Gatti, R. A., Terasaki, P. I., Hong, R., and Good, R. A.: Treatment of lymphopenic hypogammaglobulinemia and bone marrow aplasia by transplantation of allogeneic marrow. New Eng. J. Med., 281:691, 1969.
98. Middleton, G.: The incidence of follicular structures in the human thymus at autopsy. Aust. J. Exper. Biol. Med. Sci., 45:189, 1967.
99. Miller, D. G., and Karnofsky, D. A.: Immunologic factors and resistance to infection in chronic lymphatic leukemia. Amer. J. Med., 31:748, 1961.
100. Miller, J. F. A. P.: Immunological function of the thymus. Lancet, 2:748, 1961.
101. Miller, J. F. A. P., and Osoba, D.: Current concepts of the immunological function of the thymus. Physiol. Rev., 47:437, 1967.
102. Miller, R. G., and Phillips, R. A.: Sedimentation analysis of the cells in mice required to initiate an in vivo immune response to sheep erythrocytes. Proc. Soc. Exper. Biol. Med., 135:63, 1970.
103. Mitchison, N. A.: The carrier effect in the secondary response to hapten-protein conjugates. II. Cellular cooperation. Eur. J. Immunol., 1:18, 1971.
104. Mongan, E. S., Kern, W. A., and Terry, R.: Hypogammaglobulinemia with thymoma, hemolytic anemia, and disseminated infection with cytomegalovirus. Ann. Int. Med., 65:548, 1966.
105. Moore, M. A. S., and Owen, J. J. T.: Chromosome marker studies on the development of the haemopoietic system in the chick embryo. Nature, 208:956, 1965.
106. Moore, M. A. S., and Owen, J. J. T.: Experimental studies on the development of the thymus. J. Exper. Med., 126:715, 1967.
107. Mosier, D. E.: A requirement for two cell types for antibody formation in vitro. Science, 158:1573, 1967.
108. Mosier, D. E., and Coppleson, L. W.: A three-cell interaction required for the induction of the primary immune response in vitro. Proc. Nat. Acad. Sci. U.S.A., 61:542, 1968.
109. Nossal, G. J. V., Cunningham, A., Mitchell, G. F., and Miller, J. F. A. P.: Cell to cell interaction in the immune response. III. Chromosomal marker analysis of single antibody-forming cells in reconstituted, irradiated, or thymectomized mice. J. Exper. Med., 128:839, 1968.
110. Osoba, D.: Cellular cooperation in the primary immune response—the need for a uniform terminology. European J. Clin. Biol. Res., 15:929, 1970.
111. Osoba, D.: Restriction of the capacity to respond to two antigens by single precursors of antibody-producing cells in culture. J. Exper. Med., 129:141, 1969.
112. Osoba, D.: Some physical and radiobiological properties of immunologically reactive mouse spleen cells. J. Exper. Med., 132:368, 1970.
113. Osoba, D.: Unpublished observations.
114. Parrott, D. M., deSousa, M. A. B., and East, J.: Thymus-dependent areas in the lymphoid organs of neonatally thymectomized mice. J. Exper. Med., 123:191, 1966.
115. Peterson, R. D. A., Cooper, M. D., and Good, R. A.: Lymphoid tissue abnormalities associated with ataxia-telangiectasia. Amer. J. Med., 41:342, 1966.
116. Playfair, J. H. L., Papermaster, B. W., and Cole, L. J.: Focal antibody production by transferred spleen cells in irradiated mice. Science, 149:998, 1965.
117. Playfair, J. H. L., Wolfendale, M. R., and Kay, H. E. M.: The leucocytes of peripheral blood in the human foetus. Brit. J. Haematol., 9:336, 1963.
118. Raff, M. C.: Surface antigenic markers for distinguishing T and B lymphocytes in mice. Transplant. Rev., 6:52, 1971.
119. Raff, M. C.: Theta isoantigen as a marker of thymus-derived lymphocytes in mice. Nature, 224:378, 1969.
120. Reif, A. E., and Allen, J. M. V.: The AKR thymic antigen and its distribution in leukemias and nervous tissues. J. Exper. Med., 120:413, 1964.
121. Revillard, J. P., and Brochier, J.: Selective deficiency of cell-mediated immunity in humans treated with antilymphocyte globulins. Transpl. Proc., 3:725, 1971.

122. Rode, H. N., and Gordon, J.: The mixed leukocyte culture: A three component system. J. Immunol., *104*:1453, 1970.
123. Rogers, H. G., Manaligod, J. R., and Blazek, W. V.: Thymoma associated with pancytopenia and hypogammaglobulinemia. Amer. J. Med., *44*:154, 1968.
124. Roitt, I. M., Greaves, M. F., Torrigiani, G., Brostoff, J., and Playfair, J. H. L.: The cellular basis of immunological responses. Lancet, 2:367, 1969.
125. Roseman, J. M.: The X-ray resistant cell required for the induction of *in vitro* antibody formation. Science, *165*:1125, 1969.
126. Rosen, F. S., Gitlin, D., and Janeway, C. A.: Alymphocytosis, agammaglobulinemia, homografts and delayed hypersensitivity: Study of a case. Lancet, 2:380, 1962.
127. Rosen, F. S., Gottoff, S. P., Craig, J. M., Ritchie, J., and Janeway, C. A.: Further observations on the Swiss type of agammaglobulinemia (alymphocytosis). The effect of syngeneic bone-marrow cells. New Eng. J. Med., *274*:18, 1966.
128. Sanford, J. P., Favour, C. B., and Tribeman, M. S.: Absence of serum gamma globulin in adults. New Eng. J. Med., *250*:1027, 1954.
129. Schechter, G. P., and McFarland, W.: Interaction of lymphocytes and a radioresistant cell in PPD-stimulated human leukocyte cultures. J. Immunol., *105*:661, 1970.
130. Schwartz, R. S.: Immunosuppressive drugs. Progr. Allerg., *9*:246, 1965.
131. Shortman, K., Diener, E., Russell, P., and Armstrong, W. D.: The role of nonlymphoid accessory cells in the immune response to different antigens. J. Exper. Med., *131*:461, 1970.
132. Simmons, R. L., Moberg, A. W., Gewurz, H., Soll, R., and Najarian, J. S.: Immunosuppression by antihuman lymphocyte globulin: correlation of human and animal assay systems with clinical results. Transpl. Proc., 3:745, 1971.
133. Smithwick, E. M., and Berkovich, S.: The effect of measles virus on the *in vitro* lymphocyte response to tuberculin. *In* Smith, R. T., and Good, R. A., eds.: Cellular Recognition. New York, Appleton-Century-Crofts, 1969, p. 131.
134. South, M. A., Cooper, M. D., Hong, R., Wollheim, F. A., and Good, R. A.: Secretory IgA and the immunologic deficiency. *In* Good, R. A., and Bergsma, D., eds.: Immunologic Deficiency Diseases in Man. Birth Defects Original Article Series, Vol. 4. New York, National Foundation Press, 1968, p. 283.
135. South, M. A., Cooper, M. D., Wollheim, F. A., and Good, R. A.: The IgA system. II. The clinical significance of IgA deficiency. Amer. J. Med., *44*:168, 1968.
136. Starr, S., and Berkovich, S.: Effects of measles, gammaglobulin-modified measles and vaccine measles on the tuberculin test. New Eng. J. Med., *270*:386, 1964.
137. Stiehm, E. R., Ammann, A. J., and Cherry, J. D.: Elevated cord macroglobulins in the diagnosis of intrauterine infections. New Eng. J. Med., *275*:971, 1966.
138. Talal, N.: Immunologic and viral factors in the pathogenesis of systemic lupus erythematosus. Arth. Rheum., *13*:887, 1970.
139. Tan, T., and Gordon, J.: Participation of three cell types in the anti-sheep red blood cell response in vitro. J. Exper. Med., *133*:520, 1971.
140. te Velde, K., Huber, J., and Van der Slikke, L. B.: Primary acquired hypogammaglobulinemia, myasthenia and thymoma. Ann. Int. Med., *65*:554, 1966.
141. Thomas, J. W., Boldt, W., Horrocks, G., and Low, B.: Lymphocyte transformation by phytohemagglutinin: I. In Hodgkin's disease. Canad. Med. Assoc. J., *97*:832, 1967.
142. Thomas, J. W., Clements, D., and Naiman, S. C.: Lymphocyte transformation by phytohemagglutinin: IV. In acute upper respiratory infections. Canad. Med. Assoc. J., *99*:467, 1968.
143. Warner, N. L., Uhr, J. W., Thorbecke, G. J., and Ovary, Z.: Immunoglobulins, antibodies and the bursa of Fabricius: Induction of agammaglobulinemia and the loss of all antibody-forming capacity by hormonal bursectomy. J. Immunol., *103*:1317, 1969.
144. Wollheim, F. A., Belfrage, S., Coster, C., and Lindholm, H.: Primary "acquired" hypogammaglobulinemia. Clinical and genetic aspects of 9 cases. Acta Med. Scand., *176*:1, 1964.
145. Wu, A. M., Till, J. E., Siminovitch, L., and McCulloch, E. A.: Cytological evidence for a relationship between normal colony-forming cells and cells of the lymphoid system. J. Exper. Med., *127*:455, 1968.

THYMUS, IMMUNITY AND AUTOIMMUNITY*

E. J. Yunis, O. Stutman and R. A. Good

Departments of Laboratory Medicine and Pathology
University of Minnesota Medical School
Minneapolis, Minn. 55455

The thymus is essential for the establishment and maintenance of immunological competence, and it has been suggested that it influences neuromuscular transmission.[1] In this paper we will summarize the immunological functions of the thymus and the possible role of functional deficiency of thymus in the production of autoantibodies.

THE THYMUS AND THE IMMUNOLOGICALLY COMPETENT CELL

The thymic influence on peripheral lymphoid tissue is demonstrated by the effect of thymectomy. Neonatal thymectomy results in a marked deficiency of lymphocytes in the paracortical areas of the lymph nodes and the periarteriolar regions of the spleen. These regions are termed "thymus dependent" areas of the peripheral lymphoid tissue.[2] Lymphocytes in lymphatics, blood, thoracic duct lymph and the recirculating population within the peripheral lymphoid tissues represent the main pool of lymphocytes that develop under thymic influence.[3] Neonatally thymectomized mice develop lymphocytopenia, which becomes more pronounced several weeks following thymectomy and is associated with a wasting syndrome.[4,5] Mice that do not develop wasting disease following neonatal thymectomy may not show lymphocytopenia for as long as five months. On the other hand, neonatally thymectomized mice of the "autoimmune susceptible strains" (NZB, A_f, A/J, C57BL/Ks)/show moderate lymphopenia, large lymph nodes containing increased numbers of plasma cells, and have hyperactive germinal centers and many plasma cells in spleen.[5]

Cellular Immune System of Neonatally Thymectomized Mice

Neonatally thymectomized mice not only show quantitative decrease of lymphocytes but also functional deficiencies, as revealed by deficient ability of suspensions of cells containing lymphocytes to produce graft-versus-host reactions;[6] deficient ability to exercise a normal allograft rejection,[7-9] and inability to produce delayed hypersensitivity reactions.[10] In addition, their peripheral blood leukocytes transform poorly or not at all when stimulated with PHA or with allogeneic leukocytes.[11-13]

Humoral Immune Responses of Neonatally Thymectomized Mice

In neonatally thymectomized mice antibody responses against the following antigens are impaired: sheep erythrocytes, salmonella typhi O and Vi antigens, influenza A virus, T_2 coliphage, and bovine serum albumin. By contrast, re-

* Supported by United States Public Health Service grants CA03511, CA10445 and AI HD10153-01, by the Minnesota division of the American Heart Association, and by the graduate school of the University of Minnesota.

sponses to certain other antigens, e.g., salmonella H flagellar antigen, tetanus toxoid, hemocyanin, pneumococcus Type III capsular polysaccharide, ferritin, MS-2 bacteriophage and polyoma virus have been found to be normal.[14] Further, levels of all known immunoglobulins of mice are present[15,16] in normal concentrations in serum.

Miller and coworkers[17] reported experiments that suggested that the thymus exerts its influence on the development of precursors of antigen sensitive cells, and that once those cells had matured, their subsequent responses depended not on the thymus but on the presence of antigen.

Wasting Disease in Postthymectomy State

Some neonatally thymectomized mice of several strains developed wasting syndrome characterized by failure to gain weight normally or by weight loss, hypothermia with hunched posture, diarrhea, and early death.[18,19] The role of infections in wasting syndrome of postthymectomy state is strongly suggested by studies of thymectomized mice in germ-free conditions in which no wasting disease was observed,[20] and also by experiments in which we have shown that neonatally thymectomized mice developed lethal hepatitis in all animals injected with virus obtained from infected livers, while normal animals were resistant to infection.[21] By contrast, hepatitis occurred spontaneously in approximately 30% of wasting mice of several strains.[19,22,23] The hepatitis occurring either spontaneously or following virus injection in neonatally thymectomized mice can be prevented by treatment with thymus grafts, spleen cells or grafts of functional thymomas.[24] These experiments suggested that postthymic immunocompetent cells were required to prevent activation of some latent virus infections.

Variation in expression of wasting syndrome in neonatally thymectomized mice may be a function of the number of postthymic cells already present in the peripheral lymphoid tissue as the time of birth, the amount of exposure to infectious agents, and the amount of stress which has been placed on the poorly developed peripheral lymphoid system that cannot replenish itself in the absence of the differentiating influence of the thymus.

Restoration of Immune Competence by Lymphoid Cells, Thymus Grafts, Functional Thymomas and Thymus Extracts

Thymus control of development of immune competence in animals has been clarified by experiments designed to restore immunocompetence of neonatally thymectomized or thymectomized-irradiated adult animals. The restorative procedures that have been used include: (1) infusion of lymphoid cells (spleen, thoracic duct and lymph nodes) or spleen grafts; (2) thymus grafts, implantation of thymic tissue enclosed in millipore chambers, grafting of functional thymomas, implantation of functional thymomas in millipore chambers; (3) injections of thymus cells, and (4) injections of thymic extracts.

Infusion of lymphoid cells obtained from lymph nodes, spleen or thoracic duct of syngeneic mice[18,25] as well as syngeneic spleen grafts[26] resulted in prevention or reversal of wasting disease and achieved immunological reconstitution of neonatally thymectomized mice.[26] Infusion of allogeneic cells produced effects that were related to the histocompatibility differences between the donor and the host. If the neonatally thymectomized recipient and the donor were identical at the H-2 locus, prevention or reversal of wasting and immunological reconstitution attributable to donor cells was observed. If the H-2 was different, the donor cells produced an increased destruction of the host as a consequence of graft-versus-host reaction.[26,27] Large numbers of fetal liver cells or bone marrow cells did not reconstitute immunologic capacity of the neonatally thymectomized mice.[28,29]

Thymus grafting was effective and depended mainly upon the epithelial reticular tissue of the grafted thymus. The reconstitution of the animals in such experiments could be attributed almost entirely to host cells, although a thymus-derived population may be detected, and in some donor-host combinations the animals develop specific immunologic tolerance to the thymus, as judged by failure to reject skin from the donor.[25,30] Furthermore, a thymic graft restored immunological competence even if given sufficient X-ray irradiation to destroy thymic lymphocytes.[31] The humoral factor secreted by the epithelial reticular cells of the thymus does not appear to be absolutely strain-specific. Restoration of neonatally thymectomized mice with rat thymus has produced conflicting results[25,32,33] which we interpret to reflect the advantage of species-specific over nonspecific thymus. We have presented evidence showing that grafting of several syngeneic thymuses long after birth or during wasting can reconstitute neonatally thymectomized mice.[34] We suggested that this effect is mainly due to immunocompetent cells present in the thymus grafts. It appears that immunologically competent cells in the thymus are important in preventing death, while the thymic epithelial stroma influences the host precursor cells to become competent. Parental thymus grafts in thymectomized F_1 hybrids lead to graft-versus-host reactions in certain strain combinations.[35] Strong histocompatibility differences between thymus donor and thymectomized host produce host reconstitution followed by rejection of the thymus grafts and demonstration only of host immunocompetent cells and lack of tolerance to skin of the thymus donor type.[30] Experiments with thymus grafts proved that restoration depended also on a humoral activity acting on host cells. The same results can be obtained with grafting of functional thymoma and thymus grafts or thymomas enclosed in millipore chambers.[10,36-38] However, the functional activity of the thymomas appeared to depend on an interaction between two kinds of stromal cells—one clearly an epithelial cell and the other a form of spindle mesenchymal cell.[39]

It is noteworthy that our chemically induced, functional thymomas were often rejected after immunological reconstition of the allogeneic thymectomized host.[38] When neonatally thymectomized mice reconstituted with allogeneic tumor or allogeneic thymus grafts[30] are tested at 350 days, they show loss of immunocompetence as seen, for example, by feeble rejection of skin allografts.[23,40] These results indicate that the thymus not only functions to develop cellular immunity and some antibody responses in early life, but also is essential to this competence throughout life. These findings are consonant with experiments in which thymic extirpation carried out after full development of immune capacity leads to immunologic incompetence after many months.[41-43]

Dispersed thymus cells in numbers up to 10×10^6 were ineffective in restoring immune capacity in neonatally thymectomized mice.[18,25] However, $100-400 \times 10^6$ thymus cells restored immune capacity in neonatally thymectomized mice and that capacity was attributable to the cells of donor origin. These results suggested that immunologically competent cells are present within the thymus.[26,44] In addition, 400×10^6 hemiallogeneic newborn thymocytes facilitated immunologic reconstitution attributable to host cells. The possibility of a trephocytic function of the thymocytes was considered.[44] The difference between trephocytic action and humoral factor is, in the end, a difference of mechanism. Trephocytic action probably involves passage of small molecular components between cells. It is entirely possible that administration of a large number of thymocytes (including epithelial elements) in certain combinations of donors and recipients could have supplied a high concentration of trephocytic or humoral factors to expand the postthymic cells. A summary of the restoration of neonatally thymectomized mice produced by different treatments is given in TABLE 1.

Studies with thymic extracts in several laboratories have provided evidence for a thymic humoral factor which influences immunologic capacity. Restorative effects of extracts of xenogenic thymus on the peripheral lymphocyte count and prevention of the wasting syndrome of neonatally thymectomized mice have been reported.[45,46] Saline extracts of thymus also restored partially the immunological capacity of neonatally thymectomized or irradiated adult thymectomized mice.[47] In spite of these apparently telling experiments, extensive efforts in our laboratories to demonstrate action of similar thymic extracts have been most disappointing.[25,25a]

More recent studies[48] concerning action of a partially purified preparation from calf thymus also have been interpreted as evidence for the existence of a thymic hormone. Although these efforts should be intensively pursued, thus far they indicate to us that the differentiating and expanding influences of thymus may be separable and that the humoral factors are not the same as those responsible for differentiation. It seems that the humoral factors must act on an already differentiated population of postthymic cells.[28,29] Whether the expanding influence described is a true hormone or some other expanding influence, for example, antigenic stimulation still needs further clarification.

Humoral Immune Responses — The Avian Bursa of Fabricius

In birds, the thymus also controls the development of the lymphocyte population which subserves the cell-mediated immunological responses, but thymectomy in the newly hatched chick does not affect immunoglobulin synthesis.[49] The bursa of Fabricius is necessary for development of the capacity to produce immunoglobulins and specific humoral antibody.[50] Bursectomy at hatching does not affect cell-mediated responses, but results in impairment of immunoglobulin production. Extensive experimentation using irradiation and bursectomy at hatching,[51] "in ovo" bursectomy,[52] and administration of specific antiserum against μ chains just as the IgM producing cells are developing indicate that the entire

TABLE 1

Treatment	Percent Restoration			Type of Restoration
	Early (5-30)*	Late (30 to ± 50)*	Wasting (50-80)*	
Spleen cells	90–100%	80–90%	75–80%	
Lymph node cells	90–100%	—	—	adoptive donor
Thymus cells	70–80%	50–60%	30%	
Bone marrow cells	0–1 %	0	0	
Thymus grafts (1)	80–90%	5–20%	0	
Thymus grafts (5)	—	50%	10–40%	
Thymoma	70–80%	5–20%	0	mainly host
Thymoma (D.C.)	50–60%	5–20%	0	
Thymus (D.C.)	45–50%	1–5%	0	

* Days.

immunoglobulin differentiation occurs within the bursa of chickens and that differentiation to IgM and IgG producing cells is sequential.[53]

A mammalian equivalent of the avian bursa has not been identified despite several suggestions for various gut-associated lymphoid organs.[54] It has been speculated that the entire epithelium of the gut may have a bursal hormonal function,[55] but even this suggestion lacks experimental support.[56] Although the question of bursal equivalent in mammals is not settled, there seems no question that there exists in mammals an extra thymic influence responsible for differentiation of immunoglobulin producing cells. Thus, the research for and definition of the bursal equivalent for mammals and man must be continued. The bursa equivalent for mammals must be defined as that site of first appearance of lyphoid cells containing μ chains, the site of first appearance of lymphoid cells containing γ chains, the only site where cytoplasm of lymphoid cells contain both μ and γ chains at the same time, the site where antigenic stimulation does not alter the time of appearance or number of immunoglobulin producing cells, and the site where surgical extirpation sufficiently early in embryonic development yields agammaglobulinemia.

The thymus seems to control the capacity of the mouse to produce specific antibody to certain antigens. Synergy of marrow and thymus cells in x-irradiated mice in the response to sheep red cells has been demonstrated.[57] Thymus or thoracic duct cells are effective in elevating the number of host hemolysin-forming cells in spleen of neonatally thymectomized mice challenged with sheep erythrocytes.[58,59] The researchers further suspected that the thymus or thoracic duct lymphocyte recognized antigen and interacted with it, "helping" bone marrow-derived precursor cells to differentiate, since the actual cells producing antibody were found to be derived from injected bone marrow cells. The suggestion of these workers is that the thymus is responsible for generation of cells with varying immunological specificities, (antigen-sensitive cells), but that the reaction of these cells with an antigen interacting with a bone marrow cell leads to the production of effector cells derived from a thymus-independent source. Thus the antibody producing cells, according to this scheme, are thymus-independent.

More recently, the concept of interaction of thymus-dependent and thymus-independent cells through combination with antigen has become almost a fad in immunobiology.[60-62] Certain crucial data must be taken into account, however. Complete failure of development or complete elimination of the thymus and its dependent system of cells does not produce agammaglobulinemia or even hypogammaglobulinemia. Many antibody responses seem entirely independent of thymic influence.[14] It seems inescapable that antigen-sensitive cells of the thymus-independent system exist and that the thymus-dependent system contributes to immune responses of the thymus-independent system in some as yet unknown way. Perhaps this is a direct, or even an indirect, influence on the mechanism of delivery of antigen to the antigen-sensitive cells of the thymus-independent system.[63]

Definition of Prethymic and Postthymic Cells

It would seem that two factors are necessary for the normal development and continued function of the thymus: an intact reticuloepithelial framework, and a supply of "stem cells" sensitive first to the local inductive and then to the expanding humoral activity. We showed that there is a progressive decrease of restorative effectiveness of thymoma or thymus grafts when the treatment of neonatally thymectomized mice is delayed.[64] We believe that the cells capable of responding to the expanding action of the thymus represent cells that received "thymic influence" before thymectomy was performed, and the humoral function of the thymus can expand solely these "postthymic cells" in the lymphoid tissues.[24,28,64] In addition, we have shown, using a 45-day-old neonatally thymectomized mouse model, that lymphohemopoietic cells of adult and newborn origin can act in cooperation with thymus function in restoring such hosts.[28,29] Bone marrow cells, unlike lymph node and thymus lymphocytes, are capable of repopulating the thymus of lethally irradiated animals.[65,66] Experiments of this kind have suggested that bone marrow cells "home" to the thymus, from which cells emigrate to the peripheral lymphoid tissues.[65] Hemopoietic fetal liver contains cellular elements capable of thymus repopulation after lethal irradiation,[67] and such cells are also capable of producing immunological recovery of irradiated hosts.[68] Thymus grafts, but not thymus within diffusion chambers, were capable of producing maturation of the embryonic liver cells in the adult thymectomized-irradiated host.[69]

We have reported experiments that suggest the existence in the hemopoietic tissues of a "prethymic" population of partially differentiated cells insensitive to humoral activity of the thymus but requiring thymic stroma and traffic through the thymus. This population of prethymic cells can become postthymic through this process and can eventually develop into competent cells.[28,29] Postthymic cells can be detected in the liver as early as the 19th to 21st days of embryonation. The number of these cells increases at birth and is expanded in the peripheral lymphoid tissue and in the immediate postnatal period.[28]

The Thymus and Autoimmunity

That the thymus may be related to the pathogenesis of certain autoimune disorders was suggested by clinical associations of pathologic changes in the thymus with diseases having autoimmune reactivity such as: myasthenia gravis, systemic lupus erythematosus, thyrotoxicosis, rheumatoid arthritis, rheumatic fever, scleroderma, chronic hepatitis, aplastic anemia and glomerulonephritis.[1] These changes are mainly the presence of germinal centers and plasma cells within the thymic parenchyma. In addition, 10–15% of myasthenia gravis patients have thymomas composed of large, pale epithelial cells. Thymomas have also been found in association with positive LE tests and systemic lupus erythematosus and with hypogammaglobulinemia.[1] One interesting finding which is pertinent to this presentation is that of association between erythroid hypoplasia and thymoma (5% of all patients with thymoma). The plasma of two patients with erythroblastopenia, one of whom had a thymoma, inhibited erythropoiesis in mice.[70] There are at least two possibilities to explain these findings: the thymic tumor may secrete a substance which inhibits maturation of stem cells to the erythroid series, or perturbed immunologic function leads to production of an autoimmunity directed toward erythrocyte line.[71]

Genetic Susceptibility and Autoantibodies

In man, autoimmunity is found with high frequency both with genetically determined and acquired immunodeficiencies.[72,73] The possibility of genetic susceptibility to autoimmunity is suggested by the higher incidence of autoimmune phenomena in the families of patients with immune deficiencies.[74,75]

The appearance of autoantibodies against cellular antigens during aging is a propensity of certain strains of mice but not of others. There are strains of mice which are autoimmune susceptible (NZB, NZW, (NZB × NZW)F_1, A_f/Umc,

A/Umc, A/J and C57BL/Ks) or autoimmune-resistant (CBA/HDBA, and C3H$_f$/Umc, C3H/Umc). The former develop autoantibodies, while the latter do not develop autoantibodies spontaneously during aging.[23,76-82]

The best example of autoimmune susceptible mice is the NZB which, after three months of age, regularly develops hemolytic anemia associated with circulating autoantibody to red cells, detected by a positive Coombs test.[76,77] Some of these mice developed lesions in the thymus that consisted initially of germinal centers and later of expanding proliferative lesions in the thymic medulla.[83,84] Perhaps of more relevance to the NZB disease is the report of deficiency of adult type epithelial cells in the thymic medulla of NZB mice and that this change could be found even in newborn mice.[85] Immunologic aging is reflected by deficient immunologic functions, especially of the cell-mediated type in aging animals of autoimmune-susceptible strains and not in those of resistant strains.[13,86] The decrease in PHA and mixed leukocyte responses occurring with age in NZB, (NZB × A) F$_1$ and A mice is in keeping with the other declining cell-mediated immune responses.[13] In contrast, CBA/H mice which do not lose cellular immunity with age also retain their capacity to respond to phytohemagglutinin.[13]

Increasing incidence of Coombs positive tests and anti-DNP and anti-DNA antibodies are found in autoimmune-susceptible strains of mice.[13] The incidence of antiglobulin reaction of the erythrocytes develops rapidly in both sexes but, they show higher incidence in males earlier than in females. In contrast, the antinuclear antibodies occur earlier and in higher incidence in females than in males. Hemolytic anemia is accompanied by reticulocytosis, splenomegaly and normoblastosis of spleen and bone marrow.[23,76,77,82]

Other findings associated in aging autoimmune-susceptible mice include increase of plasma cells in lymph nodes and spleen accompanied by lymphocyte depletion.[23] In addition, foci of acute hepatitis, intranuclear inclusion bodies in liver cells and periportal infiltration of lymphocytes and plasma cells in the liver are seen.[23] Amyloidosis develops frequently in several organs.[23] Aging NZB and A mice show mesangial enlargement in the glomeruli, and these glomeruli contain PAS positive material as well as immunoglobulins.[13,23] The nodular type of immunoglobulin deposition along the epithelial side of the basement membrane that occurs in patients with S.L.E.[87,88] and in (NZB × NZW)F$_1$ mice[89] was not, however, observed in these aged animals. Instead, the large amounts of the immunoglobulin and complement detected in the kidneys of these mice were located in the mesangial regions of the glomerular tuft.[13,23] The basis for differences in distribution of these apparent DNA-anti-DNA complexes in the glomeruli is not known, but could reflect differences in formation of complexes of variable size and physical characteristics in the different experimental animals.[90,91]

Postthymectomy State and Autoimmunity

Association between autoimmunity and thymectomy has been reported in mice and also in rabbits subjected to neonatal extirpation of central lymphoid tissues.[5,13,92-95] Postthymectomy state was associated with autoimmune hemolytic anemia in certain strains of autoimmune-susceptible mice (A strain and C57BL/Ks).[95] These mice did not show reticulocytosis or normoblastosis, instead they showed normoblastopenia and lack of reticulocyte response in the presence of obvious hemolysis, as indicated by decreased red cell survival of Cr59 labeled erythrocytes and increased fragility of the erythrocytes in hypotonic solutions. Thymectomy is also followed by accelerated appearance of antinuclear antibodies (anti-DNP and anti-DNA) in autoimmune susceptible strains and to a lesser degree in one autoimmune resistant strain studied (CBA/H).[13] In addition, A mice with anti-DNA antibodies show glomerular lesions containing immunoglobulines and β_{1c} which are morphologically identical to those described in aging A and NZB mice.[13] Also, we described histopathological findings in autoimmune-susceptible strains: histiocytic and plasma cell infiltration of lymph nodes associated with lymphocyte depletion, ulcerative colitis, valvular and myocardial lesions of the heart, degenerative skin lesions and splenomegaly in thymectomized mice of these strains.[5] The spleens of these mice show splenomegaly with increase of normoblasts and myeloid cells.[5]

We have also described anemia associated with postthymectomy state in absence of positive Coombs tests.[23] We suggested that the anemia following thymectomy may not be due solely to hemolysis. For instance, there was a high degree of association between liver degenerative and inflammatory lesions and the anemia of A_f, C57BL/Ks and C3H neonatally thymectomized mice with wasting disease. In addition, there was normoblastic suppression of the bone marrow. These findings of hypoplasia of normoblasts and hepatitis are interesting, since it has been reported that human viral hepatitis may be associated with aplastic anemia.[96] Thus, the peculiar finding of anemia in neonatally thymectomized mice that cannot be explained or is incompletely explained by autoimmune hemolysis, and is associated with normoblastic hypoplasia, finds a reasonable explanation in the susceptibility of neonatally thymectomized mice to agents which may, in turn, depress development of red blood cells. This view is supported by experiments of depression of bone marrow colony forming units by mouse hepatitis virus (Stutman, unpublished data).

Reversibility of Wasting Disease and Autoantibodies of Postthymectomy State

In previous studies it was reported that the postthymectomy wasting in conventional mice could be reversed by supplying the neonatally thymectomized mice with a large number of spleen cells or by transplantation of number of thymuses.[26,34] TABLE 2 summarizes an experiment in which we attempted to compare the reversal of wasting and conversion of positive Coombs test to negative in A strain and (C3HxA)F_1 neonatally thymectomized mice to the reversal of wasting of neonatally thymectomized C3H$_f$ mice. All the mice included in this study had wasting disease between 38 and 51 days of age. Mice treated received 200 × 10^6 spleen cells from syngeneic, immunologically normal donors at 45- to 60 days of age. Reversal of wasting was observed in 53.8% of A_f, 66% of (C3H × A)F_1 and 75% of C3H mice. The animals with positive Coombs test became progressively negative by th age of four months and remained negative up to the age of eight months when they were sacrificed. At six months of age they received skin allografts. All C3H, some A and (C3H × A)F_1 reconstituted mice rejected these allografts in less than 13 days. Five reconstituted mice of A and (C3H × A)F_1 had delayed rejections of the allografts from 14–19 days.

Restorative Capacity of Spleen Cells of Aging Autoimmune-Susceptible and Resistant Strains

This experiment was designed to test the ability of spleen cells of autoimmune-susceptible or resistant strains of mice to reconstitute neonatally thymectomized mice. Preliminary results have been reported.[23] Neonatally thymectomized A_f and C3H were treated at two weeks with 100 × 10^6 spleen cells intraperitoneally. The donors were used in such a way that one donor was used for a maximum of

TABLE 2
REVERSAL OF POSTTHYMECTOMY WASTING AND CONVERSION OF COOMBS POSITIVE TO COOMBS NEGATIVE BY SPLEEN CELLS

Strain	Group	Pretreatment 45-60 days Positive Coombs (%)	Survivors (210 days)	Positive Coombs (%)	Skin Allograft Donor Strain	No. Mice with Prolonged Rejection*
A_t	treated	11/13 (84.5)	7/13 (53.8)	0	C3H	4/7
	untreated	10/14 (71.0)	0/14	—	—	—
$(C3H_t \times A)F_1$	treated	2/6 (33)	4/6 (66)	0	C_{68}	2/4
	untreated	3/6 (50)	0	—	—	—
C_3H_t	treated	0/8	6/8 (75)	0	A	0/6
	untreated	0/7	0	—	—	—

* Skin allografts at 6 months of age. C_3H_t in A_t, rejection time 10.8 days ± 3 (2SD), C_{68} in $(C_3H_t \times A_t) F_1$ rejection time 10 days ± 2.3 (2SD), and A in C_3H_t — 10.3 days ± 2.8 (2SD).

two recipients. Controls consisted of unoperated and untreated mice as well as mice injected with 100×10^6 spleen cells. All donors of CBA/H strains did not have antinuclear antibodies or a positive Coombs test. On the other hand, the A strain donors showed approximately 40% with positive Coombs test and 19% with anti-DNA antibodies at 12–14 months, and 58% with positive antiglobulin test and 38% with anti-DNA antibodies at 22 months of age.

The restorative capacity of A strain spleen decreases markedly with age. By contrast, the restorative capacity of the spleen cells of aging CBA/H mice decreases to a lesser degree. The cells from old A_f donors do not prevent the death of neonatally thymectomized syngeneic mice, but the CBA/H cells from donors of the same age still are capable of restoring immunological function to neonatally thymectomized syngeneic mice. In addition, spleen cells obtained from old CBA/H donors restored the neonatally thymectomized $C3H_f$ mice. These two strains differ in minor histocompatibility characteristics. The restored mice not only rejected skin allografts from an unrelated strain but showed tolerance to the CBA/H skin.

Discussion

Thymus influence on development of lymphoid tissue may be exerted through three nonexclusive mechanisms: (1) inductive influence on immigrant precursor stem cells of hemopoietic origin (prethymic cells). This influence occurs within the thymus and is a differentiating function.[24,29] (2) Proliferation of cells in the thymus, some of which emmigrate to the periphery where they may act as precursors or may interact with precursors of hemopoietic origin to produce immunocompetent cells involved in cell-mediated and humoral responses, respectively.[65] (3) Inductive and expanding influence of the thymic stroma, probably humoral, which may act within the thymus or in the periphery to expand the thymus-dependent lymphoid population of the postthymic cells.[24,28] We have shown that a special cell is present in the peripheral lymphohemopoietic tissues of the neonatally thymectomized host that is sensitive to the inductive and/or expanding humoral action of the thymus. This intermediate cell population, which we have termed postthymic,[28] requires the presence of the thymus for renewal and decreases progressively in the absence of thymic function.

Thymic involution and involution of the thymus-dependent system of cells occurs in man and in all animals which possess a thymus.[97]

Evidence from clinical and experimental analysis reveals deficiency of immune function with age in some individuals and not in others.[98,99] Neonatal thymectomy produces profound defects in cell-mediated immune responses, and the immune deficiencies observed during aging are very similar to those produced or accelerated by neonatal thymectomy.[13,23]

The association between immunological deficiency (both cell-mediated and humoral) and autoimmunity suggests that thymus-mediated immune reactions and, to some extent, immunoglobulin production constitute a surveillance mechanism against virus or other infective agents or even against mutant cells. In the development of immune deficiency and autoimmunity, the autoimmune process sometimes seems to precede demonstrable development of immune deficiency. However, this may be a very subtle relationship and more precise analytical study of immune functions may reveal selective immunodeficiency, especially in the cell-mediated functions which pave the way for development of autoimmunity.

Autoimmune phenomena in certain strains of mice increase with age and appear to be genetically determined, and it is hard to tell which is the basic perturbation.[13,99] Immune function in autoimmune susceptible strains is altered. Studies of humoral immunity in NZB mice and their hybrids indicate variable responses ranging from hypo- to hyper-responsive. This variability depends, in part, on the antigen employed.[100] In addition to observed strain differences, immunologic function in NZB, A strains and hybrids of these mice deteriorate with age.[13,86] These findings were corroborated by studies of decreased "in vitro" PHA and allogeneic cell responses of lymphoid tissues obtained from aging autoimmune-susceptible strains, suggesting a progressive quantitative or functional loss of postthymic cells.[13] In support of this concept, Denman and Denman[101] recently reported that the old NZB mice were depleted of long-lived lymphocytes when compared with young NZB or old C57BL black mice. The role of the thymus system in the prevention of autoimmune phenomena and in the decline in immunologic function is revealed by experiments which demonstrate that neonatal thymectomy accelerates the development of autoimmunity.[92,95] Conversely, the onset of autoimmunity may be delayed in older mice given injections of syngeneic cells derived from young animals.[102] Additional evidence has been presented here that postthymectomy wasting disease of autoimmune susceptible strains can also be reversed by providing the sick mice with large inocula of spleen cells obtained from young animals and that positive Coombs tests were often converted to negative. In addition, we have discussed the most direct experiments dealing with thymic and postthymic cell involution and functions. Spleen cells of autoimmune resistant strains demonstrate a higher restorative capacity of neonatally thymectomized mice than is the case with spleen cells of the autoimmune susceptible strains of the same age. These studies will be reported in detail elsewhere. Preliminary data indicate that in the autoimmune susceptible strains the decreased restorative capacity is a defect in thymus-dependent cells related to aging, independent of the autoimmune expressions themselves. These findings suggest once more that autoantibody production is secondary to immunologic deficiency.

How and/or why autoimmunity appears in patients or experimental animals cannot be answered at present. However, a relationship between thymus function, immunologic deficiency and autoimmunity is clear. Several theories have been postulated to explain this relationship. Burnet thinks that a primary function of the thymus is to maintain a hemeostasis which eliminates aberrant clones of cells. Such clones, without this influence, would be able to express potential for autoimmunity that might arise by somatic mutation.[103] Fudenberg feels that clones making autoantibodies arise continually in normal individuals and are eradicated by their immunological systems, a concept very similar to that of Burnet except that it focuses on the peripheral rather than the central immune function.[104] In contrast, such clones are not eradicated in individuals with immune deficiency, especially of the thymus-dependent function, either generalized or selective.[104] Both theories can be considered to relate basically to forbidden clones not effectively eliminated by host hemeostasis. According to both theories the forbidden clones proliferate and eventually result in autoimmune disease and/or malignancy.

Mellors and others[105,106] have linked Gross leukemia virus (MuLV) with the autoimmunity as well as with the lymphoid malignancy in the NZB strain. Viruses per se may be immunosuppressive, and the influence of such agents could account for the loss of cell-mediated immune responses with aging. These findings, as well as those of Tonietti and coworkers,[107] do not argue against our concept of genetic factors involved in the involution of the thymus-dependent system.[5,13,23] This involution can explain the increased susceptibility of certain strains of mice to certain viruses and also to the production of autoantibodies. Single or multiple infections of immunologically deficient animals could be the primary insult which results in lymphoid depletion and production of autoimmunity in both neonatally thymectomized and aging mice. The role of thymectomy and of early thymus-dependent system involution seems to be based on the reduction of normal mechanisms of resistance or surveillance.[108] The thymus-independent plasma cell system could then be excessively stimulated by antigens derived from infections and exogenous antigens. Under these conditions, and with a defective antigen recognition system, certain strains of mice reared in conventional environments are susceptible to autoimmunity because they more readily than others form antibodies resulting from infections, introducing antigens which cross-react with the host's own antigen constituents.

The fact that autoimmune resistant strains of mice also develop autoantibodies following thymectomy suggests that genetic mechanisms may control the involution of the thymus-dependent system during aging. This same surveillance system seems also to be involved in immunological mechanisms preventing cancer development in mice.

How all of this relates to the association of autoimmunity and myasthenia gravis is part of the business of this conference. We feel that the association of myasthenia with autoantibodies, autoimmune diseases and with evidence of thymic abnormality and immunodeficiency[109] is sufficiently provocative to justify further efforts to interpret the immunologic functions in myasthenic patients more definitively than has been accomplished thus far.[110,111] Further, the studies in mice would warrant both caution and concern in regard to the long-range influences of thymectomy or immune competence in man. Suggestions of progression to other serious autoimmune disease[112] have been reported following thymectomy for myasthenia gravis. One might anticipate from our findings in mice that after a sufficient period, immune deficiencies and many manifestations of autoimmunity may turn up as consequences of thymectomy treatment, which now appears to be essential in treating this disease.

REFERENCES

1. GOLDSTEIN, G. & I. R. MACKAY. 1969. The Human Thymus. Warren H. Green. St. Louis, Mo.
2. PARROT, D. M. V., M. A. B. DE SOUSA & J. EAST. 1966. Thymus-dependent areas in the lymphoid organs of neonatally thymectomized mice. J. Exp. Med. 123: 191.
3. MILLER, J. F. A. P., G. F. MITCHELL & N. S. WEISS. 1967. The cellular basis of the immunological defects in thymectomized mice. Nature 214: 992.
4. MILLER, J. F. A. P. 1962. Effect of neonatal thymectomy on the immunological responsiveness of the mouse. Proc. Roy. Soc. 156: 415.
5. YUNIS, E. J., P. O. TEAGUE, O. STUTMAN & R. A. GOOD. 1969. Post-thymectomy autoimmune phenomena in mice. II. Morphologic observations. Lab. Invest. 20: 46.
6. DALMASSO, A. P., C. MARTINEZ & R. A. GOOD. 1962. Failure of spleen cells from thymectomized mice to induce graft vs. host reactions. Proc. Soc. Exp. Biol. Med. 110: 205.
7. MILLER, J. F. A. P. 1961. Immunological function of the thymus. Lancet 2: 748.
8. GOOD, R. A., A. P. DALMASSO, C. MARTINEZ, O. K. ARCHER, J. C. PIERCE & B. W. PAPERMASTER. 1962. The role of the tyhmus in development of immunologic capacity in rabbits and mice. J. Exp. Med. 116: 773.
9. MARTINEZ, C., A. P. DALMASSO & R. A. GOOD. 1962. Acceptance of tumors homografts by thymectomized mice. Nature 194: 1289.
10. STUTMAN, O., E. J. YUNIS & R. A. GOOD. 1966. Carcinogen-induced tumors of the thymus. III. Restoration of neonatally thymectomized mice with thymomas in cell-impermeable chambers. J. Nat. Cancer Inst. 43: 499.

11. RODEY, G. E. & R. A. GOOD. 1969. The *in vitro* response to phytohemagglutinin of lymphoid cells from normal and neonatally thymectomized adult mice. Int. Arch. Allerg. **36**: 399.
12. STUTMAN, O. 1970. Hemopoietic origin of cells responding to phytohemagglutin in mouse lymph nodes. 5th Leukocyte Culture Conference. J. Harris, Ed. Academic Press. New York, N. Y.
13. TEAGUE, P. O., E. J. YUNIS, G. RODEY, A. J. FISH, O. STUTMAN & R. A. GOOD. 1970. Autoimmune phenomena and renal disease in mice. Role of thymectomy, aging, and involution of immunologic capacity. Lab. Invest. **22**: 121.
14. MILLER, J. F. A. P. & D. OSOBA. 1967. Current concepts of the immunological function of the thymus. Phys. Rev. **47**: 437.
15. HUMPHREY, J. H., D. M. V. PARROT & J. EAST. 1964. Studies on globulin and antibody production in mice thymectomized at birth. Immunology **7**: 419.
16. FAHEY, J. L., W. F. BARTH & L. W. LAW. 1965. Varied immunoglobulins and antibody response in neonatally thymectomized mice. J. Nat. Cancer Inst. **35**: 663.
17. MILLER, J. F. A. P. & G. F. MITCHELL. 1967. The thymus and the precursors of antigen reactive cells. Nature **216**: 659.
18. MILLER, J. F. A. P. 1964. Effect of thymic ablation and replacement. *In* Thymus in Immunobiology. R. A. Good & A. E. Gabrielsen, Eds. : 436. Hoeber-Harper. New York, N. Y.
19. PARROT, O. M. V. & J. EAST. 1964. Studies on a fatal wasting syndrome in mice thymectomized at birth. *In* The Thymus in Immunobiology. R. A. Good & A. E. Gabrielsen, Eds. : 523. Hoeber-Harper. New York, N. Y.
20. MCINTYRE, R. R., S. SELL & J. F. A. P. MILLER. 0000. Pathogenesis of the postneonatal thymectomy wasting syndrome. Nature **204**: 151.
21. STUTMAN, O. & E. J. YUNIS. 1970. Mouse hepatitis: Effect of neonatal thymectomy and reconstitution. Am. J. Path. **59**: 81 (abstr.).
22. EAST, J., O. M. V. PARROTT, F. C. CHESTERMAN & A. POMERANCE. 1963. The appearance of a hepatotrophic virus in mice thymectomized at birth. J. Exp. Med. **118**: 1069.
23. YUNIS, E. J., O. STUTMAN, G. FERNANDEZ, P. O. TEAGUE & R. A. GOOD. 0000. The thymus, autoimmunity and involution of the lymphoid system. *In* The Thymus, Immunity and Aging. R. A. Good & M. Sigel, Eds. In press.
24. STUTMAN, O., E. J. YUNIS & R. A. GOOD. 1969. Thymus: An essential factor in lymphoid repopulation. Transplant. Proc. **1**: 614.
25. DALMASSO, A. P., C. MARTINEZ, K. SJODIN & R. A. GOOD. 1963. Studies in the role of the thymus in immunobiology. Reconstitution of immunologic capacity in mice thymectomized at birth. J. Exp. Med. **118**: 1889.
25a. STUTMAN, O. & E. J. YUNIS. Unpublished data.
26. YUNIS, E. J., H. HILGARD, C. MARTINEZ & R. A. GOOD. 1965. Studies on immunologic reconstitution of thymectomized mice. J. Exp. Med. **121**: 607.
27. STUTMAN, O., E. J. YUNIS & R. A. GOOD. 1969. Reversal of post-thymectomy wasting in mice with immuno-competent cells: Influence of histocompatibility differences. J. Immunol. **102**: 87.
28. STUTMAN, O., E. J. YUNIS & R. A. GOOD. 1970. Studies on thymus function. I. Cooperative effect of thymic function and lymphohemopoietic cells in restoration of neonatally thymectomized mice. J. Exp. Med. **132**: 583.
29. STUTMAN, O., E. J. YUNIS & R. A. GOOD. 1970. Studies on thymus function. II. Cooperative effect of newborn and embryonic hemopoietic liver cells with thymus function. J. Exp. Med. **132**: 601.
30. STUTMAN, O., E. J. YUNIS & R. A. GOOD. 1969. Tolerance induction with thymus graft in neonatally thymectomized mice. J. Immunol. **103**: 92.
31. DUKOR, P., J. F. A. P. MILLER, W. HOUSE & V. ALLMAN. 1965. Regeneration of thymus grafts. I. Histological and cytological aspects. Transplantation **3**: 639.
32. YUNIS, E. J., C. MARTINEZ & R. A. GOOD. 1964. Failure to reconstitute neonatally thymectomized mice by successful rat thymus transplantation. Nature **204**: 604.
33. LAW, L. W. 1966. Restoration of thymic function in neonatally thymectomized mice bearing xenogeneic thymic grafts. Nature **210**: 1118.
34. STUTMAN, O., E. J. YUNIS, C. MARTINEZ & R. A. GOOD. 1967. Reversal of post-thymectomy wasting disease in mice by multiple thymus grafts. J. Immunol. **98**: 79.
35. STUTMAN, O., E. J. YUNIS & R. A. GOOD. 1969. Effect of parental strain thymus grafts in neonatally thymectomized F_1 hybrids. Transplantation **7**: 420.

36. Osoba, D. & J. F. A. P. Miller. 1963. Evidence for a humoral thymus factor responsible for the maturation of immunological faculty. Nature 199: 653.
37. Osoba, D. 1965. The effect of thymus and other lymphoid organs enclosed in millipore diffusion chambers on neonatally thymectomized mice. J. Exp. Med. 122: 633.
38. Stutman, O., E. J. Yunis & R. A. Good. 1968. Carcinogen-induced tumors of the thymus. I. Restoration of neonatally thymectomized mice with a functional thymoma. J. Nat. Cancer Inst. 41: 1431.
39. Stutman, O., E. J. Yunis & R. A. Good. 1969. Carcinogen-induced tumors of the thymus. II. Lung colonies as a means of separating different cell types of a functional thymoma. J. Nat. Cancer Inst. 142: 783.
40. Stutman, O., R. A. Good & E. J. Yunis. 1969. Decreased immune response after restoration in absence of thymic function. Fed. Proc. 28: 376 (abstr.).
41. Taylor, R. B. 1965. Decay of immunological responsiveness after thymectomy in adult life. Nature 208: 1334.
42. Metcalf, D. 1965. Delayed effect of thymectomy in adult life on immunological competence. Nature 208: 1336.
43. Miller, J. F. A. P. 1965. Effect of thymectomy in adult mice on immunological responsiveness. Nature 208: 1337.
44. Yunis, E. J., C. Martinez, J. Smith & R. A. Good. 1964. Facilitation of host lymphoid tissue development in neonatally thymectomized mice by injection of allogeneic dispersed thymus cells. Nature 204: 850.
45. DeSomer, P., P. Denys, Jr. & R. Leyten. 1963. Activity of a noncellular calf thymus extract in normal and thymectomized mice. Life Sci. 11: 810.
46. Trainin, N., A. Bejerano, M. Strahilevitch, D. Goldring & M. Small. 1966. A thymic factor preventing wasting and influencing lymphopoiesis in mice. Israel J. Med. 2: 549.
47. Trainin, N. & M. Linker-Israeli. 1967. Restoration of immunologic reactivity of thymectomized mice by calf thymus extracts. Cancer Res. 27: 309.
48. Goldstein, A. L., F. D. Slater & A. White. 1966. Preparation, assay and partial purification of thymic lymphatopoietic factor (Thymosin). Proc. Nat. Acad. Sci. U.S.A. 56: 1010.
49. Warner, N. L. & A. Szenberg. 1962. Effect of neonatal thymectomy on the immune response in the chicken. Nature 196: 784.
50. Glick, B., T. S. Chang & R. C. Jaap. 1956. The bursa of Fabricius and antibody production. Poult. Sci. 35: 224.
51. Cooper, M. D., R. D. Peterson, M. A. South & R. A. Good. 1966. The functions of the thymus system and the bursa system in the chicken. J. Exp. Med. 123: 75.
52. Van Alten, P. J., W. A. Cain, R. A. Good & M. D. Cooper. 1968. Gamma globulin production and antibody synthesis in chickens bursectomized as embryos. Nature 217: 87.
53. Kincade, P. W., A. R. Lawton, D. E. Bockman & M. D. Cooper. 1970. Differentiation of immunoglobulin class heterogeneity, effect of antibody mediated suppression of IgM synthesis in chickens. Proc. Nat. Acad. Sci. 64: 1918.
54. Cooper, M. D., D. Y. Perey, A. E. Gabrielsen, D. E. R. Sutherland, M. F. McKneally & R. A. Good. 1968. Production of an antibody deficiency syndrome in rabbits by neonatal removal of organized intestinal lymphoid tissues. Int. Arch. Allerg. 33: 65.
55. Fichtelius, K. E. 1967. The mammalian equivalent of Bursa Fabricii of birds. Exp. Cell Res. 46: 231.
56. Silverstein, A. Development of antibody production in fetal lambs subjected to complete extirpation of bowel. In preparation.
57. Claman, H. N., E. A. Chaperon & R. F. Triplett. 1966. Thymus-marrow cell combinations-synergism on antibody production. Proc. Soc. Exp. Biol. Med. 122: 1167.
58. Mitchell, G. F. & J. F. A. P. Miller. 1968. Immunological activity of thymus and thoracic duct lymphocytes. Proc. Nat. Acad. Sci. 59: 296.
59. Nossal, G. J. V., A. Cunningham, G. F. Mitchell & J. F. A. P. Miller. 1968. Cell to cell interaction in the immune response. III. Chromosomal marker analysis of single antibody-forming cells in reconstituted, irradiated, or thymectomized mice. J. Exp. Med. 128: 839.
60. Raff, M. C. 1970. Role of thymus derived lymphocytes in the secondary humoral immune response in mice. Nature 226: 1257.
61. Good, R. A. & W. A. Cain. 1970. Relationship between thymus dependent cells and humoral immunity. Nature 226: 1256.

62. MITCHISON, N. A. 1969. *In* Immunologic Tolerance. Maurice Landy & Werner Braun, Eds. : 115. Academic Press. New York, N. Y.
63. GOOD, R. A. & J. FINSTAD. Experimental and clinical models of immune deficiency and reconstitution of immunologic capacity. *In* Proc. Third Sigrid Juselius Symp. Helsinki, Finland. In press.
64. STUTMAN, O., E. J. YUNIS & R. A. GOOD. 1969. Carcinogen-induced tumors of the thymus. IV. Humoral influences of normal thymus and functional thymomas and influences of post-thymectomy period on restoration. J. Exp. Med. 130: 809.
65. FORD, C. E. 1966. Traffic of lymphoid cells in the body. *In* Thymus Experimental and Clinical Studies. G. E. W. Wolstenholme & R. Porter, Eds. : 131. Ciba Found. Symp. Churchill. London, England.
66. FORD, C. E., J. L. HAMERTON, D. W. H. BARNES & J. F. LOUTIT. 1965. Cytological identification of radiation chimaerism. Nature 177: 452.
67. TAYLOR, R. B. 1965. Pluri-potential stem cells in mouse embryo liver. Brit. J. Exp. Path. 46: 376.
68. DORIA, G. J. W., N. GOODMAN, N. GENGOZIAN & C. C. CONGDON. 1962. Immunologic study of antibody forming cells in mouse radiation chimaeras. J. Immunol. 88: 20.
69. TYAN, M. L. & L. J. COLE. 1966. Further observations on potential immunologically competent cells of fetal liver origin. Transplantation 4: 557.
70. JEPSON, J. H. & L. LOWENSTEIN. 1966. Inhibition of erythropoiesis by a factor present in the plasma of patients with erythroblastopenia. Blood 27: 425.
71. KRANTZ, S. B. & V. KAO. 1967. Studies on red cell aplasia. I. Demonstration of a plasma inhibitor to heme synthesis and an antibody to erythroblast nuclei. Proc. Nat. Acad. Sci. 58: 493.
72. GOOD, R. A. & A. E. GABRIELSEN. 1964. Agammaglobulinemia and hypogammaglobulinemia — relationship to mesenchymal diseases. *In* The Streptococcus, Rheumatic Fever and Glomerulonephritis. J. Wicks, Ed. : 368. Williams & Wilkins. Baltimore, Md.
73. HEREMANS, J. F. & P. A. CRABBE. 1968. *In* Immunologic Deficiency Diseases in Man. R. A. Good & D. Bergsma, Eds. : 298: Birth Defects Original Article Series. Vol. 4, No. 1. National Foundation Press. New York, N. Y.
74. FUDENBERG, H. H., J. J. GERMAN, III & H. G. KUNKEL. 1962. The occurrence of rheumatoid factor and other abnormalities in families of patients with agammaglobulinemia. Arthritis Rheum. 5: 565.
75. WOLF, J. K., M. GOKCEN & R. A. GOOD. 1963. Heredo-familial disease of the mesenchymal tissue: clinical and laboratory study of one family. J. Lab. Clin. Med. 61: 230.
76. BIELSCHOWSKY, M., B. J. HELYER & J. B. HOWIE. 1959. Spontaneous hemolytic anemia in mice of the NZB/BL strain. Proc. Univ. Otago Med. Sch. 37: 9.
77. HELYER, B. J. & J. B. HOWIE. 1963. Spontaneous autoimmune disease in NZB/BL mice. Brit. J. Haemat. 9: 119.
78. FRIOU, G. & P. TEAGUE. 1964. Spontaneous autoimmunity in mice. Antibodies to nucleoprotein in strain A/J. Science 143: 1333.
79. HOLMES, M. C. & F. M. BURNET. 1963. The natural history of autoimmune disease in NZB mice. Ann. Intern. Med. 59: 265.
80. NORRIS, L. C. & M. C. HOLMES. 1964. Anti-nuclear factor in mice. J. Immunol. 93: 148.
81. HELYER, B. J. & J. B. HOWIE. 1963. Renal disease associated with positive lupus erythematosus tests in a cross-bred strain of mice. Nature 197: 197.
82. EAST, J., M. A. B. DE SOUSA & D. M. V. PARROT. 1965. Immunopathology of New Zealand Black (NZB) mice. Transplantation 3: 711.
83. BURNET, F. M. & M. C. HOLMES. 1964. Thymic lesions associated with autoimmune disease in mice of strain NZB. *In* The Thymus in Immunobiology. R. A. Good & A. E. Gabrielsen, Eds. : 656. Harper & Row. New York, N. Y.
84. HOLMES, M. C. & F. M. BURNET. 1964. Experimental studies of thymic function in NZB mice and the F_1 hybrid with C3H. Aust. J. Exp. Biol. Med. Sci. 42: 589.
85. DE VRIES, M. J. & W. HIJMANS. 1966. A deficient development of the thymic epithelium and autoimmune disease in NZB mice. J. Path. Bact. 91: 487.
86. STUTMAN, O., E. J. YUNIS & R. A. GOOD. 1968. Deficient immunologic functions of NZB mice. Proc. Soc. Exp. Biol. Med. 127: 1204.
87. SVEC, K. H., J. D. BLAIR & M. H. KAPLAN. 1967. Immunopathologic studies of systemic lupus erythematosus (SLE). I. Tissue-bound immunoglobulins in relation to serum anti-nuclear immunoglobulins in systemic lupus and in chronic liver disease with LE cell factor. J. Clin. Invest. 46: 558.

88. KOFFLER, D., P. H. SCHUR & H. G. KUNKEL. 1967. Immunological studies concerning the nephritis of systemic lupus erythematosus. J. Exp. Med. 126: 607.
89. LAMBERT, P. H. & F. J. DIXON. 1968. Pathogenesis of the glomerulonephritis of NZB/W mice. J. Exp. Med. 127: 507.
90. GERMUTH, F. G., JR., L. B. SENTERFIT & A. D. POLLACK. 1967. Immune complex disease. I. Experimental acute and chronic glomerulonephritis. Johns Hopkins Med. J. 120: 225.
91. MICHAEL, A. F., A. J. FISH & R. A. GOOD. 1967. Glomerular localization and transportation of aggregated proteins in mice. Lab. Invest. 17: 14.
92. DE VRIES, M. J., L. M. VAN PUTTEN, H. BALNER & D. W. BEKKUM. 1964. Lésions suggérant une reactivité autoimmune chez des souris atteintes de la "runt disease" après thymectomie neonatale. Rev. Franc. Etud. Clin. Biol. 9: 38.
93. SUTHERLAND, D. E. R., O. K. ARCHER, R. D. A. PETERSON, E. ECKERT & R. A. GOOD. 1965. Development of "autoimmune processes" in rabbits after neonatal removal of central lymphoid tissue. Lancet 1: 130.
94. KELLUM, M. J., D. E. R. SUTHERLAND, E. ECKERT, R. D. A. PETERSON & R. A. GOOD. 1965. Wasting disease, Coombs' positivity and amyloidosis in rabbits subjected to central lymphoid tissue extirpation and irradiation. Int. Arch. Allerg. 27: 6.
95. YUNIS, E. J., R. HONG, M. A. GREWE, C. MARTINEZ, E. CORNELIUS & R. A. GOOD. 1967. Post-thymectomy wasting associated with autoimmune phenomena. I. Antiglobulin positive anemia in A and C57BL/6Ks mice. J. Exp. Med. 125: 947.
96. RUBIN, E. C. GOTTLIEB & P. VOGEL. 1968. Syndrome of hepatitis and aplastic anemia. Am. J. Med. 45: 88.
97. WALFORD, R. L. 1969. The Immunologic Theory of Aging. Munksgaard. Copenhagen, Denmark.
98. PISCIOTTA, A. V., D. W. WESTRING, C. DE PREY & B. WALSH. 1967. Mitogenic effect of phytohemagglutinin at different ages. Nature 215: 193.
99. BARNES, R. D. & M. TUFFREY. 1967. Serum antinuclear factor and the influence of environment in mice. Nature 214: 1136.
100. CEROTTINI, J. C., P. H. LAMBERT & F. J. DIXON. 1969. Comparison of the immune responsiveness of NZB and NZBxNZW F_1 hybrid mice with that of other strains of mice. J. Exp. Med. 130: 1093.
101. DENMAN, A. M. & E. J. DENMAN. 1970. Depletion of long-lived lymphocytes in old New Zealand black mice. Clin. Exp. Immunol. 6: 457.
102. TEAGUE, P. O. & G. J. FRIOU. 1969. Antinuclear antibodies in mice. II. Transmission with spleen cells. Inhibition or prevention with thymus or spleen cells. Immunology 17: 665.
103. BURNET, M. 1958. The Clonal Selection Theory of Acquired Immunity. Vanderbilt University Press. Nashville, Tennessee.
104. FUDENBERG, H. H. 1968. Are autoimmune diseases immunologic deficiency states? Hosp. Pract. 3: 43.
105. MELLORS, R. C., F. AOKI & R. J. HUEBNER. 1969. Further implication of immune leukemia-like virus in the disorders of NZB mice. J. Exp. Med. 24: 1045.
106. EAST, J. & D. M. V. PARROT. 1965. The role of the thymus in autoimmune disease. Acta Allerg. 20: 227.
107. TONIETTI, G., M. B. A. OLDSTONE & F. J. DIXON. 1970. The effect of induced chronic viral infections on the immunologic diseases of New Zealand mice. J. Exp. Med. 132: 89.
108. YUNIS, E. J., G. FERNANDES, O. STUTMAN & R. A. GOOD. Susceptibility to involution of the thymus-dependent lymphoid system and autoimmunity. Am. J. Clin. Path. In press.
109. ADNER, M. M., C. ISE, R. SCHWAB, J. D. SHERMAN & W. DAMESHEK. 1966. Immunologic studies of thymectomized and nonthymectomized patients with myasthenia gravis. Ann. N. Y. Acad. Sci. 135: 536.
110. GOOD, R. A., R. D. A. PETERSON, C. MARTINEZ, D. E. R. SUTHERLAND, M. J. KELLUM & J. FINSTAD. 1965. The thymus in immunobiology: with special reference to autoimmune disease. Ann. N. Y. Acad. Sci. 124: 73.
111. STRAUSS, A. J. L., C. W. SMITH, G. W. CAGE, H. W. R. VAN DER GELD, D. E. MCFARLIN & M. BARLOW. 1966. Further studies on the specificity of presumed immune associations of myasthenia gravis and considerations of possible pathogenic implications. Ann. N. Y. Acad. Sci. 135: 557.
112. ALARCÓN-SEGOVIA, D., R. F. GALBRAITH, J. E. MALDONADO & F. M. HOWARD. 1963. Systemic lupus erythematosus following thymectomy for myasthenia gravis — report of two cases. Lancet II: 662.

AUTHOR INDEX

Adams, Richard A., 186
Aird, Jennifer, 176
Ambrus, Julian L., 84

Bankhurst, Arthur D., 109
Battisto, Jack R., 122
Biggar, W.D., 10
Brunner, K.T., 160
Burrows, Stanley, 196

Carroll, Robert, 196

DeMuth, Jr., William E., 200

Ernström, Ulf, 99

Feldman, M., 142
Feldmann, Marc, 148

Gershon, R.K., 163
Gery, I., 163
Goldstein, Allan L., 48, 122
Good, Robert A., 10, 45, 221
Green, Ira, 72

Harris, Alan W., 148
Howe, Michael L., 122

Jeejeebhoy, H.F., 120

Knight, Stella C., 166
Kouvalainen, Kauko, 60
Krüger, J., 48

Larsson, Bengt, 99

Linna, Juhani, 99

MacLaurin, B.P., 131
Mandel, T., 25
Merk, Linda Poole, 186
Miller, J.F.A.P., 160
Mitchell, G.F., 160

Osoba, David, 204
Owen, J.J.T., 89

Raff, M.C., 89
Ritter, Mary A., 41
Rosenstreich, David L., 72
Rosenthal, Alan S., 72
Russell, Pamela J., 25, 160
Ruuskanen, Olli, 60

Shevach, Ethan, 72
Smith, James, 200
Sprent, John, 109, 160
Stavy, L., 142
Stutman, Osias, 10, 45, 221

Takada, Akikazu, 84
Takada, Yumiko, 84
Thorbecke, G. Jeanette, 166
Treves, A.J., 142

Wagner, Hermann, 148
Waksman, B.H., 48, 163
Warner, Noel L., 109

Yunis, E.J., 221

KEY-WORD TITLE INDEX

Antigens, Self, 122
Autoimmunity, 204, 221

Concanavalin A, 142

Hemopoietic Cells, Immunocompetence of, 45

Immune Response, Cell-Mediated, 148, 160
Immune Response, Thymus Dependence of, 176
Immunity, Ontogeny of Cellular, 166
Immunoglobulins, Surface, 109

Leucocytes, Peripheral, 163
Lymphocyte Interaction, Isogeneic, 122
Lymphocyte, Uropod-Bearing, 72
Lymphocytes, Maturation of, 41
Lymphocytes, Thymus-Derived, 89, 99, 109, 148
Lymphocytes, Thymus Origin of, 131
Lysis, 142

Pancytopenia, 196

Thymectomy, 120, 186
Thymocytes, Fate of, 60
Thymoma, 196, 200
Thymosin Injection in Rats, Calf, 48
Thymus, 84, 221
Thymus, Differentiation of Foetal Mouse, 25
Thymus Transplants, 10